A Rights-Based Preventative Approach for Psychosocial Well-Being in Childhood

Children's Well-Being: Indicators and Research

Volume 3

This new series focuses on the subject of measurements and indicators of children's well being and their usage, within multiple domains and in diverse cultures. More specifically, the series seeks to present measures and data resources, analysis of data, exploration of theoretical issues, and information about the status of children, as well as the implementation of this information in policy and practice. By doing so it aims to explore how child indicators can be used to improve the development and the well being of children.

With an international perspective the series will provide a unique applied perspective, by bringing in a variety of analytical models, varied perspectives, and a variety of social policy regimes.

Children's Well-Being: Indicators and Research will be unique and exclusive in the field of measures and indicators of children's lives and will be a source of high quality, policy impact and rigorous scientific papers.

For further volumes:
http://www.springer.com/series/8162

Murli Desai

A Rights-Based Preventative Approach for Psychosocial Well-Being in Childhood

Springer

Murli Desai, Ph.D. in Social Work
Former Professor at the Tata Institute
of Social Sciences
#1203 & 1204, Apollo Tower
Mahalakshmi Mandir Road, Deonar
Mumbai 400 088, India
murlidesai@gmail.com

ISSN 1879-5196 e-ISSN 1879-520X
ISBN 978-90-481-9065-2 e-ISBN 978-90-481-9066-9
DOI 10.1007/978-90-481-9066-9
Springer Dordrecht Heidelberg London New York

Library of Congress Control Number: 2010932765

Printed on acid-free paper

Springer is part of Springer Science+Business Media (www.springer.com)

To

my son Sushant
for helping me understand psychosocial
well-being in childhood in practice

Preface

Childhood is the foundational phase of human development and the most important target group for intervention. Most of the schools of human development and social work around the world have an elective course on children and some offer a concentration in this area. There are plenty of textbooks on intervention with children published by Western authors, focusing on useful theories and skills but these are mainly at the remedial level. They neither use the preventative approach nor the child rights perspective, which has been found useful in the developing nations. The books on child rights are generally published by the United Nations Children's Fund (UNICEF) and other international organisations working for children in developing nations, such as Save the Children. These books focus on the useful child rights perspective but they neither integrate theories nor use the preventative approach. Prevention approach is an imperative in the child rights approach as it is the only way to effectively deal with children's problems. The proposed book *A Rights-Based Preventative Approach for Psychosocial Well-Being in Childhood* will be the first to apply the child rights perspective and the preventative approach to intervention for children's psychosocial well-being. It attempts to integrate theories with practice and teaching relevant in different parts of the world.

The book deconstructs childhood vulnerability and re-conceptualises and traces the cycle of neglect, abuse, commercial exploitation and conflict with law in childhood with effects in childhood and implications for adult life in a longitudinal manner. In order to break this cycle, it develops a conceptual framework for a rights-based preventative approach for children's well-being based on the foundation of the child rights perspective, the prevention model of public health, theories of positive psychology, and approaches, attitudes, ethical principles, methods, techniques and skills of intervention of the social work profession.

Based on the United Nations Convention on the Rights of the Child (1989), the book identifies the objectives of a rights-based preventative approach for psychosocial well-being in childhood as achievement of child rights to family care, development, participation and protection. The child rights principles are identified as:

- Primary consideration to the dignity and the best interests of the child
- Indivisibility and interdependence of child rights and a holistic approach to children
- Universality, equality, non-discrimination and inclusion of the marginalised among children
- State and society accountable for promoting child rights

Based on the cycle of vulnerability, neglect, abuse, commercial exploitation and conflict with the law in childhood, the book uses the public health prevention model for identifying the goals of intervention as follows:

- Primary prevention of vulnerability in childhood,
- Secondary prevention of neglect of children at risk and
- Tertiary prevention of abuse, commercial exploitation and conflict with the law in childhood.

Psychosocial well-being empowers self for development and protection from vulnerability, abuse and conflict with the law in childhood. Psychosocial well-being is conceptualised in this book as being comprised of:

- Self-awareness: self-identity and self-esteem
- Proactive thinking skills: rational, realistic, flexible, creative, self-responsible and positive thinking skills
- Emotional intelligence: emotional awareness and expression, regulating negative emotions and enrichment of positive emotions
- Interpersonal relationship skills: positive perception of others, positive feelings for others, win–win goals in relationships and collaborative conflict management skills
- Interpersonal communication skills: assertive and open verbal and body language skills, sensitive listening skills and feedback skills

The rights-based preventative approach for psychosocial well-being in childhood requires the person-centred, strengths-based, participatory and empowerment-focused social work approaches; attitudes of warmth, humility and empathy; the ethical principles of self-determination, informed consent, professional boundaries and confidentiality; and the methods of psycho-educational group work and case management for intervention with children and their families.

The book is divided into the following three parts:

Part I: Introduction to A Rights-Based Preventative Approach for Psychosocial Well-Being in Childhood

Part II: Primary Prevention for Psychosocial Well-Being in Childhood

Part III: Secondary and Tertiary Prevention for Psychosocial Well-Being in Childhood

Part I introduces the rights-based preventative approach for psychosocial well-being in childhood. The teaching–learning objectives for this Part are to:

1. Critically review the theories of child development and deconstruct childhood vulnerability;
2. Understand the ecological context and cycle of vulnerability, neglect, abuse, commercial exploitation and conflict with the law in childhood and implications for adult life;
3. Understand the child's rights to family care, development, participation and protection, and the principles of child rights; and
4. Develop a conceptual framework for rights-based preventative approach for psychosocial well-being in childhood, based on the child rights perspective, prevention model of public health, theories of positive psychology, and social work approaches, attitudes, ethical principles, methods, techniques and skills of intervention.

Part II focuses on the rights-based primary prevention for psychosocial well-being in childhood. It focuses on the methodology of psycho-educational group work for development of psychosocial skills, useful also for secondary and tertiary prevention. The teaching–learning objectives for this Part are to

1. Learn the experiential methodology, group process and facilitation approach, methods, tools, discussion techniques, and programme planning for psycho-educational group work;
2. Study the theories of psychosocial skills of self-awareness, proactive thinking skills, emotional intelligence, interpersonal relationship skills, interpersonal communication skills and family life education, and learn to carry out psycho-educational group work activities for the enrichment of psychosocial skills of parents and children according to their age groups and life situations; and
3. Learn the theories of parenting education comprised of enrichment of marital relationship skills, assertive parenting skills and age-appropriate developmental tasks and interventions needed.

Part III focuses on the rights-based secondary prevention of neglect of children in at risk situations and tertiary prevention of abuse, commercial exploitation and conflict with law in childhood. The teaching–learning objectives for this Part are to

1. Learn to carry out the stages of casework process and conduct case management with children and their families with reference to direct work and system linkage;
2. Examine the types, causes and consequences of situations where children are at risk of neglect, including the emergency situations, and learn to carry out rights-based intervention with them for secondary prevention;

3. Learn to carry out child advocacy interventions for restorative justice in the juvenile justice system for tertiary prevention;
4. Learn to carry out rights-based placement of children in foster family care, child adoption and institutional childcare, aiming at tertiary prevention;
5. Examine the types, causes and consequences of abuse and commercial exploitation in childhood, and learn to carry out rights-based intervention for tertiary prevention; and
6. Examine the types, causes and consequences of conflict with law in childhood and learn to carry out rights-based intervention for tertiary prevention.

The book is planned to teach and learn two courses:

1. Primary Prevention for Psychosocial Well-Being in Childhood (comprising Part II)
2. Secondary and Tertiary Prevention for Psychosocial Well-Being in Childhood (comprising Part III)

Part I on Introduction to A Rights-Based Preventative Approach for Psychosocial Well-Being in Childhood can be included in the course that is offered first. Every chapter of the book covers the teaching–learning objectives, concepts and theories, child rights and psychosocial intervention.

This book draws considerably from a comprehensive literature review; experience of conducting workshops for adolescents and training programmes for volunteers, paraprofessionals, social work students and practitioners, and school teachers; consultation, interaction and work with several professionals from voluntary organisations, government and international organisations and academicians; and curriculum planning and teaching courses, in the United States, India, Singapore and South Korea. I am indebted to each and everyone for their inputs into my thinking that has gone into developing and organising knowledge for this book.

The primary market of this book comprises of faculty and students of Social Work and Human Development. The secondary markets comprise of faculty and students of the following institutions:

- Academic Institutions of Educational Psychology, Mental Health, Human Rights and Teacher Education
- Training Institutions run by Government and Voluntary Organisations that conduct training programmes on child rights and social work
- Social workers and counsellors in schools and child-centred government and voluntary organisations

Mumbai, India Murli Desai

Contents

List of Charts

Part I
Introduction to a Rights-Based Preventative Approach for Psychosocial Well-Being in Childhood

Introduction to Part I

Teaching–Learning Objectives

Part I introduces the rights-based preventative approach for psychosocial well-being in childhood. The teaching–learning objectives for this Part are to

1. Critically review the theories of child development and deconstruct childhood vulnerability;
2. Understand the ecological context and cycle of vulnerability, neglect, abuse, commercial exploitation and conflict with law in childhood and implications for adult life;
3. Understand the child rights to family care, development, participation and protection, and the principles of child rights; and
4. Develop a conceptual framework for rights-based preventative approach for psychosocial well-being in childhood, based on the child rights perspective, prevention model of public health, theories of positive psychology, and social work approaches, attitudes, ethical principles, methods, techniques and skills of intervention.

Chapter Plan

The chapter plan of Part I is as follows:

1. Theories of Child Development and Vulnerability in Childhood
2. The Child Rights Perspective
3. Conceptual Framework for Rights-Based Preventative Approach for Psychosocial Well-Being in Childhood

Recommended Reading

Harding, L. F. (1997). *Perspectives in Child Care Policy*. London: Prentice Hall.

Hart, R. A. (1992). *Children's Participation: From Tokenism to Citizenship*. Florence: UNICEF International Child Development Centre.

James, A. and James, A. (2004). *Constructing Childhood: Theory, Policy and Social Practice*. New York: Palgrave Macmillan.

Save the Children. (2002). *Child Rights Programming: How to Apply Rights-Based Approaches in Programming*. Stockholm: Save the Children.

Schriver, J. M. (2004). *Human Behavior and the Social Environment: Shifting Paradigms in Essential Knowledge for Social Work Practice* (4th ed.). Boston, MA: Pearson Allyn and Bacon.

United Nations Children's Fund. (2001). *Pocket Guide for a Rights-Based Approach to Programming for Children: Application in South Asia*. Kathmandu: UNICEF.

United Nations Convention on the Rights of the Child. (1989). http://www.ohchr.org/english/law/pdf/crc.pdf. Accessed 3 March 2002.

Wyness, M. G. (2006). *Childhood and Society: An Introduction to the Sociology of Childhood*. New York: Palgrave Macmillan.

Chapter 1
Theories of Child Development and Vulnerability in Childhood

1.1 Concepts of Human Development

According to Erikson (1963, cited by Newman and Newman 2006) human life is produced by the interaction and modification of three major systems: the biological system, the psychological system and the societal system. Each system can be examined for continuity and change over the life span.

1.1.1 The Biological System

The biological system includes all those processes necessary for the physical functioning of the organism: genetic, skeletal, sensory, motor, respiratory, endocrine, circulatory, waste elimination, sexual-reproductive, digestive and neurological. These processes develop and change as a consequence of the following factors:

- Genetically guided maturation
- Environmental resources: nutrition and sunlight
- Environmental toxins
- Accidents and diseases
- Lifestyle: eating, sleeping, exercises and drugs (Newman and Newman 2006).

According to Lesser and Pope (2007), neuro-behavioural disorders are a result of the linkage between brain dysfunction and behavioural manifestations. Following is the classification of neuro-behavioural disorders:

1. Learning disorders:
   - Learning disabilities (language-based learning disabilities and problems in language reception: dyslexia, etc.)
   - Attention deficit hyperactivity disorder

M. Desai, *A Rights-Based Preventative Approach for Psychosocial Well-Being in Childhood*, Children's Well-Being: Indicators and Research 3,
DOI 10.1007/978-90-481-9066-9_1,

2. Brain-based disorders:
   - Autism
   - Mental retardation
   - Genetic disorders
   - Disorders from head injuries

It is extremely important to ensure that the environment does not continue to make demands that the biological system of the individual cannot meet (Lesser and Pope 2007).

1.1.2 The Psychological System

The psychological system includes those mental processes central to a person's ability to make meaning of experiences and take action: motivation, emotion, perception, learning, memory, judgment, reasoning, problem-solving, language skills, symbolic abilities, self-awareness and reality testing. Capacity and change in psychological processes are guided by genetic factors, life experiences, and self-direction and insight (Newman and Newman 2006).

1.1.3 The Societal System

The societal system includes those processes through which a person becomes integrated into society: interpersonal relationships, social roles, rituals, cultural myths, social expectations, leadership styles, communication patterns, family organisation, social support, political and religious ideologies, patterns of economic prosperity, poverty, war or peace and patterns of intolerance and discrimination. The impact of the societal system on psychological development results largely from interpersonal relationships. Culture, age-graded role expectations, historical events and technological change affect the societal system (Newman and Newman 2006).

1.1.4 Stages of Development

Life span theories usually divide the life cycle into age-related stages. A developmental stage is a period of life that is unique and characterised by a specific underlying organisation. At every stage, some characteristics differentiate that stage from the preceding and the succeeding stages. At each stage, the accomplishments from the previous stage provide resources for mastering the new challenges. Thus, the stages form a sequence (Newman and Newman 2006).

1.2 Theories of Child Development

The main theories in child development are those of cognitive development and psychosocial development.

1.2.1 Theories of Cognitive Development

1.2.1.1 Key Concepts of Cognition

Intelligence: Intelligence denotes conceptual ability based on abstract thought and effective problem-solving and is measured by standardised intelligence quotient (IQ) tests. For Piaget, human intelligence is a type of evolutionary biological adaptation that enables people to interact successfully with the environment. According to him, intellectual development in humans is largely based on biological factors related to specific heredity of the nervous system (Robbins et al. 2006).

Alternatively, Gardener (1993, cited by Schriver 2004) posits that there are multiple intelligences of equal value and not rank ordered in terms of importance, seven of which are listed as follows: Linguistic intelligence, logical-mathematical intelligence, spatial intelligence, musical intelligence, bodily kinesthetic intelligence, interpersonal intelligence and intrapersonal intelligence.

Organisation and adaptation: Piaget proposed two inborn biologically variant functions for all species based on general heredity: organisation and adaptation. Organisation refers to the tendency to blend and coordinate physical or mental structures into more coherent, complex and higher order systems of structures (Robbins et al. 2006).

Adaptation is the ongoing process by which structures of the mind develop over time to achieve a better fit with the environment and external reality. Adaptation consists of two processes: assimilation and accommodation. Assimilation is a cognitive process through which new perceptual events and understandings of the external world are incorporated into the existing schemata. As children assimilate, they attempt to explain new information based on their current frame of reference. Accommodation is the creation of new schemata or the modification of old ones for placing new stimuli that do not fit into the already existing cognitive schemata. In doing so, the child revises old ways of thinking to fit new information and situations. Of primary importance is the ability to adapt and organise the environmental stimuli. Whereas assimilation explains the quantitative change involved in placing new input and information into existing ways of knowing, accommodation helps account for the qualitative development of new understandings (Robbins et al. 2006).

Memory: Memory involves retaining information over time and plays a crucial role in all cognitive and intellectual development (Santrock 1989, cited by Robbins et al. 2006). Piaget distinguished between two types of memory: recognition and evocation memory. Recognition occurs in the presence of an object that has previously been encountered and is one of the first types of memory that infants exhibit. Evocation (also called recall) depends on the ability to evoke a mental image of something that is not present (Robbins et al. 2006).

1.2.1.2 Cognitive Development

Factors determining cognitive development: Piaget proposed that four underlying causal factors determine cognitive development: maturation, physical experience (action with the environment), social interaction (interchange of ideas between people) and equilibrium (internal self-regulating system that operates to reconcile the roles of maturation, experience and social interaction) (Robbins et al. 2006).

Stages of cognitive development: Piaget identified four major stages of cognitive development that are universal and based on invariant sequentiality, discussed herein as reported by Robbins et al. (2006).

1. *Sensory-motor period*: From birth to about age two (infancy and toddlerhood), infants begin to gain control over their reflexes, muscles and sensory organs. They learn to reproduce pleasurable events, first in relation to their own bodies and then in relation to other people or objects. They experiment with objects, picking them up and dropping them, or pulling them, to watch the effect. As they become gradually able to follow objects visually and anticipate their positions, an awareness of the permanence of objects develops.
2. *Preoperational period*: From age 2 to 7 (preschool age), as the use of symbolic thought increases, the child is able to produce mental symbols that mediate her or his performance. Conceptual-symbolic behaviour replaces sensorimotor behaviour. Although perception still dominates over reason, behaviour sequence can now be played out mentally rather than just physically. Piaget further divided the preoperational phase into two sub-periods: the pre-conceptual period from 2 to 4 years of age and the intuitive period from 4 to 7 years of age. The pre-conceptual period is characterised by the development of language and imaginative play. During the intuitive period, there is emergence of skills in the areas of numbers, classification and interrelationships. In addition, behaviour eventually becomes less egocentric and more social.
3. *Concrete operations*: From age 7 to 11 (middle childhood), reason takes primacy over perception. Children gain two cognitive operations necessary for logical thought: reversibility and compensation. With reversibility, children gain the ability to reverse, or undo an action in their mind. When they acquire compensation, they are able to decentre their perceptions and focus on more than one aspect at a time. With these operations, logic and objectivity increase and reasoning can be applied to observable, concrete problems. As deductive thinking begins, children gain cognitive skills for

    - Conservation: the recognition that properties of an object do not change when its appearance is altered.
    - Seriation: the ability to arrange items according to their increasing or decreasing size,
    - Classification: the ability to group objects into categories and subcategories according to their characteristics and
    - Transitivity: the ability to understand reciprocal concepts.

4. *Formal operations*: From age 11 to 15 (early adolescence), abstract thought and scientific reasoning emerge. Problems are now approached using logic, reason

and combinational thought. Hypothetical reasoning and a growing appreciation of interactions among multiple factors are now possible. There is also greater importance attached to a language-based system of representation. They can operate not only on concrete objects and events but also on ideas (Shaffer 1993, cited by Robbins et al. 2006).

1.2.2 Theories of Psychosocial Development

The psychosocial theory presents human development as a product of the ongoing interaction between individual biological and psychological needs and abilities, on the one hand, and societal expectations and demands, on the other hand. The theory accounts for patterns of individual development that emerge from a bio-psychosocial process. The psychosocial theory accounts for systematic change over the life span through the concepts of stages of development, developmental tasks and psychosocial crises (Newman and Newman 2006).

1.2.2.1 Stages of Development

Freud's psychosexual stages: Freud's psychodynamic theory describes five stages of development: oral, anal, phallic, latent and genital stages. At each stage, the focus of conflict is around the expression of sexual and aggressive impulses changes. The stages reflect shifts in the body areas where pleasure is experienced and shifts in the orientation to self and social relationships (Newman and Newman 2006). Dale et al. (2006) describe the stages as follows:

Oral stage: The oral stage covers the period from birth to about 18 months. Initiated by the sucking reflex, the infant not only feeds but also derives the pleasure from the sucking process itself.

Anal stage: The anal stage starts around the 18th month. Now the anal region gets energised with libido and the child turns his or her attention to the pleasures associated with the bowel movements and the faecal products produced. Guided by id impulses, the child expresses pleasure by handling and smearing his or her faeces.

Phallic stage: The phallic stage is also known as the Oedipal stage, starting around age three and lasts until age six or so. At this time the genital area becomes the important erogenous zone. The boys take greater interest in their penis and girls in their clitoris or vulva. Mothers are the first love object for boys, who want to possess them, but the fathers are their rivals, giving the boys the Oedipal complex. Girls go through similar experiences with their fathers giving the girls the Electra complex. As boys learn that they have a penis and the girls do not, they conclude that the girls once had a penis and were castrated. As a result, they develop castration anxiety for their penis. As girls discover that they do not have a penis, they begin to feel inferior and develop penis envy (Robbins et al. 2006).

Latency stage: The latency stage begins with start of school and lasts until puberty, at 11 for girls and 13 for boys. In this stage, the child acquires a good ego-based defence structure and the power of the id-related aggressive and sexual impulses become latent. Children identify with the same-sex parent and the superego becomes strengthened as parental values continue to be incorporated (Robbins et al. 2006).

While Freud is believed to be correct in that preschoolers are highly curious about their bodies, masturbate, and engage in both same-sex and cross-sex sexual play, such activities do not occur infrequently in school-aged children. It appears that sexual experimentation, which is more common among boys than among girls, increases with age, rather than declining after the preschool period as Freud claimed. The reason for Freud being mistaken is likely to be that preschoolers, who are often unaware of society's rules of etiquette, are more likely to get caught at their sex play than are older children. Thus, even though latency-period children may be more discreet than preschoolers, they do not lose their sexual curiosity (Sigelman and Shaffer 1995).

Genital stage: The genital stage starts with the onset of puberty. Sexual feelings swell and the child is ready with the sexual organs to release their sexual impulses. Typically the resolution is accomplished by the selection of a sexual partner.

Erikson's stages and ego conflicts: Erikson (1963, cited by Newman and Newman 2006) proposed eight stages of psychosocial development, partly based on Freud's psychosexual stages. However, he does not give age groups for the stages. He also identified the main psychosocial ego conflicts of each stage.

Chart 1.1 Erikson's Stages and Ego Conflict

Development stage	Psychosocial ego conflicts
Oral sensory	Basic trust versus mistrust, depending on whether the infant's needs are appropriately met
Muscular anal	Autonomy versus shame, doubt, depending on acceptance by parents
Locomotor genital	Initiative versus guilt, leading to creativity and self-esteem
Latency	Industry versus inferiority, depending on the school environment
Puberty and adolescence	Identity versus role confusion, through experimentation
Young adulthood	Intimacy versus isolation, by becoming ready to participate in a committed long-term relationship
Adulthood	Generativity versus stagnation, by examining whether they have produced something that will outlive them
Maturity	Ego integrity versus despair, by finding meaning in life that will help them face death

1.2.2.2 Developmental Tasks

Developmental tasks, as conceptualised by Havighhurst, contribute to development at each stage of life, and increase mastery over one's environment. These tasks reflect areas of accomplishment in physical, cognitive, social and emotional development, as well as development of self-concept, as required by the society based on physical maturation for the respective age groups (Newman and Newman 2006).

1.2.2.3 Psychosocial Crises

A psychosocial crisis arises because one must make psychological efforts to adjust to the demands of the social environment at each stage of development. The word crisis in this context refers to a normal set of stresses and strains rather than to an extraordinary set of events. Mastery of the developmental tasks is influenced by the resolution of the psychosocial crisis of the previous stage and it is this resolution that leads to the development of new social capabilities. In turn, the skills learnt during a particular stage as a result of work on its developmental tasks provide the tools for the resolution of the psychosocial crisis of that stage (Newman and Newman 2006).

Newman and Newman (2006) propose the following scheme of stagewise psychosocial crises, on a continuum between opposing forces derived from Erikson's model. Most people experience both ends of the continuum, the outcome being a balance or integration of the two opposing forces.

Chart 1.2 Life Stage and Psychosocial Crisis

Life stage	Age group	Psychosocial crises
Infancy	Birth to 2 years	Trust versus mistrust
Toddlerhood	2–3 years	Autonomy versus shame and doubt
Early school age	4–6 years	Initiative versus guilt
Middle childhood	6–12 years	Industry versus inferiority
Early adolescence	12–18 years	Group identity versus alienation
Later adolescence	18–24 years	Individual identity versus identity confusion
Early adulthood	24–34 years	Intimacy versus isolation
Middle adulthood	34–60 years	Generativity versus stagnation
Later adulthood	60–75 years	Integrity versus despair
Very old age	75 until death	Immortality versus extinction

1.2.3 Critique of Theories of Child Development

Schriver (2004) notes the following criticism of the theories of child development:

- They use a medical or pathology perspective on people's problems rather than a social change or strengths perspective.
- The standards of white Eurocentric culture of the founder are considered universal. They are binary with emphasis on polarities and all the ego conflicts call for resolutions weighted towards separateness.

- They are based on masculinist and patriarchal perspectives that assume male experience as central. Female developmental experiences are described only in terms of their differences from normal or modal male experience.
- They are limited to intra-psychic structures and processes. They give no recognition to social or environmental conditions that might impinge on the individual development.

1.3 Social Construction of Childhood Vulnerability

Based on the critique of the theories of child development, the social construction of childhood vulnerability is deconstructed in this section. Burman (2008, p. 1) uses the term deconstruction, in the sense of laying bare, of bringing under scrutiny, the coherent moral-political themes and to look beyond current frameworks. This has been discussed in this section with reference to the following:

- Adultism and protective exclusion in childhood,
- Social construction of childhood and adolescence and
- Western scientific construction of "normal" childhood

1.3.1 Adultism and Protective Exclusion in Childhood

Adult control over children is often justified as necessary for their welfare. However, adult control is often a means to maintain conformity and social order across and between the generations as adults seek to preserve and recreate the childhood they remember (James and James 2004). Such behaviour is justified by adultism, which is a prejudicing ideology that refers to bias against young people, and is distinguished from ageism—which is simply prejudice on the grounds of age, not youth particularly. Adultism is used to refer to the attitudinal, cultural and systematic discrimination against children and youth. It refers to behaviours and attitudes that are based on the assumption that adults are better than young people, and entitled to act upon them without their agreement. It is characterised by disrespect towards the intelligence, judgment, emotional life, leadership or physical being of young people (Wikipedia 2005).

Adultism implies assumptions about physical and mental incapability of children, which lead to role stereotypes of dependency, hierarchy, intolerance, discrimination and also justifies violence against them. Thus, from an adultist perspective, child abuse is not an anomaly, it is built into the way in which we define childhood (Mason and Steadman 1996). According to the EU Canada Project (2003), adultism may take a number of forms including the following:

- Withholding information and access to entitlements on the basis that children are too immature or incapable or using them "properly";
- Acting "on behalf of a child or young person" using the same rationale;

- Making decisions about a child or young person based on generalised representations of children and young people rather than consulting with or treating situations on their individual merits and
- Acting as a barrier to the autonomy, independence, and empowerment of children and young people individually or collectively.

Children have been perceived as immature and imperfect by thinkers from ancient to modern times. According to Aristotle, a human child is an immature specimen of the organism type human, which, by nature, has the potentiality to develop into a mature specimen with the structure, form and function of a normal or standard adult. Aristotle regarded children as property of the father. On the ground that there can be no injustice "in the unqualified sense" towards what is one's own, he reasoned that a father cannot be unjust to his own child. John Locke viewed the child neither as inherently bad nor good but rather as a "tabula rasa" meaning a "blank slate". This idea implied that children could be shaped by all kinds of experiences during their life. Locke added that the power that parents have over their children, arises from the duty, which is incumbent on them to take care of their offspring, during the "imperfect" state of childhood (Matthews 2004). Kennedy (No date) notes that for the "civilised" Freud, the child is the voice of neurosis. The neurotic is unwilling to give up the demands of childhood, as being childish is considered being uncivilised or regressive. He described adulthood as the successful resolution of the psychosexual stages of childhood.

Even scientific wisdom on child development states that human competence is essentially a function of age. Erikson and Piaget also characterised childhood development as an orderly, linear progress from incompetence to competence, which is adulthood (Mason and Steadman 1996). Boyden and Levison (2000) noted that the overall trend in development sciences accepts transformation from an immature child to mature adult, simple to complex, irrational to rational behaviours and dependent childhood to autonomous adulthood. Children are thus understood to be immature beings in a state of development and training for competent adulthood. The concept of "developing" children into adults by "teaching" them implies that children are not developed or are incomplete and adults are "developed" or "complete". Children are not considered to have human agency, in that, they are not viewed as contributing to the accomplishment of a purpose or results (Levison 2000).

White (2003) notes that childhood is not even an area of study in social sciences such as anthropology, sociology (until recently), economics, political science and development studies. According to most economic models, children have been perceived both as a cost to society and the passive receptacles of benefits and knowledge imparted by adults. In other words, children's integration into society is portrayed, in effect, as a one-way process in which adults give and children receive (Boyden and Levison 2000). As Wyness, Harrison and Buchanan (2004) note, a political community has an exclusive adult membership with children not considered competent for entry. Children's apolitical nature is associated with family being considered their primary social environment, which is seen as the personal and private sphere, shielding the children from the public sphere of politics. In their understanding, the emphasis on rights in the United Nations Convention on the Rights of the Child (UNCRC) also locates children as welfare dependants.

White (2003) emphasises that while children and young people are of course vulnerable and in need of adult protection in some senses and situations, approaches to analysis or action which focus on vulnerability alone are likely to encourage notions of the young as passive, helpless victims, obscuring their strengths and competences, their own ideas about ways of coping with adversity, and their rights to take part as active agents in their own development. As Qvortrup (1997, cited from Haydon and Scraton 2002) noted, adultism amounts to protective exclusion, based on their alleged lack of capability and competence.

1.3.2 Social Construction of Childhood and Adolescence

1.3.2.1 Social Construction of Childhood

While adultism always existed, according to Aries (1962, cited from James and James 2004), childhood did not exist in the medieval society, as the younger members of the society were not granted a special or distinctive social status. They participated in the society according to their abilities, just as adults did. The institution of childhood is the product of culture and politics, varying not only between societies but also within societies, between genders and over time (White 2003). Biology does not determine childhood or adolescence, but provides a context for it (O'Neill 2000, cited from White 2003), just as biology (sex) does not determine but provides the context for the gendered lives of girls and women. Industrial capitalism has led to and science, policies and programmes have shaped the social construction of childhood.

According to Jans (2004), until the eighteenth century, children were protected and cherished till they were 6 or 7 years old. Later they were considered to be pocket-sized adults, who were mostly involved in employment. The eighteenth century philosopher Rousseau is credited with inventing the modern notion of childhood as a distinct period of human life with particular needs of stimulation and education. This model upheld the innocence of the child and their freedom of contamination with the ugly lessons of civilization (Burman 2008).

Ruddick (2003) noted that the modern childhood and youth that emerged at the turn of the last century in Europe and North America had strong links to the anxieties of a growing middle class in western industrialising nations. According to her, for this class, the rise of industrial capitalism required a shift in strategies of social reproduction towards an increasingly educated (male) progeny, as the path into clerical and managerial work was directed increasingly through the classroom and away from the "shop floor". With the advent of compulsory education, a separation was realised between environment of children and that of adults. According to Jans (2004), the position of children has evolved from a strong social participation with minimal protection during the eighteenth and nineteenth centuries, to a strong protection with minimal participation during the twentieth century. As a result, children spend most of their time among themselves, secluded from the rest of society, in a psychosocial moratorium (Dasberg 1965, cited from Jans 2004).

According to Burman (2008, p. 74), the outrage over the conditions of child labourers in the late eighteenth century had less to do with exploitation than with fears of unruly and potentially undesirable activities made possible by an independent income. A national childhood was constructed through schooling, justifying making children dependent, imposing a middle-class ideal of childhood as a period of helplessness (Hendrick 1990, cited by Burman 2008). Although schooling was officially classless, it rendered the child (and therefore the family) always available for reformation of their working-class morals. Childhood thus emerged as a domain to be colonised and civilised (Burman 2008). Immigrant and economically disadvantaged families fought this new construction of childhood because it served to limit their family income (Jiminez 2010).

Education as the distinguishing factor for childhood has changed with the growing emphasis on lifelong learning. As Jans (2004) notes, learning no longer exclusively belongs to the domain of the school and no longer is restricted to the youth phase. It is changing the classic relation between children as those who need to learn and adults who need to teach. As Hengst (2001) states, childhood is being liberated from modernity's educational project.

According to Lavalette and Cunningham (2002), the New Sociology of Childhood has developed an approach based on post-modern perspectives, which comprises of four central claims:

1. Childhood is not merely a biological phenomenon, but a social construction, affected and shaped by wider social and cultural elements, within concrete, historical circumstances.
2. Children occupy and conduct themselves in worlds that are full of meaning for them, but about which adults are, at least partially, ignorant. It has led to an emphasis on listening to children's voices.
3. Politically children are powerless and disadvantaged. The new sociology is a theory of advocacy, sociology for children rather than sociology of children. This approach has closely tied into children's rights agenda.
4. Children are an identifiable social group. It is a universal category, as a result of which, children have a common set of needs and rights.

In this perspective, children are not the passive output of child-rearing practices nor their social development envisaged as the product of a simple biological determinism, but as social agents in shaping their own childhood experiences (James et al. 1998).

1.3.2.2 Social Construction of Adolescence

Baethge (1989, cited by Saraswathi 1999) noted that adolescence emerged as a life stage in the twentieth century, under the following conditions: learning process that is divorced from practice, delayed experience of one's own social usefulness, later choice of job or career, prolonged economic dependence on parents, more leisure time that can be spent with the same age group members and longer time spent in individual development rather than in collective code of performance. The prolonged emotional, psychological and economic dependency led to a century-long enduring mythology of adolescence, depicted as a period of storm and stress subject to hormonally induced mood swings. Those, who did not meet these norms of dependency in this stage, got to be termed "juvenile delinquents" (Ruddick 2003).

With the social construction of adolescence, and extension of childhood to age 18, more persons are covered under adultism. A report commissioned by the European Union that calls for a substantive European children's policy recommends the reduction of the age of majority to 16 in member countries (Ruxton 1999, cited from Wyness et al. 2004).

1.3.3 Western Scientific Construction of "Normal" Childhood

Childhood is largely studied by the disciplines of developmental psychology, child/human development and social work. These sciences have developed standards of "normal" childhood development according to age, based on Western, white, middle class, male constructs of normality. This western scientific construction of "normal" childhood has led to the following problems:

- Universal chronologisation negating variations in movement through childhood
- Discontinuity of childhood
- Confusion over adolescence as a stage in childhood as well as in youth
- Social construction of deviance

1.3.3.1 Universal Chronologisation Negating Variations in Movement Through Childhood

In different cultures, the movement of individual children through childhood is not followed with much precision and age is frequently treated as only an approximate benchmark. Many different kinds of criteria – although seldom age – are used to demarcate childhood (Boyden and Levison 2000). There is no universal agreement as to when childhood ceases and adulthood begins, as age is merely a rough indicator of his or her level of development. Sigelman and Shaffer (1995) observed that age means what a society chooses it to mean. While all societies treat age as a significant human attribute, each has its own ways of dividing the life span and of treating the individuals who fall into different age groups.

Universal biological markers like age at walking, emergence of speech, or onset of puberty can facilitate the demarcation of life stages. However, even such biological markers do not emerge at a uniform age for everyone, since they are dependent on genetic variations in different racial and ethnic groups, and on environmental factors such as nutrition, or socialisation practices. In addition to biological markers, societies use role transitions, which involve assuming new responsibilities and duties, to divide the life span (Craig 1996).

Earlier, puberty marked the end of childhood and the beginning of adulthood. In many societies puberty is a critical milestone, celebrated often by rites of passage, such as schooling, work, criminal responsibility, and sexual maturity. Children's tasks tend to change systematically at around puberty, the balance between education, unpaid and paid work shifting radically, with gender determining the appropriate roles, dress codes and patterns of social behaviour (Boyden and Levison 2000).

While the age of puberty as the beginning of adolescence varies, the age at which adolescence is supposed to end and adulthood starts is even more variable, depending on the criteria used. These criteria include the commencement of work, end of schooling, betrothal and marriage, among others. Normally the criteria that are applied differ according to gender and class. For street or working children, or girls married off in their mid-teens, adolescence may end even earlier. On the other hand, during the early years of adulthood, the tasks of adulthood may yet be in the process of being completed for those going through higher studies. Thus, it is essential to bear in mind that the experience of adolescence can differ considerably for individuals going though this stage, as a result of differences in socio-economic class and cultural practices, rural, urban, or semi-urban environment, involvement in labour force instead of the formal educational system and so on (Boyden and Levison 2000).

As Hockey and James (1996, cited from James and James 2004) noted, the precise chronologisation of ageing in relation to life course identities is a relatively recent phenomenon of modernity.

1.3.3.2 Discontinuity of Childhood

Chronologisation has created an artificial dichotomy between childhood and adulthood, as though they are distinctly different from one another. The distinction between childhood and adulthood at the age of 18 is arbitrary, fixed first by the sciences and then the UNCRC, negating childhood as a social construct. The prevalent adultist perspective of children considers children dependent, incomplete, changing, ignorant, becoming and, therefore, rendered powerless; and adults as independent, complete, stable, knowledgeable, being and, therefore, given power over the other, alienating one from the other. The former is given rights and the latter is given duties to protect these rights. In fact, as James and James (2004) emphasise, it is the supposed differences between children and adults that underpin the institution of childhood.

Benedict (1938) noted way back that

> ... our [modern Western] culture goes to great extremes in emphasizing contrasts between the child and the adult. The child is sexless, the adult estimates his virility by his sexual activities; the child must be protected from the ugly facts of life, the adult must meet them

> without psychic catastrophe; the child must obey, the adult must command this obedience. ... a good son is tractable, and does not assume adult responsibilities; a good father provides for his children and should not allow his authority to be flouted .... The individual in one role must revise his behavior from almost all points of view when he assumes the second role. ... adults in our culture put all the blame on the child when he fails to manifest spontaneously the new behavior or, overstepping the mark, manifests it with untoward belligerence.

According to Benedict (1938), such discontinuities in cultural conditioning contribute to maladjustment and personality upheavals. The "storm and stress", for which adolescence is known, is a manifestation of such discontinuous cultural institutions and dogmas rather than a physiological necessity. Operationally, it raises the need and problems with reference to age verification as two different sets of norms and laws apply to those below and those above 18.

1.3.3.3 Confusion over Adolescence as a Stage in Childhood and in Youth

"Youth" is a construct that has further confused the chronologisation of childhood. During the International Youth Year, in 1985, the United Nations General Assembly defined "youth" as those persons falling between the ages of 15 and 24 years inclusive. Thus, "childhood" as well as "youth" includes adolescence. Within the category of "youth", the UN distinguishes between teenagers (13–19) and young adults (20–24), since the sociological, psychological and health problems they face may differ (Youth at the United Nations No date). Thus, "childhood" as well as "youth" includes adolescence, but children's documents, policies and programmes are different than those for youth.

1.3.3.4 Social Construction of Deviance

The Western standards of normal childhood are based on adultist notions of childhood as a basically biologically driven "natural" phenomenon in which children are distinguished from adults by specific physical and mental (as opposed to social) characteristics. Children are seen as separated from the world of work and devoting their time to learning and play and thus economically worthless, apolitical and asexual. Another feature of this model is the emphasis on the child as individual (rather than a member of a social group), and on parents and nuclear family as the "natural" immediate vehicles of protection, socialisation and control. Globalisation is transferring these mythical norms of childhood to the world's children, a majority of whom are growing up in poverty groups of the developing nations. The transfer of these "normal" standards to them makes their life seem deviant, inferior or pathological (White 2003). The UNCRC is also critiqued of doing the same (Wyness et al. 2004). Thus, deviance is socially constructed by western norms and the world's children are vulnerable to services that control and work on them to attain measures that bring them inside the bands of "normal" (EU Canada Project 2003).

1.3.4 Conclusion

In conclusion, vulnerability in childhood is socially constructed and it can be prevented by

- Challenging adultism and achieving age-based equality and participatory inclusion;
- Challenging homogenisation of childhood by advocating the life-cycle approach, that perceives life as divided into stages of early childhood, middle childhood, adolescence, youth, middle adulthood and old age;
- A contextualised "normalisation" of children's behavior and
- Abandoning derogatory labels for children such as "illegitimate", "delinquent", "disabled" (Desai 2007).

1.4 Ecological Context of Childhood Vulnerability

1.4.1 Ecological Perspective on Childhood

The ecological perspective enhances a holistic view to understand the entirety of the social, psychological and physiological organism and enlarges an appreciation of the creative and adaptive potentialities, not only within the people but also within the environment in which they function (Goldstein 1973). Bronfenbrenner (1979, cited from Newman and Newman 2006) defined the environment as an interlocking system of micro-, meso-, exo- and macro-systems.

Family is the micro-system for most of the children. It is an inseparable part of children's birth, identity, name, language, ethnicity, religion and nationality. The family's composition, structure and interaction patterns are major factors in children's survival, health, education, development and protection. The ecological perspective views the child in the context of his/her family and the family in the context of its environment as these constantly interact with and, therefore, influence one another. The child's meso-system is the family's immediate environment, comprising of the ethnic/kinship community, neighbourhood, natural environment, work place, school/college, friends, media and so on. The state, corporate sector and the market influence the family indirectly as the exo-system. The macro-system is the larger international eco-political contexts in which these systems are embedded. Diversity in the environment brings variations in family life, which, in turn, explains differences in children's well-being to a large extent. Similarly, changes in the environment influence the family life, which affects the children (Desai 1994).

In the ecological social work perspective, children's problems are seen as deficits in the environment, as dysfunctional transactions between systems, rather than a disease located within the child. Problems are not viewed as an attribute of children; these are viewed as an attribute of their social situation (Hartman and Laird 1983). The embeddedness of children's problems from micro- to macro-systems and linkages between these systems are understood. Oppression and discrimination issues are identified based on ethnicity, gender, class, age and sexual orientation (Parsons et al. 1994). Such ecological perspective implies that intervening only with the children does not go very far in improving their situation, unless the micro-, meso-, exo- and also the macro-factors influencing children are understood and dealt with.

This section will examine the following ecological factors influencing children:

- Patriarchal family which form the children's micro-systems; and
- Modern factors of development and liberalisation and emergency situations which form children's meso-, exo- and macro-systems.

1.4.2 Childhood Vulnerability in Patriarchal Family

The societal evolutionary theory indicates that the primeval practice was group living, based on the sharing of partners and children within a group. Later this gave way to a matrilineal system as children were biologically attached to their mothers. In the agriculture and horticulture phase, paternity was discovered through domestication of animals. This led to the development of patriliny and patriarchy (Pandhe 1989). Marriage became a basic societal requirement for controlling women's sexuality and reproduction to ensure paternity of the child. In patriliny, identity and property are handed down from the father to the "legitimate" son. Children born out of wedlock, before or after marriage, are considered "illegitimate". Thus, the concept of "legitimacy" of the child linked to child's identity is rooted in the concept of sexual morality of their mothers, controlled by the institution of marriage. Children of unmarried mothers are often abandoned, due to the stigma of the "illegitimacy".

Child bearing is institutionalised in marriage for perpetuation of the patrilineal lineage. Although child bearing is considered extremely important in the patriarchal family, children have not been considered important as it is an adultist, age-conscious structure. Roles and responsibilities and control and distribution of resources are strictly determined by hierarchies of age, gender and generation. Control over resources and assumption of superiority give the man the authority to make decisions about his dependents, which mainly include women and children. Children are supposed to be obedient to elders and have little say in decisions, which are made for them. Kinship orientation or the community expectations and family unity are considered more important than individual desires. If a child asserts himself or herself, in the process of disagreeing with the elderly or making his or her own life choices, the family's unity and stability are perceived to be threatened. Familism or the belief that individuals have to make some sacrifices for the benefit of all is fostered. Thus, by age, children are made vulnerable to subordination and control in patriarchal families.

Parents are given the authority to control their children for disciplining them, thus child abuse gets institutionalised in the family. However, there is an aura of silence about this aspect, as the family is considered a very private matter.

1.4.3 Development, Liberalisation and Globalisation Aggravating Childhood Vulnerability

Although children are vulnerable to neglect and abuse in the traditional patriarchal families, traditionally children did grow up among family and community support. Development and liberalisation have not only aggravated patriarchy but have made families and communities weaker. Experiences from across the world have shown that children are among the most vulnerable when local economies are opened up to global market forces without making adequate investments and putting safeguards for the susceptible sections of population (Hukku 2004).

The liberal paradigm of development adopted by most of the world, has led to a profit and production-oriented society, ignoring people and their needs. Liberalism has substituted economic relations for traditional communal bonds, neglecting such values as solidarity, love, affection and a sense of community (Fink 1981). It has created a world of possessive individualism. It assumes the existence of individuals and abstract rules without a society that shapes them (Marshall 1994). Individualism became essential for the economic growth, social values being considered secondary to the creation and satisfaction of wants. The unlimited pursuit of pleasure is considered the ultimate right of every person, thus transmitting selfishness into a universal virtue (Pereira 1997).

Globalisation is the natural outcome of the neo-liberalist ideology, which promotes minimum government interference and considers market as the sole social regulator (George et al. 1997). The global economy arranges its global operations to produce products where costs are lowest, sell them where markets are more lucrative, and shift the resulting profits to where tax rates are least burdensome. This weakens the bargaining power of any given locality and shifts the balance of power from the local human interest to the global corporate interest. It weakens the community to free the market, eliminates livelihoods to create wealth and destroys life to increase unneeded and often unsatisfying consumption (Korten 1999). Thus, consumerism has increased among the few rich, which has resulted in ecological degradation, migration and displacement among a large number of poor. This causes loss of livelihood, urban ghettoisation, expansion of slums and pavement dwelling.

Globalisation has led to increased migration together with increased unemployment among men due to replacement by automatic machines. It has resulted in a major expansion of the unprotected, unorganised labour force. This force is also joined by an increasing number of women and children. The unorganised sector does not provide social security and scope for unionisation or application of anti-discrimination laws and so on. This has led to increased poverty among the female-headed families or feminisation of poverty. As Ilich (1983) put it, higher labour force participation by women implies that more women have been incorporated into the population that is economically discriminated against on the ground of sex. According to Luxton (2002), what causes child poverty are gendered division of labour, labour market segregation and segmentation, pay inequalities, the lack of public support for care-giving and men's widespread reluctance to pay child support. It is these social practices which result in women's poverty and, by extension, impoverish their children.

1.4.4 Conclusion

The environmental factors impinging childhood may be dealt with by aiming at prevention of patriarchy and poverty by working towards achieving the United Nations Millennium Goals of eradication of extreme poverty and hunger, promotion of gender equality and empowerment of women and ensuring environmental sustainability (Desai 2007).

1.5 Concepts and Cycle of Problems in Childhood and Adult Life

1.5.1 Need to Redefine Concepts

The growing global studies on children, across the developed and developing countries, have thrown up the need to redefine the concepts used in different parts of the world, rather than make everything fit into the existing concepts.

The trend in the western countries is to use the terms "child abuse" and "child neglect" together in knowledge development, laws and the child protection programmes. For example, the International Society for Prevention of Child Abuse and Neglect publishes an international journal called *Child Abuse and Neglect.* According to the Child Abuse Prevention and Treatment Act of 1974 (amended in 2003), "the term 'child abuse and neglect' means, at a minimum, any recent act or failure to act on the part of a parent or caretaker, which results in death, serious physical or emotional harm, sexual abuse or exploitation, or an act or failure to act which presents an imminent risk of serious harm" (United States Department of Health and Human Services 2003, p. 44). Then the Child Welfare Information Gateway (2006) defines *neglect* as the failure to provide for a child's basic needs. The reasons for failure to provide for children's basic needs and reasons for causing intentional harm to children are significantly different so the interventions needed in these two situations are also different.

Some authors use the term "child abuse" to include commercial exploitation of children, when they examine child abuse across the globe (for example Schwartz-Kenney et al. 2000).

1.5.2 Cycle of Problems in Childhood

Child welfare and child rights literature generally discuss a list of problems of children without any attempt to see linkages among them, which results in fragmentation of services. These linkages are necessary to examine as they would help prioritise services that can prevent problems. Today all children are vulnerable to neglect and abuse due to adultism and patriarchy. However, some individual, parental and situational characteristics put children at a greater risk of neglect. Neglected children are more vulnerable to abuse or commercial exploitation. Abused children are more vulnerable to commercial exploitation. Commercially exploited children are more vulnerable to conflict with the law (Desai 2007). It is important to understand this cycle of problems as well as the differential causes, manifestations and consequences in each problem situation, as elaborated in this section.

1.5.3 Neglect in Childhood

Since parents are the main caretakers of children, child neglect takes place when parents are incapacitated, unavailable or unwilling to carry out their parental role or are facing conflicts (adapted from Kadushin and Martin 1988). Children at risk are more vulnerable to neglect also due to individual and/or situational characteristics. Thus, the following children are at risk of vulnerability to neglect

- Children with special needs
    - Children with neuro-behavioural disorders
    - Children with disability and/or chronic illness
- Parental characteristics
    - Children of incapable parents
        - Children of substance users
        - Children of HIV/AIDS-infected/terminally ill parents
    - Children of Parents Facing Conflict
        - Children of battered women
        - Children of divorce
    - Children of unavailable parents
        - Children of single-parent families
        - Children of prisoners
        - Child-headed households
        - Street children
    - Children of unwilling parents
        - Children born out of wedlock
        - Abandoned children

- Situational characteristics
  - Children in poverty groups
  - Children of migrants
  - Children in emergency situations

Neglected children are vulnerable to abuse, commercial exploitation and conflict with law.

1.5.4 Abuse in Childhood

Child abuse is

- Any intentional non-accidental physical, emotional and psychological or sexual harm done to a child, that endangers or impairs the child's physical, emotional and psychological or sexual health and development;
- By older children, parents, relatives, caretakers, neighbours, teachers, employers, police or strangers; in family, neighbourhood, street, school, institutions, site of occupation or police custody;
- Because of adult–child power imbalance due to adultism and patriarchy, psychosocial problems or socio-economic problems, and cycle of abuse.

The commercially exploited children and those in conflict with law are more vulnerable to abuse and the abused children are vulnerable to commercial exploitation and conflict with law.

1.5.5 Commercial Exploitation in Childhood

In the context of increased consumerism among the rich and poverty among the poor, children from the poverty groups are commodified for begging, labour, sexual exploitation, adoption, marriage and entertainment to meet the needs of their poor parents and for consumption of the rich adults. Vitit Muntarbhorn, the Special Rapporteur on Sale of Children, Child Prostitution and Child Pornography, stated in his report (1994) that poverty alone does not lead to commercial exploitation of children. It relates to the supply side of the problem. The global demand is explained by customers and the criminal networks which benefit from it and by collusion and corruption in many national settings. Globalisation has also led to expansion of the international organised crime, enlarging the scope for exploitation of children. Rehabilitation of the rescued children has become the most challenging issue for child protection due to the global nexus.

Thus, in commercial exploitation of children

- Child abuse that is connected with cash or in-kind profit for the child and/or a third party;

- The third party who make profit, that is the procurers/agents, are part of the commercial and/or criminal nexus comprising largely of men, also women;
- The child victims are generally neglected school dropouts from the poverty groups who are commodified mainly for labour or sexual consumption of the rich adults;
- The result is impairment of not only the child's physical, emotional and psychological or sexual health and development but also child right to health and nutrition, housing, education, rest and recreation, and participation (adapted from UNESCAP 1999, cited from UNICEF 2001).

Commercial exploitation of children comprises of

1. Trafficking and sale of children: gender and age-specific, rural to urban, interstate and international, for begging, labour, prostitution, adoption, entertainment, sale of organs and marriage
2. Exploitation of children for labour: in organised hazardous industries and unorganised begging, domestic and hotel sector; trafficked and bonded, unpaid or under-paid
3. Commercial sexual exploitation of children: Child prostitution, sex tourism and pornography
4. Substance abuse among children

Commercial exploitation of children is a crime and often the victims of this crime are criminalised. Commercially exploited children are thus more vulnerable to conflict with the law.

1.5.6 Conflict with Law in Childhood

"Child in conflict with law" is a broad term that describes the situation in which the child is rather than describing the child himself/herself. Children in conflict with law thus include the following children:

- Status offenders
- Children who commit property crimes
- Children who commit violent crimes

The characteristics of the children in conflict with law comprise of

- Poverty
- Neuro-behavioural disorders
- Neglect
- Abuse
- Commercial exploitation

1.5.7 Effects in Childhood

Neglect, abuse, commercial exploitation or conflict with law in childhood can lead to the following problems, amounting to loss of childhood and further vulnerability to neglect, abuse, commercial exploitation and conflict with law:

- Loss of self-respect and dignity, leading to submissiveness and tolerance to more abuse and exploitation.
- Problems with mental and emotional health and social relationships.
- Problems with physical health and development.
- Disruption of education, recreation and cultural life.

1.5.8 Implications for Adult Life

Children's well-being is crucial not only for their well-being in childhood but for their well-being as adults and that of their children as well. It is, therefore, vulnerability in childhood as a stage of human life that we are concerned with, for the well-being in subsequent life stages and subsequent generations. The implications of neglect, abuse, commercial exploitation or conflict with law in childhood for adult life are

- Submissiveness and tolerance to more abuse and exploitation.
- Recycling of ideology of adultism, protective exclusion and patriarchy.
- Survivor turning abuser/criminal and abusing and exploiting their own or others' children and other vulnerable groups.

Chart 1.3 Cycle of Problems in Childhood and Adult Life

Factors leading to vulnerability in childhood

Social construction of childhood vulnerability:	Ecological factors affecting childhood vulnerability:
• Adultism and protective exclusion in childhood • Social construction of childhood and adolescence • Western scientific construction of "Normal" childhood	• Patriarchy • Development, liberalisation and globalisation

↓

Chart 1.3 (continued)

Factors leading to risk of neglect in childhood

Children characteristics:
- Neuro-behavioural Disorders
- Disability and/or chronic illness

Parental characteristics:
- Incapable parents
- Parents facing Conflict
- Unavailable parents
- Unwilling parents

Situational characteristics:
- Poverty
- Migration
- Emergency situations

↓

Abuse in childhood

Types:
- Physical
- Emotional
- Sexual

Characteristics of the abuser:
- Adultist
- Patriarchal
- Facing psychosocial problems
- Facing socio-economic problems
- Abused in childhood

Characteristics of the Abused children:
- Commercially Exploited
- Conflict with law

↑↓

Commercial exploitation in childhood

Types:
- Trafficking and sale of children
- Child labour
- Commercial sexual exploitation of children
- Substance abuse among children

Characteristics of the Exploiter:
- Paedophiles
- Commercial networks
- Criminal networks

Characteristics of the Exploited children:
- Poverty
- Migration
- Emergency situations
- Abused
- Conflict with law

Conflict with law in childhood

Types:
- Status offenders
- Children who commit property crimes
- Children who commit violent crimes

Characteristics of the children in conflict with law:
- Poverty
- Neuro-behavioural Disorders
- Neglect
- Abuse
- Commercial Exploitation

↑↓

↑↓

Effects in childhood

- Loss of self-respect and dignity, leading to submissiveness and tolerance to more abuse and exploitation
- Problems with mental and emotional health and social relationships
- Problems with physical health and development
- Disruption of education, recreation and cultural life

↓

Implications for adult life

- Submissiveness and tolerance to more abuse and exploitation
- Recycling of ideology of adultism, protective exclusion and patriarchy
- Survivor turning abuser/criminal and abusing and exploiting their own or others' children and other vulnerable groups

Note

This chapter is further development of parts of the following articles by the author:

- 'Towards a comprehensive cross-national conceptual framework for child protection', in a special issue on "Child protection: Challenges worldwide". *Social Development Issues*, 2007, 29(3), 1–18; and
- 'Towards a rights-based approach to child protection', Inaugural issue of *Rajagiri Journal for Social Development*, 2006, 1(1), 66–86.

References

Benedict, R. (1938). Continuities and discontinuities in cultural conditioning. *Psychiatry*, 1, 161–167.

Boyden, J. and Levison, D. (2000). *Children as Economic and Social Actors in the Development Process*. Stockholm: Ministry of Foreign Affairs.

Burman, E. (2008). *Deconstructing Developmental Psychology* (2nd ed.). London: Routledge Taylor and Francis Group.

Child Welfare Information Gateway. (2006). *What Is Child Abuse and Neglect?* http://www.childwelfare.gov/pubs/factsheets/whatiscan.cfm. Accessed 8 May 2007.

Craig, G. J. (1996). *Human Development*. Upper Saddle River, NJ: Prentice Hall.

Dale, O., Smith, R., Norlin, J. M. and Chess, W. A. (2006). *Human Behavior and the Social Environment: Social Systems Theory* (5th ed.). Boston, MA: Pearson Allyn and Bacon.

Desai, M. (1994). Concepts and conceptual frameworks for understanding family. In *Enhancing the Role of the Family as an Agency for Social and Economic Development*. Bombay: Tata Institute of Social Sciences.

Desai, M. (2007). Towards a comprehensive cross-national conceptual framework for child protection, for the special issue on "Child protection: Challenges worldwide". *Social Development Issues*, 29(3), 1–18.

EU Canada Project. (2003). *Child Welfare Across Borders*. www.sws.soton.ac.uk/cwab/index.htm. Accessed 3 March 2004.

Fink, H. (1981). *Social Philosophy*. London: Methuen.

George, V., Ramakrishnan, A. K. and Cheriyan, G. (1997). Ecumenical response to globalisation. *Lokayan Bulletin*, 13(5), 61–64.

Goldstein, H. (1973). *Social Work Practice: A Unitary Approach*. Columbia, SC: University of South Carolina Press.

Hartman, A. and Laird, J. (1983). *Family-Centered Social Work Practice*. New York, NY: The Free Press.

Haydon, D. and Scraton, P. (2002). Sex education as regulation. In B. Goldson, M. Lavalette and J. McKechnie (Eds.) *Children, Welfare and the State* (pp. 152–168). London: Sage Publications.

Hengst, H. (2001). Rethinking the liquidation of childhood. In M. Du Bois-Raymond, H. Süncker and H. H. Krüger (Eds.) *Childhood in Europe* (pp. 13–41). New York, NY: Peter Lang.

Hukku, I. (2004). Globalisation – Will our children pay the price? *Combat Law*, 3(1).

Ilich, I. (1983). *Gender*. London: Marion Boyars.

James, A. and James, A. (2004). *Constructing Childhood: Theory, Policy and Social Practice*. New York, NY: Palgrave Macmillan.

James, A., Jenks, C. and Prout, A. (1998). *Theorising Childhood*. Cambridge: Polity Press.

Jans, M. (2004). Children as citizens: Towards a contemporary notion of child participation. *Childhood*, 11(1), 27–44.

Jiminez, J. (2010). *Social Policy and Social Change: Toward the Creation of Social and Economic Justice*. London: Sage.

Kadushin, A. and Martin, J. A. (1988). *Child Welfare Services* (4th ed.). New York, NY: Macmillan Publishing Co. http://linc.nus.edu.sg:2084/record=b1220699.

Kennedy, D. (No date). *Notes on the Philosophy of Childhood and the Politics of Subjectivity*. Massachusetts: The Paedia Project On-Line. www.bu.edu/wcp/Papers/Chil/ChilKenn.htm. Accessed 18 April 2004.

Korten, D. C. (1999). When corporations rule the world. *Humanscape*, 6(2), 8–13.

Lavalette, M. and Cunningham, S. (2002). The sociology of childhood. In B. Goldson, M. Lavalette and J. McKechnie (Eds.) *Children, Welfare and the State* (pp. 9–28). London: Sage Publications.

Lesser, J. G. and Pope, D. S. (2007). *Human Behavior and the Social Environment: Theory and Practice*. Boston, MA: Pearson Allyn and Bacon.

Levison, D. (2000). Children as economic agents. *Feminist Economics*, 6(1), 125–134. http://www.hhh.umn.edu/img/assets/3737/Levison%20(2000)%20Children%20As%20Economic%20Agents.pdf. Accessed 18 April 2004.

Luxton, M. (2002). *Feminist Perspectives on Social Inclusion and Children's Well-Being*. Toronto, ON: Working Paper Series of Laidlaw Foundation.

Marshall, G. (Ed.) (1994). *The Concise Oxford Dictionary of Sociology*. New York, NY: Oxford University Press.

Mason, J. and Steadman, B. (1996). *The Significance of the Conceptualisation of Childhood for Promoting Children's Contributions to Child Protection Policy*. Paper presented at the fifth Australian Family Research conference, organised by the Australian Institute of Family Studies, Brisbane.

Matthews, G. (2004). The philosophy of childhood. In E. N. Zalta (Ed.) *The Stanford Encyclopedia of Philosophy*. www.plato.stanford.edu/archives/fall2002/entries/childhood/. Accessed 25 February 2005.

Muntarbhorn, V. (1994). Report of the Special Rapporteur on sale of children, child prostitution and child pornography.

Newman, B. M. and Newman, P. R. (2006). *Development Through Life: A Psychosocial Approach* (10th ed.). Belmont, CA: Brooks/Cole.

Pandhe, S. (1989). *Women's Subordination* (Its Origins). New Delhi: Kanak Publications.

Parsons, R. J., Jorgensen, J. D. and Hernandez, S. H. (1994). *The Integration of Social Work Practice*. Belmont, CA: Brooks/Cole.

Pereira, W. (1997). *Inhuman Rights: The Western System and Global Human Rights Abuse*. Mapusa, Goa: The Other India Press.

Robbins, S. P., Chatterjee, P. and Canda, E. R. (2006). *Contemporary Human Behavior Theory: A Critical Perspective for Social Work* (2nd ed.). Boston, MA: Pearson Allyn and Bacon.

Ruddick, S. (2003). The politics of aging: Globalization and the restructuring of youth and childhood. *Antipode: A Radical Journal of Geography*, 35(2), 334–362.

Saraswathi, T. S. (1999). Adult-child continuity in India: Is adolescence a myth or an emerging reality? In T. S. Saraswathi (Ed.) *Culture, Socialization and Human Development* (pp. 213–232). New Delhi: Sage Publishers.

Schriver, J. M. (2004). *Human Behavior and the Social Environment: Shifting Paradigms in Essential Knowledge for Social Work Practice* (4th ed.). Boston, MA: Pearson Allyn and Bacon.

Schwartz-Kenney, B. M., McCauley, M. and Epstein, M. A. (Eds.) (2000). *Child Abuse a Global View*. Westport, CT: Greenwood Press.

Sigelman, C. K. and Shaffer, D. R. (1995). *Life-Span Human Development*. Pacific Grove, CA: Brooks/Cole.

United Nations Children's Fund. (2001). *Pocket Guide for a Rights-Based Approach to Programming for Children: Application in South Asia*. Kathmandu: United Nations Children's Fund.

United States Department of Health and Human Services: Administration for Children and Families. (2003). *Child Abuse Prevention and Treatment Act*. http://www.acf.hhs.gov/programs/cb/laws_policies/cblaws/capta03/sec_I_111.htm. Accessed 6 March 2007.

White, B. (2003). *A World Fit for Children?* Dies Natalis address delivered on the occasion of the 51st anniversary of the Institute of Social Studies, The Hague, The Netherlands.
Wikipedia. (2005). *Adultism*. www.//en.wikipedia.org/wiki/Adultism. Accessed 15 January 2006.
Wyness, M., Harrison, L. and Buchanan, I. (2004). Childhood, politics and ambiguity: Towards an agenda for children's political inclusion. *Sociology*, 38(1), 81–99.
Youth at the United Nations. (No date). *Frequently Asked Questions*. //www.un.org/esa/socdev/unyin/qanda.htm. Accessed 5 May 2007.

Chapter 2
The Child Rights Perspective

2.1 Pre-rights Policy Perspectives for Children

2.1.1 Laissez-faire and Patriarchy Perspective

According to Harding (1991), the laissez-faire and patriarchy perspective was essentially the position that the patriarchal power in the family should not be disturbed by the state except in very extreme circumstances, such as criminality. It implied that the state should not interfere with the power of adults over children and men over women within the family.

2.1.2 State Paternalism and Child Protection Perspective

The state paternalism and child protection perspective is the most popular perspective today. James and James (2004) emphasise that law and policies work to ground, control and legitimatize the power imbalance between children and adults. Children are segregated into schools, children's hospitals and young offenders' institutions and are not permitted access to the adult spaces of the workplace and public house.

According to Harding (1991), in the juvenile justice system, extensive state intervention to protect and care for children is legitimatize by the paternalistic perspective, but state intervention itself is authoritarian and the child's biological family (which will be referred to as the "natural family" in this book) bonds are undervalued. In this perspective, much greater faith is placed in the value of the beneficent state action to protect children's welfare. Substitute care is favoured when the care of the natural family is found to be inadequate.

2.1.3 Defence of the Birth Family and Parents' Rights Perspective

Harding (1991) notes that the defence of the birth family and parents' rights perspective encapsulates the idea that birth or biological families are important for both children and parents and should be maintained wherever possible. The role of

M. Desai, *A Rights-Based Preventative Approach for Psychosocial Well-Being in Childhood*, Children's Well-Being: Indicators and Research 3,
DOI 10.1007/978-90-481-9066-9_2, © Springer Science+Business Media B.V. 2010

the state is seen as supportive of families, providing various services that they need to remain together. There is an emphasis on the rights of parents as people in their own right, with an explanation of poor quality childcare, which is sympathetic to parental difficulties. Placing children in substitute care is seen as generally undesirable. Where children do have to come into state care, considerable intervention should be devoted to helping their families and maintaining links with them so that the children can return home again. It points out the class element in state care where middle-class decision-makers pass judgement on working-class parents and children from deprived homes who are placed in somewhat better-off ones.

2.2 The Child Rights Perspective

2.2.1 History of the United Nations Convention on the Rights of the Child

In 1924, the League of Nations endorsed the first Declaration on the Rights of the Child. In 1948, the General Assembly adopted a second Declaration of the Rights of the Child, a brief seven-point statement that built on the 1924 Declaration. It stated that "... men and women of all nations, recognising that mankind owes to the child the best that it has to give, declare and accept it as their duty to meet this obligation in all respects ...". The same year, the United Nations (UN) adopted and proclaimed the Universal Declaration of Human Rights (UDHR), comprised of values of human dignity drawn from secular humanism; freedom drawn from liberalism; participation drawn from democracy and equality drawn from socialism. All the articles of the UDHR are applicable to all human beings including children, except for Article 16, which is in reference to rights within marriage. Article 25 in particular, states that motherhood and childhood are entitled to special care and assistance. This Article further states that all children, whether born in or out of wedlock, shall enjoy the same social protection. Article 26 states that parents will have the prior right to choose the kind of education that shall be given to their children. In 1959, a more detailed third Declaration of the Rights of the Child was adopted by the UN General Assembly. However, a Declaration is not a binding instrument and does not impose specific obligations on Member States.

Boyden and Levison (2000) noted that the United Nations International Year of the Child (1979) provided considerable momentum internationally for childhood issues. A multitude of new child-focused organisations – national, regional and international – were founded during and immediately after 1979. Conferences and workshops on a variety of childhood topics encouraged the exchange of field experience across continents and disciplines. Research, advocacy and networking on childhood issues led to revised definitions and understanding of existing problems, highlighted new concerns and raised general awareness of the magnitude of the threat to child well-being globally. Studies of hazardous work and child abuse, for example challenged previous notions that physical deprivation – in terms of clean water, nutrition, rest and so on – is the only major threat to children globally and suggested that such social violations may also be extremely common and severe. At the same time, traditional responses to social distress, such as the institutionalisation of children separated from their families, were found inadequate: they did not reach enough children, nor did they have consistently positive impacts on the children that they did reach. This implied the need for new ideas and new approaches.

According to Boyden and Levison (2000), children's rights advocates began to gather evidence pointing to political causes of much childhood deprivation and suffering. They showed that the State could imperil children just as much as protect and nurture them, sometimes even under the guise of protection. They uncovered instances not just of inaction by the state but, more seriously, of acts of commission against children, such as their arrest, detention and torture. Practitioners and advocates in children's rights argued for the urgency of defining more precisely the responsibilities of the modern nation state in relation to children and, especially, the need to make more explicit its protective roles in regards to children deprived of family or community support. The UN Commission on Human Rights eventually began to consider a proposal advanced by the Polish government for a Convention on the Rights of the Child (CRC), a Convention being more binding on State Parties than a Declaration. The main idea was, essentially, to make the State accountable for its effects on children.

In 1989, the United Nations General Assembly unanimously adopted the Convention on the Rights of the Child (UNCRC). Its Preamble states the following:

> Considering that the child should be fully prepared to live an individual life in society, and brought up in the spirit of the ideals proclaimed in the Charter of the United Nations, and in particular in the spirit of peace, dignity, tolerance, freedom, equality and solidarity;
> Bearing in mind that, as indicated in the Declaration of the Rights of the Child, the child, by reason of his physical and mental immaturity, needs special safeguards and care, including appropriate legal protection, before as well as after birth;
> Recognizing that, in all countries in the world, there are children living in exceptionally difficult conditions, and that such children need special consideration;
> Taking due account of the importance of the traditions and cultural values of each people for the protection and harmonious development of the child.

The UNCRC is the most universally and speedily signed and ratified convention in the UN's history. White (2003) posits the question of whether this is because governments, power-holders and societies take young people's needs and rights seriously or precisely because they do not take them seriously and therefore do not mind committing themselves to obligations which they do not intend to fulfil, and which cannot be enforced. According to white, the latter is more likely to be true.

2.2.2 Needs Versus Rights Approach

According to Save the Children (2002), the rights-based approach to development is often defined by contrasting it with the child welfare or the needs-based approach. They are both based on a desire to help people survive and develop to their full potential. They both seek to identify a range of assistance and actions that are needed to achieve this. Where they differ is in their underlying assumptions and the implications of these assumptions for programming. The box that follows lays out the key features of both the approaches, demonstrating how the approaches can be placed at different ends of the same continuum.

Chart 2.1 Comparison of Needs Approach and Rights Approach

Needs approach	Rights approach
• Each programme has its own goal but there is no unifying overall purpose	• There is an overarching goal to which all programmes contribute
• Specific projects targeting specific groups of children	• Holistic approach
• Hierarchy of needs as some needs are considered more important than others	• Rights cannot be divided, they are indivisible and interdependent
• Address symptoms	• Address root causes
• Short-term perspective	• Long-term perspective
• Aims at welfare	• Aims at legal entitlements, claims, guarantees justice, equality, freedom
• Providing welfare services as object of needs	• Empowering rights holders as subject of rights to claim their rights
• Service provision	• Awareness-raising (of parents, children, decision-makers)
• Private charity	• Public, political, moral and legal responsibility, obligation, duty
• Voluntary	• Mandatory
• Needs vary according to the situation, the individual and the environment	• Rights are universal
• Determination of needs is subjective	• Rights are based on international standards
• Governments ought to do something but nobody has definite obligations	• Governments have binding legal and moral obligations
• Given scarce resources some children may be left out	• All children have the same right to fulfil their potential
• Children are recipients of services	• Children are active participants in the service delivery

2.2.3 *Concepts of Child Rights*

According to UNICEF (2001), children justify special arrangements and special attention to protect, promote and fulfil their human rights, for the following reasons:

- Children are initially totally dependent – they can grow towards independence only with the help of adults;
- Childhood is the most formative period in life. The developmental state of children makes them particularly susceptible to the conditions under which they may live – whether it be poor food, environmental pollution, violence or a supportive, loving and stimulating environment;

- Children's survival, development and active participation are crucial to the progress of any society; and it makes good sense to invest in the growth and development of the child;
- Adolescence is a critical period in a child's life – positive and negative behaviours adopted during this period will have impact on the adult life;
- Children play no part in the formal political process and it is difficult for them to use the legal system – therefore, special arrangements are required to ensure that, children's rights and interests are properly represented in all decision-making which affects them.

2.2.4 Review of the United Nations Convention on the Rights of the Child

The new paradigm in childhood studies questions the understanding that children need rights because they are dependent and in the formative period, that they are an investment with a goal for outcome as adults, and children's interests are to be represented. Sentimentality towards children's vulnerability is no substitute for the recognition of their entitlement to the right to equal concern and respect as adults (Freeman 1983, cited from Boyden and Levison 2000).

Wyness, Harrison and Buchanan (2004) note that the UNCRC is based on the norms of a "normal" childhood development, based on western, white, middle class, male constructs of normality. These are based on adultist notions of childhood as a basically biologically driven "natural" phenomenon in which children are distinguished from adults by specific physical and mental (as opposed to social) characteristics. Children are seen as separated from the world of work and devoting their time to learning and play and thus economically worthless, apolitical and asexual. UNCRC is transferring these mythical norms of childhood to the world's children. The transfer of these "normal" norms to them makes their life seem deviant, inferior or pathological (White 2003). The world's children are then vulnerable to services that control and work on them to attain measures that bring them inside the bands of "normal" (EU Canada Project 2003).

White (2003) further notes that the UNCRC rights to expression of views, communication of information and freedom do not adequately amount to right to participation. These do not deal with the blanket exclusion of children from social, economic, or political processes for which appropriate age for specific responsibilities may be worked out.

The UNCRC focuses on children rather than childhood as a life stage, implying that children are a never-changing separate group. According to James and James (2004), the identity of "the child" is a transient identity for the individual, simply a passing through en route to adulthood. A life-cycle approach is needed to understand childhood as a life stage, the experiences of which have a bearing on future phases, either immediate or long term (UNICEF 2001). The definition of children as those up to the age of 18 years also suffers from conceptualisation of children as an agewise homogenous group. This age is arbitrarily fixed as the distinction between childhood and adulthood. Operationally, it raises the need and problems with reference to age verification as two different sets of norms and laws apply to those below and those above 18. Moreover, the UNCRC definition of children as those up to the age of 18 years is applied across the world, negating childhood as a social construct (James and James 2004).

There is a need to consider adolescence as a stage of transition between childhood and adulthood, rather than a stage within childhood. Rights in adolescence need to be dealt with differently than those in childhood. The former would have emphasis on the following:

- Sexual rights and responsibilities
- Right to vocational guidance and selection
- Citizens' rights and responsibilities
- Right to selection and preparation for marriage

2.3 Categories of Child Rights

Like the UDHR, the UNCRC also broadly comprises of the economic, social and cultural rights, which are the positive rights, and the civil and political rights, which are the negative rights. Article 4 of the UNCRC emphasises the economic, social and cultural rights, as follows: "With regard to economic, social and cultural rights, States Parties shall undertake such measures to the maximum extent of their available resources and, where needed, within the framework of international co-operation." These rights are the contribution of the socialist lobby, which recommends state intervention for redistribution of resources. They emphasise the child right to adult provision for basic necessities, which adults can do better than children themselves. They specifically include right to family care and right to development. The state and the society need to fulfil these rights. The civil and political rights are the capitalist contribution to UNCRC that focuses on the liberal ideology, comprising of participation and protection rights. Unlike the adult scenario, in child rights, the economic, social and cultural rights dominate the civil and political rights, probably as children are not considered capable of participation as adults are.

2.3.1 Child Right to Family Care

According to the UNCRC, the child rights to family care include

- Child right to family care and relations,
- Child right to parenting by both parents and family right to assistance for childcare,
- Child right not to be separated from parents and
- Child right to reunification with parents.

2.3.1.1 Right to Family Care and Relations

The Preamble of the UNCRC states that "Recognizing that the child, for the full and harmonious development of his or her personality, should grow up in a family environment, in an atmosphere of happiness, love and understanding."

Article 5 of the UNCRC emphasises that "States Parties shall respect the responsibilities, rights and duties of parents or, where applicable, the members of the extended family or community as provided for by local custom, legal guardians or other persons legally responsible for the child, to provide, in a manner consistent with the evolving capacities of the child, appropriate direction and guidance in the exercise by the child of the rights recognized in the present Convention."

Article 7.1 states that the child shall be registered immediately after birth and shall have the right from birth to a name, the right to acquire a nationality and, as far as possible, the right to know and be cared for by his or her parents.

Article 8.1 states that States parties shall undertake to respect the right of the child to preserve his or her identity, including nationality, name and family relations as recognised by law without unlawful interference.

2.3.1.2 Child Right to Parenting by Both Parents and Family Right to Assistance for Childcare

The Preamble of the UNCRC emphasises that "Convinced that the family, as the fundamental group of society and the natural environment for the growth and well-being of all its members and particularly children, should be afforded the necessary protection and assistance so that it can fully assume its responsibilities within the community." This implies that the family has the right to livelihood, housing, health, child day care and community support so that it can fully assume its responsibility for children within the community.

Article 18 of the UNCRC states the following:

1. States that the states parties shall use their best efforts to ensure recognition of the principle that both parents have common responsibilities for the upbringing and development of the child. Parents or, as the case may be, legal guardians, have the primary responsibility for the upbringing and development of the child. The best interests of the child shall be their basic concern.
2. For the purpose of guaranteeing and promoting the rights set forth in the present convention, states parties shall render appropriate assistance to parents and legal guardians in the performance of their child-rearing responsibilities and shall ensure the development of institutions, facilities and services for the care of children.
3. States parties shall take all appropriate measures to ensure that children of working parents have the right to benefit from childcare services and facilities for which they are eligible.

2.3.1.3 Child Right Not to Be Separated from Parents

Article 9 of the UNCRC emphasises the child right not to be separated from his or her parents, as follows:

1. States parties shall ensure that a child shall not be separated from his or her parents against their will, except when competent authorities subject to judicial review determine, in accordance with applicable law and procedures, that such separation is necessary for the best interests of the child. Such determination may be necessary in a particular case such as one involving abuse or neglect of the child by the parents, or one where the parents are living separately and a decision must be made as to the child's place of residence.
2. In any proceedings pursuant to paragraph 1 of the present chapter, all interested parties shall be given an opportunity to participate in the proceedings and make their views known.
3. States parties shall respect the right of the child who is separated from one or both parents to maintain personal relations and direct contact with both parents on a regular basis, except if it is contrary to the child's best interests.
4. Where such separation results from any action initiated by a state party, such as the detention, imprisonment, exile, deportation or death (including death arising from any cause while the person is in the custody of the state) of one or both parents or of the child, that state party shall, upon request, provide the parents, the child or, if appropriate, another member of the family with the essential information concerning the whereabouts of the absent member(s) of the family unless the provision of the information would be detrimental to the well-being of the child. States parties shall further ensure that the submission of such a request shall of itself entail no adverse consequences for the person(s) concerned.

2.3.1.4 Child Right to Reunification with Parents

Article 10 of the UNCRC emphasises the child right to reunification with his/her parents, as follows:

1. In accordance with the obligation of states parties under Article 9, paragraph 1, applications by a child or his or her parents to enter or leave a state party for the purpose of family reunification shall be dealt with by states parties in a positive, humane and expeditious manner. States parties shall further ensure that the submission of such a request shall entail no adverse consequences for the applicants and for the members of their family.
2. A child whose parents reside in different states shall have the right to maintain on a regular basis and save in exceptional circumstances personal relations and direct contacts with both parents. Towards that end and in accordance with the obligation of states parties under Article 9, paragraph 1, states parties shall respect the right of the child and his or her parents to leave any country, including their own, and to enter their own country. The right to leave any country shall

be subject only to such restrictions as are prescribed by law and which are necessary to protect the national security, public order (ordre public), public health or morals or the rights and freedoms of others and are consistent with the other rights recognized in the present convention.

2.3.2 Child Right to Development

Article 6 of the UNCRC emphasises the rights to life, survival and development as follows:

1. States parties shall recognize that every child has the inherent right to life.
2. States parties shall ensure to the maximum extent possible the survival and development of the child.

Article 27 of the UNCRC emphasises the right to development, as follows:

1. States parties recognize the right of every child to a standard of living adequate for the child's physical, mental, spiritual, moral and social development.
2. The parent(s) or others responsible for the child have the primary responsibility to secure, within their abilities and financial capacities, the conditions of living necessary for the child's development.
3. States parties, in accordance with national conditions and within their means, shall take appropriate measures to assist parents and others responsible for the child to implement this right and shall in case of need provide material assistance and support programmes, particularly with regard to nutrition, clothing and housing.
4. States parties shall take all appropriate measures to secure the recovery of maintenance for the child from the parents or other persons having financial responsibility for the child, both within the state party and from abroad. In particular, where the person having financial responsibility for the child lives in a state different from that of the child, states parties shall promote the accession to international agreements or the conclusion of such agreements, as well as the making of other appropriate arrangements.

Child's development rights include child rights to health and nutrition, clothing, housing, education and rest, recreation and cultural life which are discussed below.

2.3.2.1 Health and Nutrition Rights

Article 24 of the UNCRC emphasises the right to health, as follows:

1. States parties recognize the right of the child to the enjoyment of the highest attainable standard of health and to facilities for the treatment of illness and rehabilitation of health. States parties shall strive to ensure that no child is deprived of his or her right of access to such health care services.

2. States parties shall pursue full implementation of this right and, in particular, shall take appropriate measures:

   (a) To diminish infant and child mortality;
   (b) To ensure the provision of necessary medical assistance and health care to all children with emphasis on the development of primary health care;
   (c) To combat disease and malnutrition, including within the framework of primary health care, through, inter alia, the application of readily available technology and through the provision of adequate nutritious foods and clean drinking water, taking into consideration the dangers and risks of environmental pollution;
   (d) To ensure appropriate pre- and post-natal health care for mothers;
   (e) To ensure that all segments of society, in particular parents and children, are informed, have access to education and are supported in the use of basic knowledge of child health and nutrition, the advantages of breastfeeding, hygiene and environmental sanitation and the prevention of accidents;
   (f) To develop preventive health care, guidance for parents and family planning education and services.

3. States Parties shall take all effective and appropriate measures with a view to abolishing traditional practices prejudicial to the health of children.

2.3.2.2 Education Rights

Article 28 of the UNCRC emphasises the right to education, as follows:

1. States parties recognize the right of the child to education, and with a view to achieving this right progressively and on the basis of equal opportunity, they shall, in particular:

   (a) Make primary education compulsory and available free to all;
   (b) Encourage the development of different forms of secondary education, including general and vocational education, make them available and accessible to every child and take appropriate measures such as the introduction of free education and offering financial assistance in case of need;
   (c) Make higher education accessible to all on the basis of capacity by every appropriate means;
   (d) Make educational and vocational information and guidance available and accessible to all children;
   (e) Take measures to encourage regular attendance at schools and the reduction of dropout rates.

2. States parties shall take all appropriate measures to ensure that school discipline is administered in a manner consistent with the child's human dignity and in conformity with the present convention.

3. States parties shall promote and encourage international cooperation in matters relating to education, in particular with a view to contributing to the elimination of ignorance and illiteracy throughout the world and facilitating access to scientific and technical knowledge and modern teaching methods. In this regard, particular account shall be taken of the needs of developing countries.

Article 29 of the UNCRC emphasises the goals of education, as follows:

1. States parties agree that the education of the child shall be directed to:

    (a) The development of the child's personality, talents and mental and physical abilities to their fullest potential;
    (b) The development of respect for human rights and fundamental freedoms, and for the principles enshrined in the charter of the United Nations;
    (c) The development of respect for the child's parents, his or her own cultural identity, language and values, for the national values of the country in which the child is living, the country from which he or she may originate, and for civilizations different from his or her own;
    (d) The preparation of the child for responsible life in a free society, in the spirit of understanding, peace, tolerance, equality of sexes and friendship among all peoples, ethnic, national and religious groups and persons of indigenous origin;
    (e) The development of respect for the natural environment.

2.3.2.3 Rest, Recreation and Cultural Rights

Article 31 of the UNCRC emphasises the right to rest, recreation and cultural life, as follows:

1. States parties recognize the right of the child to rest and leisure, to engage in play and recreational activities appropriate to the age of the child and to participate freely in cultural life and the arts.
2. States parties shall respect and promote the right of the child to participate fully in cultural and artistic life and shall encourage the provision of appropriate and equal opportunities for cultural, artistic, recreational and leisure activity.

2.3.3 Child Right to Participation

The UNCRC includes the child rights to expression of views, communication of information and freedom, as listed below.

2.3.3.1 Right to Expression of Views

Article 12 of the UNCRC emphasises child right to expression of one's views, as follows:

1. States parties shall assure to the child who is capable of forming his or her own views the right to express those views freely in all matters affecting the child, the views of the child being given due weight in accordance with the age and maturity of the child.
2. For this purpose, the child shall in particular be provided the opportunity to be heard in any judicial and administrative proceedings affecting the child, either directly, or through a representative or an appropriate body, in a manner consistent with the procedural rules of national law.

2.3.3.2 Right to Communication of Information

Article 13 of the UNCRC emphasises child right to communication for information, as follows:

1. The child shall have the right to freedom of expression; this right shall include freedom to seek, receive and impart information and ideas of all kinds, regardless of frontiers, either orally, in writing or in print, in the form of art, or through any other media of the child's choice.
2. The exercise of this right may be subject to certain restrictions, but these shall only be such as are provided by law and are necessary:
   (a) For respect of the rights or reputations of others; or
   (b) For the protection of national security or of public order, or of public health or morals.

2.3.3.3 Rights to Freedom

Article 14 of the UNCRC emphasises child right to freedom, as follows:

1. States parties shall respect the right of the child to freedom of thought, conscience and religion.
2. States parties shall respect the rights and duties of the parents and, when applicable, legal guardians, to provide direction to the child in the exercise of his or her right in a manner consistent with the evolving capacities of the child.
3. Freedom to manifest one's religion or beliefs may be subject only to such limitations as are prescribed by law and are necessary to protect public safety, order, health or morals, or the fundamental rights and freedoms of others.

Article 15 of the UNCRC emphasises child right to freedom, as follows:

1. States parties recognize the rights of the child to freedom of association and to freedom of peaceful assembly.

2. No restrictions may be placed on the exercise of these rights other than those imposed in conformity with the law and which are necessary in a democratic society in the interests of national security or public safety, public order, the protection of public health or morals or the protection of the rights and freedoms of others.

2.3.4 Child Right to Protection

Article 19 of the UNCRC deals with right to protection from neglect, abuse and exploitation, as follows:

1. States parties shall take all appropriate legislative, administrative, social and educational measures to protect the child from all forms of physical or mental violence, injury or abuse, neglect or negligent treatment, maltreatment or exploitation, including sexual abuse, while in the care of parent(s), legal guardian(s) or any other person who has the care of the child.
2. Such protective measures should, as appropriate, include effective procedures for the establishment of social programmes to provide necessary support for the child and for those who have the care of the child, as well as for other forms of prevention and for identification, reporting, referral, investigation, treatment and follow up of instances of child maltreatment described heretofore, and, as appropriate, for judicial involvement.

Article 39 of the UNCRC emphasises recovery and reintegration of child victims of neglect, abuse and exploitation, as follows:

> States Parties shall take all appropriate measures to promote physical and psychological recovery and social reintegration of a child victim of any form of neglect, exploitation, or abuse; torture or any other form of cruel, inhuman or degrading treatment or punishment; or armed conflicts. Such recovery and reintegration shall take place in an environment, which fosters the health, self-respect and dignity of the child.

2.4 Principles of Child Rights

Child rights principles comprise of the principle of the best interests of the child and the principles of human rights as applied to child rights. Thus, child rights principles include the following:

- Primary consideration to dignity and the best interests of the child,
- Indivisibility and interdependence of child rights and holistic approach,
- Universality, equality, non-discrimination and inclusion of vulnerable among children and
- State and societal accountability.

2.4.1 *Primary Consideration to Dignity and the Best Interests of the Child*

The primary consideration has to be the child's right to dignity. Article 16 of the UNCRC states the following:

1. No child shall be subjected to arbitrary or unlawful interference with his or her privacy, family, home or correspondence, nor to unlawful attacks on his or her honour and reputation.
2. The child has the right to the protection of the law against such interference or attacks.

The UNCRC not only accepts that children are subjects of the same rights as adults, it also acknowledges the special status of childhood by providing specific rights only to those under the age of 18 years, such as the "best interest principle". Article 3 of the UNCRC states the following:

1. In all actions concerning children, whether undertaken by public or private social welfare institutions, courts of law, administrative authorities or legislative bodies, the best interests of the child shall be a primary consideration.
2. States parties undertake to ensure the child such protection and care as is necessary for his or her well-being, taking into account the rights and duties of his or her parents, legal guardians, or other individuals legally responsible for him or her, and, to this end, shall take all appropriate legislative and administrative measures.
3. States parties shall ensure that the institutions, services and facilities responsible for the care or protection of children shall conform with the standards established by competent authorities, particularly in the areas of safety, health, in the number and suitability of their staff, as well as competent supervision.

According to UNICEF (2001), these rights imply the following:

- The best interest of a child principle must govern all decisions and actions affecting children.
- Governments, public and private bodies must ascertain the impact on children of their activities in order to ensure that the best interest of the child are a primary consideration.
- Children's own views are a key component in determining their best interests, and should be considered according to the child's age and maturity.
- There must be a first call for children in times of conflict and emergencies.
- The best solution for the individual child must be sought and be of basic concern to parents and caregivers.
- Children should be given primary consideration when resources are mobilised and allocated.

- The child's best interests should serve as a mediating principle in conflicts between the child/children and others, and between conflicting rights of the individual child.

2.4.2 *Indivisibility and Interdependence of Child Rights and Holistic Approach*

All rights are inter-related, indivisible and have equal status. One group of rights is not more important than another and all rights – whether civil, political, economic, social or cultural – must be equally respected. Children should first and foremost be seen as whole human beings and not be labelled as a certain category. According to UNICEF (2001), it implies the following for child rights:

- Child development is a holistic concept, demanding consideration of the whole child – physical, cognitive, emotional, social, cultural and spiritual development.
- Child rights are indivisible and inter-related, it means that we need to take a holistic approach to programming, considering the full range of inter-related rights of children, although action might be specific.
- Implementation of one right of the child has to take other rights into account and be promoted in the spirit of human rights principles.
- Although rights have equal status not all rights may have equal importance at all times. Resources are also limited so priorities have to be identified.
- Programmes have to be built on holistic assessment and multidisciplinary analysis, multi-sectoral approaches, inter-sectoral coordination and a range of convergent actions.

2.4.3 *Universality, Equality, Non-discrimination and Inclusion of the Marginalised Among Children*

Human rights are universal and must be equally applied to all people – regardless of culture or traditions. According to Article 1 of the UNCRC, a child means every human being below the age of 18 years.

Article 2 of the UNCRC deals with right to non-discrimination as follows:

1. States parties shall respect and ensure the rights set forth in the present convention to each child within their jurisdiction without discrimination of any kind, irrespective of the child's or his or her parent's or legal guardian's race, colour, sex, language, religion, political or other opinion, national, ethnic or social origin, property, disability, birth or other status.
2. State parties shall take all appropriate measures to ensure that the child is protected against all forms of discrimination or punishment on the basis of the status, activities, expressed opinions or beliefs of the child's parents, legal guardians or family members.

According to UNICEF (2001), it implies the following:

- Each and every child has equal and inalienable rights.
- While the well-being of all children is important, a rights-based approach also means that priority must be given to the most disadvantaged children like girls, low caste children, children in remote areas and children with disabilities and children who are refugees/internally displaced persons or returnees.
- Disaggregation of data by age, ethnic group, gender and geographic area is essential for identifying and targeting these discriminated groups.
- Everybody must be treated with respect. It means that children brought up in brothels, prisons or in families with HIV/AIDS have an equal right to be treated with respect.
- All rights apply everywhere at all times – including in times of austerity, conflict and natural disaster. Rights apply to illegal immigrants, refugees, children belonging to minority groups and children without citizenship or documents.
- Challenging discrimination will involve identifying discriminatory attitudes and practices, which may have their roots in religious, social, cultural or economic norms.
- Gender and caste equity must be promoted and gender and caste sensitive approaches applied to reveal discriminatory practices in families.

A gender-sensitive approach means identifying major phenomena of inequality and discrimination due to sex and to address such discrimination, if required through affirmative action (giving special benefits to the disadvantaged sex or group). A gender-sensitive approach also means that the same problem may need to be addressed in different ways for boys and girls taking the distinct social roles and domains of males and females into account; and the impact of most programme activities will be different for boys and girls (UNICEF 2001).

2.4.4 State and Societal Accountability

Once a state has adopted a particular international convention it is obliged to respect, protect, promote and fulfil the human rights covered by that convention (UNICEF 2001). The UN Committee on children, an elected Committee of international experts, was established under Article 43 of the CRC to monitor implementation of the CRC. Article 44 of the convention requires states parties to report on measures they have adopted to give effect to child rights within 2 years of their adherence to the convention and thereafter every 5 years. Governments that ratify the convention are under an obligation to submit regular and detailed reports on their national situations related to children's rights to the Committee for examination. The Committee reviews countries' reports and urges all levels of governments to use the convention as a guide in policy-making and implementation to undertake the following tasks:

- Develop a comprehensive national agenda for children.
- Develop permanent bodies or mechanisms to promote coordination, monitoring and evaluation of activities throughout all sectors of government.
- Ensure that all legislation is fully compatible with the convention.
- Make children visible in policy development processes throughout government by introducing child impact assessments.
- Carry out adequate budget analysis to determine the portion of public funds spent on children and to ensure that these resources are being used effectively.
- Ensure that sufficient data are collected and used to improve the plight of all children in each jurisdiction.
- Raise awareness and disseminate information on the convention by providing training to all those involved in government policy-making and working with or for children.
- Involve civil society – including children themselves – in the process of implementing and raising awareness of child rights.
- Set up independent statutory offices – ombudspersons, commissions and other institutions – to promote children's rights.

One of the key differences between the needs and the rights approaches is that a needs-based approach does not come with accountability. Many rights have developed from needs, but a rights-based approach adds legal and moral obligations and accountability. According to UNICEF (2001), human rights add the notion of accountability and social justice to the development agenda. To have rights is to have claims on institutions and people that they should help in ensuring the realisation of these rights. Human rights have traditionally focused on the conduct of official institutions, and the special accountability of those responsible for ensuring justice. When states ratify human rights instruments, they become accountable to all citizens, including children, and to the international community.

If children are the holders of rights and have a legal entitlement that their rights are secured, then it is essential that those responsible for delivering on these rights are identified and made accountable and responsive. States are the primary duty-bearers. Their duty means that they have to ensure implementation also when it comes to private institutions like private schools, religious centres and work places. They have obligations towards all children within their jurisdiction (for example refugees) and not just their own citizens. States have the obligation to respect, protect, promote and fulfil child rights in terms of result and process. They are obliged to take deliberate action to ensure progressive fulfilment of rights and the transparent assessment of progress.

Families and parents have the major responsibility to recognise and implement the human rights of children. The UNCRC recognises them as primary caregivers, protectors and guides of children. The state is required to support and empower them in these roles – in particular those in poverty and suffering stress. Societal accountability includes responsibility of schools, neighbourhoods and civil society organisations to promote and protect the rights of children (UNICEF 2001).

References

Boyden, J. and Levison, D. (2000). *Children as Economic and Social Actors in the Development Process*. Stockholm: Ministry of Foreign Affairs.

EU Canada Project. (2003). *Child Welfare Across Borders*. www.sws.soton.ac.uk/cwab/index.htm. Accessed 1 May 2004.

Harding, L. F. (1991). *Perspectives in Child Care Policy*. London: Longman.

James, A. and James, A. (2004). *Constructing Childhood: Theory, Policy and Social Practice*. New York, NY: Palgrave Macmillan.

Save the Children. (2002). *Child Rights Programming: How to Apply Rights-Based Approaches in Programming*. Stockholm: Ministry of Foreign Affairs.

United Nations Children's Fund. (2001). *Pocket Guide for a Rights-Based Approach to Programming for Children: Application in South Asia*. Kathmandu: United Nations Children's Fund.

United Nations Convention on the Rights of the Child. (1989). http://www.ohchr.org/english/law/pdf/crc.pdf. Accessed 3 March 2002.

White, B. (2003). *A World Fit for Children?* Dies Natalis address delivered on the occasion of the 51st anniversary of the Institute of Social Studies, The Hague, The Netherlands.

Wyness, M., Harrison, L. and Buchanan, I. (2004). Childhood, politics and ambiguity: Towards an agenda for children's political inclusion. *Sociology*, 38(1), 81–99.

Chapter 3
A Conceptual Framework for Rights-Based Preventative Approach for Psychosocial Well-Being in Childhood

3.1 Conceptual Framework for Rights-Based Preventative Approach for Psychosocial Well-Being in Childhood

3.1.1 Foundation

A conceptual framework for rights-based preventative approach for psychosocial well-being in childhood is developed based on the foundation of:

- The child rights perspective,
- Prevention model of health care,
- Theories of positive psychosocial development and behaviour and
- Social-work profession.

3.1.2 Objectives and Principles from the Child Rights Perspective

3.1.2.1 Objectives of Child Rights

The objectives of rights-based preventative approach for children's psychosocial well-being are

- Achievement of child right to family care
- Achievement of child right to development
- Achievement of child right to participation
- Achievement of child right to protection

3.1.2.2 Principles of Child Rights

The principles of rights-based preventative approach for psychosocial well-being in childhood are

- Primary consideration to the dignity and the best interests of the child
- Indivisibility and interdependence of child rights and holistic approach to children

M. Desai, *A Rights-Based Preventative Approach for Psychosocial Well-Being in Childhood*, Children's Well-Being: Indicators and Research 3,
DOI 10.1007/978-90-481-9066-9_3,

- Universality, equality, non-discrimination and inclusion of the marginalised among children
- State and society accountable for promoting child rights

3.1.3 Goals from the Prevention Model of Health Care

The rights-based preventative approach for psychosocial well-being in childhood uses the public health prevention model of goals of intervention as follows:

- Primary prevention of vulnerability in childhood,
- Secondary prevention of neglect of children at risk and
- Tertiary prevention of abuse, commercial exploitation and conflict with law in childhood.

3.1.4 Definition of Psychosocial Well-Being from the Theories of Positive Psychology

Psychosocial well-being is comprises of:

- Self-awareness: self-identity and self-esteem
- Proactive thinking skills: rational, realistic, flexible, creative, self-responsible and positive thinking skills
- Emotional intelligence: emotional awareness and expression, regulating negative emotions and enrichment of positive emotions
- Interpersonal relationship skills: positive perception of others, positive feelings for others, win–win goals in relationships and collaborative conflict management skills
- Interpersonal communication skills: assertive and open verbal and body language skills, sensitive listening skills and feedback skills

Psychosocial well-being empowers self for development and protection from vulnerability, abuse and conflict with law in childhood.

3.1.5 Intervention Aspects from Social Work Profession

3.1.5.1 Social-Work Approaches

The rights-based preventative approach for psychosocial well-being in childhood uses the following social-work approaches:

- Person-centred approach
- Strengths-based approach

Chart 3.1 Psychosocial Well-Being

Self-awareness

Self-identity
- Individual-level Self-identity for uniqueness
- Group-level Self-identity for connectiveness

Self-esteem
- Self-acceptance
- Self-worth
- Self-love
- Self-confidence
- Assertiveness

↓

Reframing reactive thinking with proactive thinking skills

Reframing irrational thinking with rational and critical thinking skills

Reframing rigid thinking with realistic, flexible and creative thinking skills

Reframing protective thinking with self-responsibility

Reframing negative thinking with positive thinking skills

↓

Emotional intelligence

Emotional awareness and expression
- Awareness and expression of emotions in self
- Awareness of emotions in others/empathy

Regulating negative emotions
- Regulating anger and hurt
- Forgiveness and letting go
- Regulating sadness
- Regulating fear and anxiety

Enrichment of positive emotions
- Enrichment of love
- Enrichment of joy and happiness
- Enrichment of smiles and laughter

↓

Interpersonal relationship skills

Interdependence with others
- Separated and connected cohesion
- Structured and flexible adaptability

Positive perception of others
- Egalitarian perception
- Recognition of strengths
- Acceptance and respect
- Celebration of differences

Positive feelings for others
- Warmth
- Humility
- Empathy

Win–win goals in relationships
- Mutual benefits
- Co-operativeness
- Third alternative

Collaborative conflict management skills
- Attitude adjustment
- Reducing defensiveness in others
- Understanding the other Person's perception of the conflict
- Win–win goals

↓

Chart 3.1 (continued)

Interpersonal communication skills		
Open communication skills	*Sensitive listening skills*	*Feedback skills*
• Non-judgmental • Permissive • Spontaneous • Empathic • Equal • Provisional	• Just listen • Observe body language • Express concern • Express understanding and acceptance • Preserve and promote self-esteem	• Giving negative feedback directly and clearly, requesting behaviour change • Receiving negative feedback without being defensive • Giving genuine and unconditional positive feedback • Accepting positive feedback

- Participatory approach
- Empowerment-focused approach

3.1.5.2 Social-Work Attitudes

The rights-based preventative approach for psychosocial well-being in childhood requires the following attitudes in the worker:

- Warmth
- Humility
- Empathy

3.1.5.3 Social-Work Ethical Principles

The rights-based preventative approach for psychosocial well-being in childhood uses the following social-work ethical principles:

- Self-determination
- Informed consent
- Professional boundaries
- Confidentiality

3.1.5.4 Psychosocial Methods and Techniques of Social Work

The rights-based preventative approach for psychosocial well-being in childhood uses the following psychosocial methods and techniques of social work:

- Psycho-educational group work
- Case management
    - Direct intervention for giving information and advice, teaching and training in psychosocial skills and counselling

  - Linking with natural support systems, self-help groups, flexitime supplementary childcare and other formal systems of state and voluntary organisations
  - Advocacy intervention for restorative justice through the juvenile justice system and integrated substitute childcare

3.1.5.5 Organisational Setup

The organisations working for rights-based preventative approach for psychosocial well-being in childhood need to be planned as follows:

- The policies should be formulated according to clearly articulated child rights-based missions, goals and ethical principles.
- The programmes should be planned for child rights-based intervention for primary, secondary and tertiary prevention.
- The physical setting should be planned for privacy and as a friendly, comfortable, relaxed and a safe place for the child to be (Thompson and Henderson 2007).
- The staff should be recruited with reference to their qualifications for working with children. Those who work directly with children should preferably have an ethnic background similar to that of the children who come to the organisation.
- Board members and staff at all the levels may be provided with in-service training in child rights and psychosocial skills.

3.2 Preventative Framework for Well-Being in Childhood

3.2.1 Current Classification of Child Welfare Services

Child welfare means the well-being of children and child welfare services are services that promote the well-being of children. These services were defined by the United States Department of Health, Education and Welfare in 1960 as

> ...those social services that supplement or substitute for parental care and supervision for the purpose of protecting and promoting the welfare of children and youth, preventing neglect, abuse and exploitation, helping overcome problems and result in dependency, neglect or delinquency and, when needed, providing adequate care for children and youth away from their own homes, such care to be given in foster family homes, adoptive homes, childcare institutions, or other facilities.

Since the family is regarded as the primary child welfare system and parents as the primary caretakers, when family or parents have problems that affect their role of providing for the care and well-being of the child, the state or voluntary organisations need to support, supplement or substitute childcare. Kadushin and Martin (1988) categorised child welfare services into supportive, supplemental and substitutive.

In recent years, due to the attention on the problems of child abuse and neglect, the term child welfare has become almost synonymous with child protection. This trend has resulted in resources being diverted away from needed supportive and developmental services for children to only for those who are in crisis (Popple and Vecchiolla 2007). Moreover, child protection services deal with "child abuse and neglect" (Depanfilis 2005), whereas the neglected children need childcare or welfare and not protection in the same sense as what the child victims of abuse need. The services for the two need to be separated and made more appropriate.

Child protection is the residual approach or the deficit model in child welfare, which is the most prevalent child welfare orientation. A residual orientation in child welfare is criticised for leaving the child without protection until much harm is done as it is remedial rather than preventative. Defining child welfare as the well-being of children and child welfare services as all of the measures designed to protect and promote the well-being of children, these services cannot focus only on child protection and remain residual or remedial. What is needed is the institutional or developmental or preventative orientation in child welfare that would be available to all children (Kadushin and Martin 1988).

3.2.2 Preventative Framework for Well-Being in Childhood

The prevention approach is an imperative in the child rights approach as it is the only way to effectively deal with children's problems. It is:

- Grounded in the ecological perspective
- Oriented to the future
- Empowerment-focused
- Developmental (adapted from Downs et al. 2009)
- Cost-effective

The redefinition of problems faced by children and the linkages among these problems provide the basis for a preventative approach for well-being in childhood. The services can be planned to sequentially prevent children's problems with the goals and interventions depicted in the following table.

3.3 Approaches of Intervention with Children

3.3.1 Person-Centred Approach

The person-centred concept is based on concepts from humanistic psychology, many of which were articulated by Carl Rogers in the early 1940s (Corey 2005). In the person-centred perspective, people:

- Have worth and dignity in their own right and therefore deserve respect
- Have the capacity and right to self-direction and, when given the opportunity, make wise judgements

Chart 3.2 Preventative Framework for Well-Being in Childhood

Level of prevention	Target group	Goal	Systems	Interventions
Primary prevention	All children	Prevent vulnerability	• Family • School • Health • Recreation and cultural life	Psycho-educational group work with children, parents and teachers
Secondary prevention	Children at risk	Prevent neglect	• Professional voluntary organisations	Case management with children and their families: • Direct intervention for giving information and advice, teaching and training in psychosocial skills and counselling • Linking with natural support systems, self-help groups, flexitime supplementary childcare and other formal systems
Tertiary prevention	Children facing abuse, commercial exploitation and conflict with law	Prevent abuse, commercial exploitation and conflict with law	• Police • Juvenile/other courts • Foster family care • Child adoption • Institutional childcare	Child advocacy intervention for restorative justice through: • The juvenile justice system and • Integrated substitute childcare

- Can select their own values
- Can learn to make constructive use of responsibility
- Have the capacity to deal with their own feelings, thoughts and behaviour
- Have the potential for constructive change and personal development towards a full and satisfying life (Thompson and Henderson 2007)

According to Rogers, the following practitioner attributes can create a growth-promoting climate in which individuals can move forward and become what they are capable of becoming:

- Congruence (genuineness)
- Unconditional positive regard (acceptance and caring)
- Accurate empathic understanding (an ability to deeply grasp the subjective world of another person) (Corey 2005)

The person-centred approach aims towards the client achieving a greater degree of independence and integration. Its focus is on the person and not the person's presenting problem. It aims to assist clients in their growth process so they could better cope with their current and future problems (Corey 2005). The person-centred practitioners refrain from giving advice or solutions, diagnosis, interpreting, moralising and making judgements. Instead, they use the methods of active and listening, reflection of thoughts and feelings, clarification, summarisation, confrontation of contradictions and general or open leads that help client self-exploration (Thompson and Henderson 2007).

The person-centred approach, as modified by Carkhuff (1973, cited by Thompson and Henderson 2007), involves three general stages through which the client proceeds:

1. Self-exploration: people examine exactly where they are in their lives;
2. Understanding: people begin to understand the relationship between where they are in life and where they would like to be; and
3. Action: goal-directed action to reach the point where they want to be.

3.3.2 Strengths-Based Approach

The deficit/problem orientation in social-work encourages the following individual rather than ecological accounts of psychosocial functioning:

- The person is the problem
- There are fixed, inevitable, critical and universal stages of human development
- Childhood trauma invariably leads to adult psychopathology
- The disease linear module is used with reference to causes and solutions (Saleeby 2006).

In the strengths-based approach, the social worker builds on client strengths for achieving positive and lasting change instead of trying to eliminate his or her problems or deficiencies. The strengths-based perspective is an important counterbalance to the preoccupation with client problems, pathology and deficits that is so pervasive in the service delivery system and inherent in many of the practice theories and models used by social workers (Sheafor and Horejsi 2006).

According to Saleeby (2006), the major principles of the strengths perspective include the following:

- Every individual, group, family and community has strengths that are assets, resources, wisdom and knowledge.
- Trauma and abuse, illness and struggle may be injurious but they may also be sources of challenge and opportunity.
- Assume that we do not know the upper limits of the capacity to grow and change and take individual, group and community aspirations seriously.

- We best serve clients by collaborating with them and using less political elements of helping such as paternalism, victim-blaming and pre-emption of client views.
- Every environment is full of resources such as informal systems and associations, groups and institutions.

The social worker should help the client identify his/her strengths and build upon them. Because clients are true experts on their situation, in this perspective the professional role is mostly that of facilitator or consultant (Sheafor and Horejsi 2006). Sheafor and Horejsi (2006) provide the following guidelines to maintain a focus on strengths, drawing on suggestions made by Cowger (1994, cited by Sheafor and Horejsi 2006):

- Believe the client. Assume that he or she is honest and trustworthy unless it is proven otherwise.
- Display an interest in strengths. Listen for and call to the client's attention all indicators of the client's competence, skills, resourcefulness and motivation to make his or her situation better.
- Assume that the client is an expert on his or her behaviour, life and situation, and knows best what will and will not work in a change effort or treatment plan. Give primary attention to the client's own perceptions and understanding of his or her situation.
- View the assessment and the service planning as joint worker–client activity.
- Assess but do not diagnose. Avoid the use of diagnostic labelling as for it draws attention away from client strengths and places the focus on pathology and deficits.
- Avoid discussion of blame and what the client or others should or should not have done previously. Time is better spent on here-and-now problem-solving.
- Assume that within the client's family, social network and community, there is an oasis of potential resources, both formal and informal, that can be drawn into the helping process.

3.3.3 Participatory Approach

According to Poulin (2005), the strengths perspective can be adopted by maximising client collaboration and empowerment. The collaborative approach with children needs the child participatory approach. Boyden and Levison (2000) note that supporting children's best interests requires the perspective that they have valid insights into their well-being, valid solutions to their problems and a valid role in implementing those solutions. Such an approach acknowledges children not merely as beneficiaries of intervention by adults, or a future societal asset, but as competent social agents in their own right.

The principle of participation is the practical manifestation of individual equality and personal autonomy. A rights-based approach to programming requires participation of stakeholders and empowerment of the people concerned throughout the programming cycle. In this approach, efforts to achieve outcomes should be balanced by attention to participatory processes. A perspective that allows for children to have the right to participate and be involved in decisions affecting them emphasises children's capabilities rather than their limitations. It moves us away from the objectification of children and from parental control as paramount (EU Canada Project 2003).

3.3.3.1 Child Right to Communication of Information

Article 13 of the UNCRC emphasises child right to communication for information, by stating that the child shall have the freedom to seek, receive and impart information and ideas of all kinds, regardless of frontiers, either orally, in writing or in print, in the form of art, or through any other media of the child's choice.

Often the issue is not that children are incapable of making decisions, but that their decisions are based on poor information, partial information or information that they have not been able to interpret well for lack of experience. Then, because children are poorly informed in the first place, we criticise their choices. Even when they have been informed, children may not be able to make the right judgements because they do not have the power to make choices. Children often have sound ideas about their problems and needs and the possible solutions to these, and are better able to protect themselves when properly informed and given some say in decisions and processes affecting them (Boyden and Levison 2000).

3.3.3.2 Child Right to Expression of Views

Article 12 of the UNCRC emphasises child right to expression of one's views, by stating that the States Parties shall assure to the child who is capable of forming his or her own views the right to express those views freely in all matters affecting the child, the views of the child being given due weight in accordance with the age and maturity of the child.

3.3.3.3 Child Right to Freedom

Article 14 of the UNCRC emphasises that the States Parties shall respect the right of the child to freedom of thought, conscience and religion. Article 15 of the UNCRC emphasises that the States Parties recognise the rights of the child to freedom of association and to freedom of peaceful assembly.

3.3.3.4 Children as Resourceful

Even in adversity, children are active survivors. Because children's responses to adversity are neither direct nor predictable, but subtle and complex, children in difficult situations should not be conceptualised merely as susceptible victims. Representing children as passive victims rather than active survivors undermines the possibility of them acting on their situation and thereby further threatens their self-esteem and self-efficacy. The view of children as resourceful suggests that children may be better served by assuming an active role in their own protection and at least some degree of responsibility for their own safety, insofar as this is possible (Boyden and Levison 2000).

3.3.3.5 Children's Agency

Boyden and Levison (2000) argued that children are not passive recipients of adult investment and training, but social agents in their own right. Children's agency is a key contributor to their development and hence children should play a part in defining what is in their own best interests. For adults to better understand children's problems and needs, they require children to explain and interpret their childhoods, only children can provide real insight into their feelings and experiences.

3.3.3.6 Child Responsibilities

White (2003) notes that the UNCRC rights to expression of views, communication of information and freedom do not adequately amount to right to participation. These do not deal with the blanket exclusion of children from social, economic or political processes for which appropriate age for specific responsibilities may be worked out. Pupavac notes that it is important to remember that rights are not simple entitlements, powers, absolute and isolated from the manner in which they are exercised, namely, with rights come responsibilities through participation. According to Boyden and Levison (2003, cited from White 2003), growing up without responsibility is not necessarily the most effective way to promote children's well-being and best interests. A sense of responsibility develops only with participation.

3.3.3.7 Benefits of Child Participation

According to Council of Europe (2004), following are the benefits of child participation for children:

- They are taken seriously by adults. Ideally, they become acquainted with a culture of democratic decision-making, in which children and adults are equals.
- They participate actively in areas of life, which are normally off-limits to children, such as decisions making on a local policy level. This gives children a sense of importance and builds up their self-confidence.
- They are educated for democratic citizenship, by directly learning how democracy works.
- Participating in a decision-making culture can increase respect for property and goods held in common. For example, children report that they handle new equipment and installations more carefully if they have participated in the

decision-making process on what equipment should be bought and how it should be installed.

- They learn from each other. In mixed age groups, younger children learn from the older ones who serve as role models in demonstrating self-confidence, for example by giving speeches to adult audiences. Older children learn to treat younger ones thoughtfully, with respect and consideration, and, when necessary, give them protection. Generally speaking, participation projects are opportunities for peer education in both directions, enhancing the development of mutual respect between different age groups.
- They learn to work as part of a team, which has a positive effect on relationships between children. In mixed groups, gender equality is reinforced.
- They learn that, in well-implemented projects, participation can be fun, lively and enjoyable.
- They develop important personal and social skills, such as methods of conflict resolution, decision-making and communication. In some projects, they learn to speak in public in front of adults, and to explain why they hold a certain opinion or why they reject or dislike something.

3.3.3.8 Participatory Approach to Intervention

According to Hart (1997), participatory approaches can range from adult-initiated, shared decisions with children to child-initiated, shared decisions with adults. Rather than social worker being the problem-solver the client becomes the problem solver. The social worker's primary function is to help the client recognise, strengthen and marshal his or her inherent strengths and abilities. Self-determination requires workers and clients to collaborate in all decisions and aspects of their work together. The collaborative relationship recognises the client as the expert increases clients' ownership of their decisions. The worker helps the client expand the repertoire of choices. Only through direct participation can children develop a genuine appreciation of a sense of their own competence and responsibility to participate.

3.3.3.9 Child-Friendly Participatory Process

According to the Council of Europe (2004), participation with children can be managed adequately only if the whole process is designed in a child-friendly way, with due attention to the age of the children. The role of the involved adults is to create a child-friendly practice, by playing a supportive and not an intervening role. It is the children who are the real experts. They make the following suggestions to make the participatory process child-friendly:

- Treat children with the same respect as adults, and take their views and interests seriously. This will help them feel important.

- Involve children as early as possible ideally, during the preparation phase – as this strengthens their motivation and identification with the social worker's objectives.
- Try to guarantee easy access to information on the project and its outcomes for the children involved, as well as outsiders.
- Keep the organisational structures and procedures transparent, including schedules, and session rules.
- Create an open, tolerant and nurturing environment that encourages the children to say what they think.
- Use the type of language that children can understand, and listen carefully to what they have to say.
- All written material should take into account the ages of the children.
- Use child-friendly settings, methods and techniques, such as amusing games, varied materials, colourful photos, paintings, symbols, such as animals, flowers, and smiling faces.
- Be careful to not overstrain children, for example involving them in a long conversation.
- Be honest and explain to children, giving concrete reasons, when you think that their ideas are not realistic.
- Take into account that children and adults have different time horizons. It is motivating for children to achieve at least some results promptly. Visibility of results is a main factor of success in children's views.
- Be self-critical and flexible. If some methods, tools or approaches turn out to be not child-friendly enough, you need to adapt your original ideas to the children's needs and requirements.

3.3.4 Empowerment-Focused Approach

The person-centred, strengths-based and participatory approach of intervention with children empowers them. Fook (2007) emphasises that power involves the potential to control and restrict, to form and transform. According to Batliwala (1993) power is the ability to develop the potential of oneself. Powerlessness is then the absence of the ability to develop the potential of oneself to control and restrict, to form and transform and empowerment is the gaining of the ability to develop the potential of oneself to control and restrict, to form and transform. Empowerment can thus be the goal, the process as well as the outcome of social-work intervention.

Parsons et al. (1994) recommend that the following practice components must be present in empowerment-based social-work practice:

- Power-shared relationship
- Competency-based assessment
- Collectivity for mutual aid
- Education for critical thinking, and knowledge and skills for finding resources and taking action.

Parsons et al. (1994) cite Torre's components of the empowerment process:

- Positive perceptions of personal worth, efficacy, and internal locus of control
- Recognition, by self and others, that some of one's perceptions about one's self and the surrounding world are indeed valid, and therefore legitimate to voice
- The ability to think critically about macro-level social, political and economic systems as well as about one's position within such systems
- Knowledge and skills necessary to more successfully influence micro-, mediating- and macro-systems.

Children's empowerment seeks to activate, support and honour children's ability to know their own knowing. Practice is based on children's strengths rather than problems and value-based rather than method-based (adapted from Weick 1994). Children's empowerment may also be enhanced by enrichment of their psychosocial skills.

3.4 Attitudes in Intervention with Children

The worker requires to developing the attitudes of warmth, humility and empathy when intervening with children and their families.

3.4.1 Warmth

According to Shebib (2003, pp. 72–73), warmth is an expression of non-possessive caring. It is demonstrated by showing sincere interest in the comfort of the other person. Kirst-Ashman and Hull (2006) noted that displaying warmth involves genuinely conveying a feeling of interest, concern, well-being and affection to another individual. It is a vehicle for acceptance. Alberti and Emmons (1998) have observed that positive, caring feelings are more difficult for many people to express than assertiveness. Embarrassment, fear of rejection or ridicule, the idea that reason is superior to emotion are excuses for not expressing warmth, caring and love spontaneously. Warmth can be expressed by eyes, smile, touch and words.

3.4.2 Humility

According to Stauffer (1988), humility opens our mind to perceive accurately the needs of others as they see them and to desire to meet those needs when it is practical to do so. Without humility, the needs of others, as they see them, are blocked from our mind. The one who practices humility, develops the ability to listen, to hear the needs of others. The one who is humble also sees value in others. The humble person not only senses the sometimes-unexpressed needs of others, but also relates to the one in need in an appropriate manner.

3.4.3 Empathy

Empathy is the capacity to understand the feelings and views of another person. Its practice makes one other-centred. Sympathy merely mirrors another person's trouble, empathy discovers the causes of the trouble with the searchlight of insight (Peterson 1961). An empathic attitude is characterised by one's willingness to learn about the world of another and begins with suspending judgement (Shebib 2003, p. 73). Kadushin and Kadushin (1997) noted that empathy is the expression of placing of credence on what the other feels and experiences. By being empathic, we share the emotions of another person – excitement, sadness, joy, exhilaration and so on. We particularly need to understand needs of others that may be different from ours. In doing so, we are able to achieve a subjective understanding of what the other person is experiencing.

According to Cartledge and Milburn (1995), empathy leads to acceptance or appreciation of the individuality and dignity of persons. It provides accessibility, a pre-condition for the emergence of relationships that are free of constraining obligation and conformity.

3.5 Skills for Intervention with Children

3.5.1 Barriers in Communication

We often talk to children in the following ways which Hepworth et al. (2006) identified as barriers to communication in social-work interviews:

- Reassuring, sympathising, consoling or excusing
- Advising and giving suggestions or solutions prematurely
- Using sarcasm or employing humour that is distracting or makes light of their problems
- Judging, criticising or placing blame
- Trying to convince them about the right point of view through logical arguments, lecturing, instructing or arguing
- Analysing, diagnosing, or making dogmatic interpretations
- Interrupting inappropriately
- Dominating the interaction
- Responding infrequently
- Parroting or overusing certain phrases or cliches
- Threatening, warning or counterattacking.

Intervention with children requires open communication, feedback skills and use of play and humour.

3.5.2 Open Communication

We need to have open communication with children. According to Humphreys (2002), open communication is non-judgmental and not judgemental, permissive and not controlling, spontaneous and not strategic, empathic and not neutral, equal and not superior, and provisional and not certain.

3.5.2.1 Asking Questions

Questions are important adjuncts to empathy because they allow workers to explore, clarify and define emotions (Shebib 2003). Open-ended questions are advantageous because they give the child greater control over the interview and more discretion in introducing significant material. Interviewers may also use closed questions to obtain greater clarity and focus, to obtain more definite or detailed information (Kadushin and Kadushin 1997).

Shebib (2003) identified the following errors in asking questions to clients in general, all the more applicable to children:

- Jargon in the language may not be understood by children.
- Leading questions manipulate them to choose what appears to be the preferred answer.
- Excessive questioning makes them feel interrogated and bombarded.
- Two or more questions asked at the same time can bombard them with complex and conflicting demands.
- "Why" questions are threatening for them as they tend to ask for justification, and their tone often suggests judgment, disapproval or embedded advice.

Egan (2002) recommended that a mix of statements – open-ended questions, prompts and requests should be used for probing and not questions alone. The client should not be engaged in a question–answer session. Following are the Don'ts of asking questions according to Smith and Delahaye (1987):

- Don't use long, involved questions. Do not use leading questions. These you can often identify because they can start or end in "don't you?"
- Do not overuse yes/no questions. These give limited response variety and have a 50/50 chance of being answered correctly. You can effectively use a yes/no question to get a "sleeper" involved initially. Then you can ask the sleeper to justify his or her answer.
- Don't use ambiguous questions. These are questions that are open to different interpretations. They usually generate confusion and/or argument.

3.5.2.2 Use of Non-discriminatory Language

Our language may tend to reflect our biases or stereotypes on the basis of gender, ethnicity, disability or age, either intentionally or accidentally. This should be avoided and replaced with non-discriminatory language. Consider some of the following examples:

- An ethnic group should not be trivialised by describing it with words such as "culturally backward".
- A family situation should not be denigrated with words such as broken family.
- It is advisable to describe the situation of people instead of using words that label them.

Avoid	Prefer
Servant	Domestic worker
Aged	Elderly/older persons
Delinquent	Child in conflict with law
Disabled	Person with disability
Illegitimate	Born out of wedlock
Divorcee	Person after divorce
Prostitute	Woman in prostitution

3.5.2.3 Sensitive Listening

Kadushin and Kadushin (1997) provide the following guidelines for effective listening in a social-work interview:

1. A clear idea about the purpose of the interview is an important filter for selectivity in listening.
2. The worker should listen for recurrent dominant themes rather than focus on detail.
3. Effective interviewers suspend closure, holding everything they listen to tentatively and subject to revision because of what the client might say next.
4. Good listening requires an assumption and acceptance of ignorance.

According to Egan (2002), full listening means listening actively, listening accurately and listening for meaning. Listening to child's words includes:

- Listening to the child's stories that include experiences, behaviour and feelings, emotions and moods
- Listening to child's point of view
- Listening to child's decisions
- Listening to child's intentions or proposals
- "Hearing" opportunities and resources.

Covey (1997) points out that one should listen not only with ears, but also with eyes and most importantly with the heart with the intent to understand, not just the words that are spoken, but also the feelings and the body language. Following are some suggestions to enhance sensitive listening:

(1) *Just listen*: Allow the child to complete speaking and listen with interest and an intent to understand. Do not rush or get preoccupied with replying. Often a person reaching out to us may not particularly want answers/solutions to his/her problems, but may simply want to be heard out.
(2) *Observe body language*: Read non-verbal cues and try to understand.
(3) *Express concern*: Ask open-ended questions for more information, opinion and feeling by asking where, who, how and why.
(4) *Express understanding and acceptance*: Restate or interpret the speaker's ideas and feelings in our own words, instead of repeating their exact words. Allow others to have their own opinions even if one does not agree.
(5) *Preserve and promote self-esteem*: Preserve their self-esteem even if we think they have made a mistake. Promote their self-esteem by reminding them of their strengths. Give opinion or suggestions only if asked or ask before giving opinion or suggestions.

According to Egan (2002), the social worker needs to process what he or she hears in the following ways:

- Identify key messages and feelings.
- Understand the context.
- Hear the slant or spin.
- Muse on what is missing.

3.5.3 Feedback Skills

3.5.3.1 Paraphrasing

Paraphrasing is the act of restating what another person has said. According to Shebib (2003), paraphrasing involves restating the client's thoughts in your own words to clarify the essence of what he or she has said. It is a way of stating thoughts from a different angle. In the process, paraphrasing can help clients organise disjointed thoughts. Rees (1998) provides the following guidelines for paraphrasing:

- Paraphrase only to check for understanding.
- Do not paraphrase to improve upon the speaker's wording.
- Avoid adding to or changing what the speaker said.
- Paraphrase when a person is having difficulty expressing ideas more clearly.

3.5.3.2 Probing

The following goals of probing are identified by Egan (2002) and adapted for children:

- Help non-assertive or reluctant children tell their stories and engage in other behaviours related to managing their problems and developing their opportunities.
- Help children identify experiences, behaviours, and feelings that give focus to their stories.
- Open up new areas for discussion.
- Help children explore and clarify points of view, decisions and proposals.
- Help children be as concrete and specific as possible.
- Help children remain focused on relevant and important issues.
- Help children move on to further stages or steps in the helping process.
- Mildly challenge children to examine the way they think, behave and act both within helping sessions and in their daily lives as they try to manage problems and develop opportunities.

According to Hepworth et al. (2006), people are inclined to think and talk in generalities. Clients are more prone to focus on others or on content, or to speak of themselves as a part of a group rather than to personalise their statements by using "I" or other self-referent pronouns. To communicate one's feelings and experiences so that they are fully understood, a person must be able to respond concretely, that is with specificity. They recommend the following ways to facilitate specificity of expression by clients:

- Checking out perceptions
- Clarifying the meaning of vague or unfamiliar terms
- Exploring the basis of conclusions drawn by clients
- Assisting clients to personalise their statements
- Elicit specific feelings
- Focusing on the here-and-now, rather than on the distant past
- Eliciting details related to clients' experiences
- Eliciting details related to interactional behaviour.

3.5.3.3 Responding with Empathy

Egan (2002) emphasises that probing should be done in the spirit of empathy. If a probe helps a client reveal relevant information, follow it up with an empathic highlight rather than another probe.

Change of subject, arguing, giving advice prematurely and lecturing convey low level of empathy. When social workers relate at this low level, clients often become confused or defensive. They may react by discussing superficialities, arguing, disagreeing, changing the subject or withdrawing into silence (Hepworth et al. 2006). According to Shebib (2003), following responses also should be avoided:

- Cutoffs such as "don't feel" or "you should feel" or "this is not important" inhibit further expression of feelings.
- Empty responses such as "I hear what you are saying" or "I understand what you mean" convey no real confirmation that the social worker has understood.

- Sympathy refers to concern for other people's problems and emotions and is related to our emotional and behavioural reactions. It is our reaction and though it is intimately connected to others' feelings, it is not empathy.

According to Egan (2002), the social worker needs to:

- Respond accurately to clients' feelings, emotions and moods
- Respond accurately to the key experiences and behaviours in clients' stories
- Respond with highlights to clients' points of view, decisions and proposals
- After responding, attend carefully to cues that either confirm or deny the accuracy of your response. Note signs of client stress or resistance; try to judge whether these arise because you are inaccurate or because you are too accurate in your responses.

3.5.4 Use of Play and Humour

3.5.4.1 Play

According to UNICEF (2002), play is a serious business for children as described below.

Play in early childhood: Play gives children the stimulation and physical activity they need to develop their brains for future learning. Through play, children explore, invent and create. They develop social skills and ways of thinking, learn how to deal with emotions, improve their physical abilities, and find out about themselves and their capabilities. A child's play forms a solid foundation for a life of learning.

Play in school-age: Games with rules and formal teamwork play an important role in helping school-aged children develop their physical skills and practise cooperation, mutual understanding and logical thinking. They learn about taking turns with their teammates, sharing, respecting their peers and valuing rules.

Play in adolescence: The search for identity becomes the major development task of adolescents. Organised sport and physical recreation provide adolescents opportunities for self-expression, critical to this discovery process. They help adolescents to develop skills in communication, negotiation and leadership and to test and improve their abilities, which increase confidence. They allow young people a way to bond with adults and with one another, creating a sense of community and belonging.

3.5.4.2 Humour

Kadushin and Kadushin (1997) identified the following values of humour in social-work interview that can be applied to intervention with children:

- Helps to establish and maintain positive relationships.
- Can be used to stimulate client's insights.
- Reduces the negative aspects of confrontation.
- Increases egalitarian feelings among interview participants.

- Helps us recognise that we all face common problems.
- Reduces feelings of frustration, anxiety, stress and defensiveness.
- Permits the acceptable release of hostility.
- Helps interviewees to accept that which is difficult.
- Helps reduce the discomforting aspects of the formal interview.
- Helps clients to learn the information offered in the interview.
- Reduces inhibitions about disclosing sensitive material.

Loomans and Kolberg (2002, p. 16) note that when humour and play are used for teaching they spread joy that heals, affirms, uplifts and inspires. Humour can heal, affirm, uplift, inspire and give joy to the other person through merriment or through wordplay. They (p. 32) further note that when "learners gather together in the spirit of play, the walls expand, the ceiling lifts, differences begin to dissolve, and a tremendous sense of mental mobility abounds. Risks become adventures and the most timid students may answer questions or surprise everyone by revealing hidden talents."

The child-centred social worker will therefore most likely be a person who is playful, and has fun-loving attitude and willingness to use play as communication tools (adapted from Kottman 2001, cited by Thompson and Henderson 2007).

3.6 Ethical Principles of Intervention with Children

The following ethical principles of intervention with children are based on the person-centred, strengths-based, participatory and empowerment-focused approaches of intervention with children.

3.6.1 Self-Determination

Self-determination embodies the belief that depending on their age, children have the capacity to develop solutions to their difficulties, as well as the right and capacity to exercise free choice responsibly. Such a positive perspective engenders hope and courage on the child's part and nurtures self-esteem. These factors, in turn, enhance the child's motivation, which is indispensable to achieving a successful outcome. If social workers provide solutions and advices, they foster dependency and demean children by failing to analyse and affirm their strengths (Hepworth et al. 2006).

3.6.2 Informed Consent

According to the NASW (1996) Code of Ethics, "Social workers should use clear and understandable language to inform clients of the purpose of the services, risks related to the services, limits to services because of the requirements of a third-party payer, relevant costs, reasonable alternatives, clients' right to refuse or withdraw consent, and the time frame covered by the consent."

3.6.3 Professional Boundaries

The social worker should maintain professional boundaries, that is clear lines of difference with the client, in order to focus on the working relationship and prevent conflicts of interests (Hepworth et al. 2006).

3.6.4 Confidentiality

Social workers are expected to respect clients' privacy, to gather information only for the purpose of providing effective services, and to disclose information only with client's consent. There are limits to this principle when seeking supervision or consultation, when clients waive confidentiality, when the client presents danger to self or others, for reporting suspicion of abuse and when presented with subpoena or court order (Hepworth et al. 2006). The privacy and confidentiality of the child need to be ensured in the following matters:

(1) Access to case records or other personal records
(2) Sharing personal background
(3) Interviews, photographs or "observation" of activities by press persons or others
(4) Unrequested entry into children's "private space" and access to their personal possessions
(5) Meetings and conversations with parents and family (Frederick 2005).

References

Alberti, R. and Emmons, M. (1998). *Complete Guide to Assertive Living*. Mumbai: Jaico Publishing House.

Batliwala, S. (1993). *Empowerment of Women in South Asia: Concepts and Practices*. Colombo: Asian-South Pacific Bureau of Adult Education.

Boyden, J. and Levison, D. (2000). *Children as Economic and Social Actors in the Development Process*. Stockholm: Ministry of Foreign Affairs.

Cartledge, G. and Milburn, J. F. (1995). *Teaching Social Skills to Children: Innovative Approaches* (2nd ed.). New York: Pergamon.

Corey, G. (2005). *Theory and Practice of Counseling and Psychotherapy* (8th ed.). South Melbourne, VIC: Thomson Brooks Cole.

Council of Europe. (2004). *Children, Participation, Projects – How to Make It Work!* Germany: Council of Europe.

Covey, S. R. (1997). *The 7 Habits of Highly Effective People*. London: Simon and Schuster.

Depanfilis, D. (2005). Child protective services. In G. P. Mallon and P. M. Hess (Eds.) *Child Welfare for the Twenty-First Century: A Handbook of Practices, Policies, and Programs*. New York, NY: Columbia University Press.

Downs, S. W., Moore, E. and McFadden, E. J. (2009). *Child Welfare and Family Services: Policies and Practice* (8th ed.). Boston, MA: Pearson Allyn and Bacon.

Egan, G. (2002). *The Skilled Helper: A Problem-Management and Opportunity-Development Approach to Helping* (7th ed.). Pacific. Grove, CA: Brooks/Cole.

EU Canada Project. (2003). *Child Welfare Across Borders*. www.sws.soton.ac.uk/cwab/index.htm. Accessed 1 May 2004.

Fook, J. (2007). *Social Work: Critical Theory and Practice*. London: Sage.

Frederick, J. (2005). *Guidelines for the Operation of Care Facilities for Victims of Trafficking and Violence Against Women and Girls: Rationale, Basic Procedures and Requirements for Capacity Building*. Kathmandu: Planète Enfants. http://www.childtrafficking.com/Docs/planete_enfants_2005_guidelines_for_the_operation_of_care_facilities_20060223.pdf. Accessed 26 July 2009.

Hart, R. A. (1997). *Children's Participation: The Theory and Practice of Involving Young Citizens in Community Development and Environmental Care*. London: UNICEF.

Hepworth, D. H., Rooney, R. H., Rooney, G. D., Strom-Gottfried, K. and Larson, J. A. (2006). *Direct Social Work Practice: Theory and Skills* (7th ed.). Belmont, NY: Thomson Higher Education.

Humphreys, T. (2002). *Self-Esteem: The Key to Your Child's Future*. Dublin: Newleaf.

Kadushin, A. and Kadushin, G. (1997). *The Social Work Interview: A Guide for Human Service Professionals* (4th ed.). New York, NY: Columbia University Press.

Kadushin, A. and Martin, J. A. (1988). *Child Welfare Services* (4th ed.). New York, NY: Macmillan Publishing Co. http://linc.nus.edu.sg:2084/record=b1220699.

Kirst-Ashman, K. K. and Hull, G. H., Jr. (2006). *Understanding Generalist Practice* (4th ed.). Belmont, CA Brooks/Cole.

Loomans, D. and Kolberg, K. (2002). *The Laughing Classroom: Everyone's Guide to Teaching with Humor and Play. Novato,* CA: New World Library.

National Association of Social Workers. (1996, revised in 1999). *The Code of Ethics*. http://www.socialworkers.org/pubs/code/code.asp. Accessed 4 January 2007.

Parsons, R. J., Jorgensen, J. D. and Hernandez, S. H. (1994). *The Integration of Social Work Practice*. Belmont, CA: Brooks/Cole.

Peterson, W. A. (1961). *The New Book of the Art of Living*. New York: Simon and Schuster Publishers.

Popple, P. R. and Vecchiolla, F. (2007). *Child Welfare Social Work: An Introduction*. Boston, MA: Pearson Allyn and Bacon.

Poulin, J. (2005). *Strengths-Based Generalist Practice*. Belmont, CA: Brooks/Cole.

Rees, F. (1998). *The Facilitator Excellence Handbook: Helping People Work Creatively and Productively Together*. San Francisco, CA: Jossey-Bass Pfeiffer.

Saleeby, D. (2006). Introduction: Power in the people. In D. Saleeby (Ed.) *The Strengths Perspective in Social Work Practice* (4th ed., pp. 1–24). Boston, MA: Pearson.

Sheafor, B. W. and Horejsi, C. R. (2006). *Techniques and Guidelines for Social Work Practice* (7th ed.). Boston, MA: Allyn and Bacon.

Shebib, B. (2003). *Choices: Counseling Skills for Social Workers and Other Professionals*. New York, NY: Allyn and Bacon.

Smith, B. J. and Delahaye, B. L. (1987). *How To Be an Effective Trainer: Skills for Managers and New Trainers*. New York, NY: John Wiley and Sons.

Stauffer, E. R. (1988). *Unconditional Love and Forgiveness*. Whittier, CA: Triangle Publishers.

Thompson, C. L. and Henderson, D. A. (2007). *Counseling Children* (7th ed.) . South Melbourne, VIC: Thomson Brooks/Cole.

United Nations Children's Fund. (2002). *Sports, Recreation and Play*. Florence: United Nations Children's Fund.

Weick, A. (1994). Reconstructing social work education. In J. Laird (Ed.) *Revisioning Social Work Education: A Social Reconstructionis Approach* (pp. 11–30). New York, NY: The Haworth Press.

White, B. (2003). *A World Fit for Children?* Dies Natalis address delivered on the occasion of the 51st anniversary of the Institute of Social Studies, The Hague, The Netherlands.

Part II
Primary Prevention for Psychosocial Well-Being in Childhood

Introduction to Part II

Introduction to Primary Prevention

Goals of Primary Prevention

Primary prevention is prevention of vulnerability in childhood that is based in adultism and patriarchy. Primary prevention may aim at:

- Promotion of psychosocial skills of children, parents and teachers and
- Promotion of age-appropriate developmental opportunities and promotion of child rights to family care, development and participation in families and schools.

Psychosocial Skills

According to a document on *Partners in Life Skills Education: Conclusions from a United Nations Inter-agency Meeting* (World Health Organization 1999), "life skills" refers in particular to psychosocial skills, such as self-awareness, problem-solving, critical thinking and interpersonal skills. It does not necessarily include physical or motor skills or skills for livelihood/job.

In this book, psychosocial life skills are based in positive psychology. Positive psychology uses psychological theory, research and intervention techniques to understand the positive, the adaptive, the creative and the emotionally fulfilling elements of human behaviour. The dimensions of positive psychology are

- At the subjective level, positive subjective states or positive emotions, constructive thoughts about self and future, and feelings of energy, vitality and confidence;

- At the individual level, positive individual traits such as courage, persistence, honesty, and wisdom, aesthetic sensibility and creativity; and
- At the group or societal level, development, creation and maintenance of positive institutions such as the civic virtues, the creation of healthy families, work environments and communities (Compton 2005).

The objectives of positive psychosocial development and behaviour for rights-based psychosocial intervention with children are a combination of the positive psychological development of self-awareness, thinking skills and emotional intelligence and the social development of relationships, communication and family life.

Importance of Psychosocial Skills

The World Health Organization document (1999) considers life skills as essential for the promotion of healthy child and adolescent development; the primary prevention of some key causes of child and adolescent death, disease and disability; socialisation in general; and preparing young people for changing social circumstances. Psychosocial skills are essential for preventive mental health and children and adolescents with good mental health are able to achieve and maintain optimal psychological and social functioning and well-being. They have a sense of identity and self-worth, sound family and peer relationships, an ability to be productive and to learn, and a capacity to tackle developmental challenges and use cultural resources to maximise growth. Moreover, the good mental health of children and adolescents is crucial for their active social and economic participation (World Health Organization 2005).

Psychosocial Skill Education

According to the World Health Organization document (1999), "Life skills education is designed to facilitate the practice and reinforcement of psychological skills in a culturally and developmentally appropriate way; it contributes to the promotion of personal and social development, the prevention of health and social problems, and the protection of human rights." Besides life-skill education, various other streams of non-formal education have emerged in the last few decades. A vast amount of literature has been developed on human resource development, with organisational management as the goal. Self-help literature for college students has been developed by the counselling centres of several American universities.

The South Asia Strategy against Commercial Sexual Exploitation of Children and Child Abuse (UNICEF 2001) recommended introducing training in life skills in schools and out of schools for young girls and boys. Knowledge building and skills such as negotiation, conflict resolution, critical thinking, decision making and communication are essential for young people to protect themselves. What is needed is a comprehensive approach to knowledge building for psychosocial skills, based in the theories of positive psychosocial development and behaviour, for mainstreaming it through PEGs in the school syllabus or through co-curricular and extra-curricular activities, parent–teachers associations, and voluntary organisations.

Psycho-educational Group Work for Development of Psychosocial Skills

Psycho-educational groups (PEGs) are structured by some central theme, aiming at imparting information and self-development through skill-building exercises (Corey 2008). A literature review done by Thompson and Henderson (2007, p. 512) show that PEGs focus on such topics as attitudes, beliefs, working together, communicating and building friendship skills. PEGs could be planned to help children investigate their identity concerns, developmental transitions, academic matters and career planning (cited from Bergin, 2004). The social interaction in the group helps the members gain a sense of well-being that can lead to preventing future problems (cited from Boutwell and Myrick 1992).

PEGs are short-term groups, suited to all age groups. They can be used for development of psychosocial skills of children, parents and teachers, at primary, secondary and tertiary prevention levels. At the secondary and tertiary prevention levels also, the participants are treated as students who are learning rather than patients who need to be treated.

Delucia-Waack (2006, p. 14) notes that with children and adolescents, the PEG activities need to be of duration appropriate to their attention span. They also need more structure and focused and specific activities and directive facilitation compared to adults.

Teaching–Learning Objectives

Part II focuses on the rights-based primary prevention for psychosocial well-being in childhood. It focuses on the methodology of psycho-educational group work for development of psychosocial skills, useful also for secondary and tertiary prevention. The teaching–learning objectives for this Part are to:

1. Learn the experiential methodology, group process and facilitation approach, methods, tools, discussion techniques and programme planning for psycho-educational group work;
2. Study the theories of psychosocial skills of self-awareness, proactive thinking skills, emotional intelligence, interpersonal relationship skills, interpersonal communication skills and family life education, and learn to carry out psycho-educational group work activities for enrichment of psychosocial skills of parents and children according to their age groups and life situations; and

3. Learn the theories of parenting education comprising of enrichment of marital relationship skills, assertive parenting skills and age-appropriate developmental tasks and interventions needed.

Chapter Plan

The Chapter Plan of Part II comprises of

4. Methodology of Psycho-educational Group Work
5. Enrichment of Self-Awareness
6. Enrichment of Proactive Thinking Skills
7. Enrichment of Emotional Intelligence
8. Enrichment of Interpersonal Relationship Skills
9. Enrichment of Interpersonal Communication Skills
10. Family Life Education
11. Parenting Education

Tutorial Plan

The tutorial plan for this course will comprise of planning and implementing a Group Assignment on a Psycho-educational Group Work Programme. The procedure for this assignment comprises of the following steps:

1. **Form Assignment Groups**
   Students may be divided into five assignment groups among whom the following target groups will be allocated:
   (1) Parents of Children in Early Childhood
   (2) Children in Middle Childhood
   (3) Parents of Children in Middle Childhood
   (4) Children in Adolescence
   (5) Parents of Children in Adolescence
2. **Identify Assignment Theme**
   Each assignment groups may select a theme from any one of the modules for a psycho-educational group work programme relevant to their target group:
3. **Plan Part I of the Assignment**
   (1) Make a tentative group plan for Part I with the following format:
   Background for planning:
   - Age group of children in a life situation and their local demographics
   - Developmental and situational needs of these children/parents
   - Relevant theme

- Theoretical/conceptual framework of the theme
- Relevant local agency for carrying out the programme

Planning the overall programme:

- Objectives
- Topicwise sessions according to the number of students in the group (a 2-h session per student)
- Schedule of the programme
- Composition of the group selected: age, sex and the number
- Organisational plan: venue, equipment, posters and budget
- Baseline assessment of the group with reference to the theme
- Planning the opening session
- Icebreaker
    - Objectives
    - Procedure and tool
    - Questions for processing the activity
    - Estimated time
- Planning the closing session: summarising and review
- References
- Allocation of tasks among the group members

(2) Visit the agency and have a consultation session with the social worker that deals with the developmental programmes for children at the setting to ground the plan in the local reality. The consultation may include

- Profile of the children in terms of age and life situations and the purpose for which they or their parents come to the agency.
- Psychosocial skills training programmes for children carried out in the setting
- The timings the children come into the agency.
- The social worker's feedback on the relevance and practicality of the plan.

(3) Revise Part I based on the consultation and submit to the professor for consultation.

4. Plan Part II of the Assignment
Each student to plan a topicwise session for Part II in the following format:

- Topic and its theoretical/conceptual framework
- Objectives
- Plan for posters
- Activities:
    - Initiating the sub-topic
    - Activities for learning new skills

- For each activity:
  - Objectives
  - Procedure and tool
  - Questions for processing the activity
  - *Estimated time*
- Concluding the sub-topic:
  - Discussion on integration and application of new skills
  - Self-assessment
  - Homework activity
- References

5. Consult the Professor and Make a Class Presentation of the Assignment Plan and Finalise Based on Suggestions Received

6. Conduct the Programme in the Agency

7. Write the Report of the Programme Including Its Review by the Participants and Reflections by the Students and Submit

Recommended Reading

Anderson, S. A. and Sabatelli, R. M. (2007). *Family Interaction: A Multigenerational Developmental Perspective* (4th ed.). Boston, MA: Pearson.

DeLucia-Waack, J. L. (2006). *Leading Psychoeducational Groups for Children and Adolescents*. Thousand Oaks, CA: Sage.

Duncan, S. F. and Goddard, H. W. (2005). *Family Life Education: Principles and Practices for Effective Outreach*. Thousand Oaks, CA: Sage.

Ford, L. (2006). *Human Relations: A Game Plan for Improving Personal Adjustment* (4th ed.). Upper Saddle River, NJ: Prentice Hall.

Gordon, T. (2000). *Parent Effectiveness Training: The Proven Program for Raising Responsible Children*. New York: Three Rivers Press.

Hanbury, C. (2002). *Life Skills: An Active Learning Handbook for Working with Street Children*. London: VSO and Macmillan Publishers.

Johnson, D. W. and Johnson, F. P. (2009). *Joining Together: Group Theory and Group Skills* (10th ed.). Columbus, OH: Pearson.

Marion, M. (2007). *Guidance of Young Children* (7th ed.). Upper Saddle River, NJ: Pearson/Merrill/Prentice Hall.

Miller, D. F. (2007). *Positive Child Guidance* (5th ed.). Pyrmont, NSW: Thomson.

Webster-Stratton, C. (1999). *How to Promote Children's Social and Emotional Competence*. London: P. Chapman and Thousand Oaks, CA: Sage.

References

Compton, W. C. (2005). *An Introduction to Positive Psychology*. Southbank, VIC: Thomson Wadsworth.

Corey, G. (2008). *Theory and Practice of Group Counselling* (7th ed.). South Melbourne, VIC: Brooks/Cole.

DeLucia-Waack, J. L. (2006). *Leading Psychoeducational Groups for Children and Adolescents*. Thousand Oaks, CA: Sage.

Thompson, C. L. and Henderson, D. A. (2007). *Counseling Children*. South Melbourne, VIC and Belmont, CA: Thomson/Brooks/Cole.

UNICEF. (2001). *Pocket Guide for a Rights-Based Approach to Programming for Children: Application in South Asia*. Kathmandu: UNICEF.

World Health Organization. (1999). *Partners in Life Skills Education: Conclusions from a United Nations Inter-Agency Meeting*. Geneva: World Health Organization.

World Health Organization. (2005). *Child and Adolescent Mental Health Policies and Plans*. Geneva: World Health Organization.

Chapter 4
Methodology of Psycho-educational Group Work

4.1 Concepts of Psycho-educational Group Work

Psycho-educational groups (PEGs) are structured by some central theme, aimed at imparting information and self-development through skill-building exercises (Corey 2008). A literature review done by Thompson and Henderson (2007, p. 512) show that PEGs focus on such topics as attitudes, beliefs, working together, communicating and building friendship skills. PEGs could be planned to help children investigate their identity concerns, developmental transitions, academic matters and career planning. The social interaction in the group helps the members gain a sense of well-being that can lead to prevent future problems.

PEGs are short-term groups, suited to all age groups. They can be used for development of psychosocial skills of children, parents and teachers, at primary, secondary and tertiary prevention levels. At the secondary and tertiary prevention levels also, the participants are treated as students who are learning rather than patients who need to be treated.

Delucia-Waack (2006, p. 14) notes that with children and adolescents, the PEG activities need to be of duration appropriate to their attention span. They also need more structure and focused and specific activities and directive facilitation compared to adults.

4.2 Methodologies

According to a UNICEF report (2000), what most clearly defines a "life skill approach" from other health promotion initiatives is it's teaching and learning approach. In life skill programmes, the emphasis is more on process rather than on content; on how something is learnt rather than on what is learned; on how to think, not what to think. Moreover, life skills need to be dealt with holistically, taking into account the social, cultural and economic context of the learners' lives, with application to life concerns (UNICEF 2000). The methodology of PEG work is discussed in this section as a process of reflecting and rethinking of one's assumptions,

M. Desai, *A Rights-Based Preventative Approach for Psychosocial Well-Being in Childhood*, Children's Well-Being: Indicators and Research 3,
DOI 10.1007/978-90-481-9066-9_4, © Springer Science+Business Media B.V. 2010

attitudes and skills, through the experiential methods, with the use of humour and the spirit of play, leading to the development of psychosocial life skills.

4.2.1 Experiential Learning

Following are the principles of the experiential learning process based on the theories of Kurt Liwen (cited by Johnson and Johnson 2009, pp. 50–51):

1. Effective experiential learning affects the learner's cognitive structures, attitudes and values, perceptions and behavioural patterns.
2. People believe more in knowledge they have discovered themselves than in knowledge presented by others.
3. Learning is more effective when it is an active rather than a passive process.
4. New action theories, attitudes and behavioural patterns cannot be accepted using a piecemeal approach; one's entire cognitive-affective behavioural system has to change.
5. It takes more than information to change action theories, attitudes and behavioural patterns.
6. It takes more than first-hand experience to generate valid knowledge.
7. Behavioural changes are temporary unless the action theories and attitudes underlying them are changed.
8. Perceptions of oneself and one's social environment must change before changes in action theories, attitudes and behaviour can take place.
9. The more supportive, accepting and caring the social environment, the freer a person is to experiment with new behaviours, attitudes and action theories.
10. In order for changes in behaviour patterns, attitudes and action theories to be permanent, both the person and the social environment have to change.
11. It is easier to change a person's action theories, attitudes and behavioural patterns in a group context than in an individual context.
12. A person accepts a new system of action theories, attitudes and behavioural patterns when he or she accepts membership in a new group.

Johnson (1986) suggests a four-stage cycle in experiential learning:

1. Concrete personal experiences are followed by:
2. Observation of, reflection on and examination of one's experiences which leads to:
3. Formulation of abstract concepts and generalisations, which leads to:
4. Hypotheses to be tested in future action.

Thus, experiential learning results in personal theories about effective behaviour and continuously recurs as a person tests out and confirms or modifies his or her personal theories (Johnson 1986).

4.2.2 Group Process

Group process is at the core of the methodology of PEG work. Kirst-Ashman and Hull (2009) identify the following benefits of groups that go beyond those available in one-to-one relationships:

- Mutual assistance;
- Connecting with others;
- Testing new behaviours in a safer environment;
- Greater ability for goal achievement and
- Wisdom of many for decision-making.

4.2.2.1 Self-Awareness and Complementarity

One of the keys to building an effective group is an understanding that each member brings unique perspectives, talents and skills to the group, which needs to be valued and fostered so that the group diversity flourishes and grows. This approach requires significant self-awareness. When a person is aware of one's limitations, it instills humility sufficient to seek another's strengths to compensate for it. Then that weakness becomes strength because it enables complementariness to take place. However, when people are unaware of their weaknesses, and act as if their strengths are sufficient, their strengths become their weaknesses – and their very undoing for lack of complementariness (Covey 1997).

4.2.2.2 Requirements of Effective Teamwork

According to Johnson and Johnson (2009), effective teamwork requires the following:

- Face-to-face interaction;
- Positive interdependence that promotes working together to maximise joint benefits, sharing resources, providing mutual support and celebrating joint success; and
- Individual accountability that requires procedures for determining the quality and quantity of each member's contribution.

According to Tillman (2000), teamwork requires cooperation, that is governed by the principle of mutual respect, recognising the value of everyone's part and keeping a positive attitude

4.2.2.3 Democratic Decision-Making

According to *A Manual for Participatory Training Methods in Development* (1998), decision-making within a group takes place in one or more of the following manners:

Self-authorised: A decision is made by the individual who assumes authority.
A plop: A decision is suggested by one individual to which there is no response and the decision is adopted by default.
Pairing: A decision is made by two individuals joining forces, one floats the idea, the other seconds it and the decision is made on behalf of the group.
Minority group: The decision is made by a clique and the rest accept it.
Vote: The decision depends upon the number of people adhering to it.
Consensus: In true consensus, there is open discussion, everyone has contributed to the discussion, all angles have been considered and everyone is in full agreement and is prepared to act on the decision taken.

At the heart of group processing is democratic decision-making, which is the affirmation of each participant's dignity, worth and welfare. All the members should be encouraged to participate in the group discussion, no matter how different their contributions might be. All the members, in turn, have a responsibility to contribute their best for the betterment of the group functioning. When genuine respect is received from others, each person feels comfortable in revealing his or her ideas, confident that no one will ridicule or condemn them. Even if a solution is not finally adopted as a solution or plan, the one who offered it still retains dignity and a sense of worth if given a respectful and courteous hearing (Khavari and Khavari 1989).

In teamwork, each person should avoid becoming attached to his or her own ideas or preferences. Once expressed, the idea no longer belongs to an individual, but becomes the property of the group, which means that the contributor can then look at the idea just as objectively as the other members. This leaves the group free to accept or reject the idea without fear of hurting the feelings of the one who suggested it. All members should fully understand that rejection of an idea is not a rejection of its originator (Khavari and Khavari 1989). In teamwork, sometimes an idea is needed, and sometimes we need to let go of an idea. Sometimes we need to lead, sometimes we need to follow (adapted from Tillman 2000).

4.2.3 Facilitation Approach

The PEG facilitator has to be good at facilitation techniques besides the theoretical content of psychosocial skills. Facilitation is based in the person-centred, strengths-based, participatory and empowerment-focused approaches. It is extremely essential that the facilitator creates an atmosphere of unconditional positive regard, transmitted in a context of empathic understanding, facilitating development of self-esteem, through repeated emphasis on the strengths and positive traits of the participants (Elkins 1983).

The facilitators need to facilitate the process of self-discovery, in the following ways:

- Link scientific knowledge to day-to-day experiences.
- Combine structure with freedom, so that the group can be trained with maximum flexibility and creativity, within realistic boundaries (Rees 1998).

- Map the participants' world, meet them where they are, talk their language and they will listen (Smith and Delahaye 1987).
- Facilitate learning from the group's life experiences.
- Provide a range of learning experiences and activities.
- Give the learners choices (Smith and Delahaye 1987).
- Use simple language.
- Use humour and the spirit of play.
- Maintain continuity and sustained interest from introduction to conclusion and objectives to review.
- Monitor the group's understanding and involvement with the programme.

4.3 Methods

A combination of the following experiential methods may be planned to meet different units/objectives of a PEG programme and vary pace and rhythm:

- Lecturette;
- Pairing and sharing, small and large group activities;
- Role-plays and simulations;
- Rounds and brainstorming;
- Workshops and
- Self-reflection and expression.

4.3.1 Lecturettes

The facilitator may provide small lectures or lecturettes to introduce the theme or the sub-themes. This can be done with the help of a slideshow.

4.3.2 Pairing and Sharing, Small and Large Group Activities

According to the Lions Quest (no date) *Skills for Adolescence* Manuals, when groups are newly formed or lack cohesion, participants may be asked to pair and share with a partner. This method takes less time and requires everyone to participate. It stimulates a high energy level in the room. Pairing may be done between participants sitting next to each other, making sure that everyone is covered.

Small groups are very useful for several activities, such as discussion of case studies, situations or newspaper/magazine cuttings, creative work and preparing role-plays, for presentation to the large group. In small groups, participants learn from being part of a developing team, which carries out an activity during the programme. It is particularly useful when the subject of the programme relates closely to interpersonal skills or teamwork. Six to eight is an ideal size of a small group; the exact size may depend upon the task. The simplest way to form groups is to number the participants serially, according to the number of the small groups to be formed.

Small groups may be formed afresh for every task so that there are no permanent small groups (Staley 1982).

In large group activities such as brainstorming, rounds, games, exercises, songs and energisers, all the participants can participate. Other large group activities such as role-plays and simulations, and so on, involve all the members at the level of thinking but only some may participate verbally or behaviourally.

4.3.3 Role-Plays and Simulations

The following functions of role-play method is taken from *A Manual for Participatory Training Methods in Development* (1998).

4.3.3.1 Practice Psychosocial Skills

The facilitator may demonstrate skills by first acting out the general mistakes that we make and then doing it in the right way. The first demonstration of the right skill may be done at the normal speed. The second time it may be done slowly, stating the key points at each step. Demonstration by the facilitator should be followed by practice by the participants, under supervision. The prime methods of learning here is by practicing and receiving feedback from participants and facilitators after that practice (Kroehnert 1995).

4.3.3.2 Stimulate Discussion on Complex Issues

A brief enactment by facilitators or participants or both can be used to stimulate further group discussion on similar issues and experiences that participants share. This method of learning is essentially group discussion where role-play merely acts as a stimulant or catalyst for the discussion that follows. The scripting can be done completely or partly by the organisers or totally left to the participants.

4.3.3.3 Re-enact Past Experiences

In this sense, all participants are involved to enact an issue or a situation about which they are familiar in their past. Since all the participants share this experience and all of them are involved in re-enactment, learning occurs here through the twin steps of preparation and re-enactment.

In whichever way role-play is used, real consolidation of learning through role-play occurs through the steps of preparation, re-enactment, discussion, processing and analysis with generalisation to real life situation. Simulations are mock-ups of the real thing that include role-plays with props (Kroehnert 1995).

4.3.4 Rounds and Brainstorming

Round is a method by which every participant has an opportunity to say something quickly, in turns, in answer to a question or to report an opinion or feeling. Rounds are useful quick monitoring exercise to give a sense of individual and group learning. It is particularly useful if you have uneven participation in the group (Williams et al. 1994).

Brainstorming is a structured process that encourages the generation of a large quantity of ideas in a group setting. All ideas are recorded, and no judgements or evaluations are made, while recording. These are clarified and discussed later. It fosters creativity by encouraging people to think beyond the conventional and leads to synergy (Rees 1998).

4.3.5 Workshops

The workshop method is useful for generating creativity and synergy for team consensus in a short amount of time. The Institute of Cultural Affairs (1991b) recommends five steps for the workshop method as described below:

1. *Setting the stage*: Setting the stage includes highlighting a focus question and outlining the process and timeline.
2. *Generating new ideas*: First ask the group to brainstorm individually, and put down their three best ideas. Let them put each idea boldly on a card and send to the facilitator. Read the card aloud and place randomly on the board. Accept and acknowledge all responses. Indicate that there are no wrong answers. Only clarification may be sought from the person who suggests the idea. Ask for any additional ideas.
3. *Forming new relationships*: Ask the group to develop clusters of similar ideas displayed.
4. *Discerning the consensus*: Discuss each cluster with reference to what it means. Accordingly, give it a title. Border title cards to distinguish them from other cards.
5. *Confirming the resolve*: Arrange the clusters according to their relationships to each other. Discuss the steps undertaken, where did the group get most involved, what breakthroughs did the group have, what is the significance of the work done and what are the next steps.

4.3.6 Self-Reflection and Expression

Self-reflection and expression may be facilitated through diary keeping, anonymous disclosure, sentence completion, statement ranking, quizzes, guided fantasy or visualisation and creative expressions and homework.

- Sentence completion, statement ranking and quizzes stimulate thinking and expression.
- Guided fantasy or visualisation can be used for private reflection and shared with the group. It is useful to start with general relaxation to enable individuals to free their imaginations.

- Creative work includes collage, drawing, painting, modelling and composing songs, poems, stories or plays. These can be done individually or as a group. It is important to stress that these activities are vehicles for ideas, not a test of people's talents or abilities (Williams et al. 1994).
- Anonymous disclosure allows for individuals to share honest opinions with reference to controversial topics and for the group to identify the range of opinions on the subject. The individuals should not be sought to own their opinions (Spinks and Clements 1999).
- Diary keeping is an important method for PEG programmes as it allows the group members to reflect and talk to themselves, at the beginning, during or at the end.

4.4 Tools

The tools to be used for PEG work may include case studies/newspaper cuttings, local stories, songs and games, games and exercises, energisers and audio-visual aids.

4.4.1 Case Studies

According to *A Manual for Participatory Training Methods in Development* (1998), in the case study method, others' experiences are provided to the group in the form of a case study. These experiences are reflected upon and analysed by the learners to then extract or arrive upon new principles. The learners' own experiences, values, feelings form the basis for analysing others' experiences. This method can be used to convey complex theoretical concepts in a simple way. It allows the group to reflect on its appropriateness in their milieu/life, allows discussions/sharing on potentially threatening situations, on which the learners will not be willing to share if asked directly, sharpens the participants' analytical and diagnostic skills, exposes them to situations they might not ordinarily experience in their own lives, exposes them to similar experiences elsewhere to enable them to feel a sense of solidarity and validation and helps in creating new knowledge through collective reflection, analysis and synthesis (*A Manual for* ... 1998).

4.4.2 Local Stories and Songs

Relevant local stories/folk tales/songs/popular movies/television serials/games are valuable aids that can be used to discuss the issues on the agenda.

4.4.3 Games and Exercises

A game or an exercise is normally simple and brief, requires all the participants to participate, is relaxing and enjoyable, inexpensive, predictable and adaptable to a variety of situations. The well-known games such as dumb charade, passing the parcel, Chinese Whisper and so on can be adapted for the theme. Similarly, well-known television game shows can also be adapted to the theme. Sentence completion, statement ranking, quizzes are other forms of exercises. These need to be followed by discussion for the group to see the connection with the theme. The common games are energisers.

4.4.4 Energisers

The Lions Quest (no date) *Skills for Adolescence* Manuals have described energisers as brief activities that can help a group get acquainted, spark a discussion, change the pace, or bring closure to an activity. They make the following suggestions:

- Begin by briefly describing the activity, its basic rules and purpose.
- Then demonstrate it with some volunteers, adding rules and explanations as you go.
- Play yourself. Be a positive model for fair play and cooperation.
- Allow participants to observe if they choose.
- Adapt activities whenever necessary. Change the rules, materials, boundaries, size of teams or anything else to make the activity more fun for the groups.
- Talk about the energiser afterward. Point out the cooperative behaviours participants used. Talk about working towards a common goal and helping one another. Ask what they learned, how they solved a problem, or whether the activity turned out differently than they expected.

Icebreakers are energisers that are used in the beginning of a programme or a session in order to:

- Allow the participants to introduce themselves to each other in a playful manner;
- Orient the members to the norms and processes of the programme that helps overcome the initial anxiety related to the programme;
- Lead into the topic matter, in a relaxed manner and bring the major issue to the fore of the group consciousness and
- Do on the spot assessment of the relevant awareness, attitudes and skills of the participants.

4.4.5 Audio-Visual Aids

The audio-visual aids useful for PEG work are verbal and visual symbols on blackboards, flip charts, charts, posters, flash cards and handouts; newspaper/magazine cuttings; radios and tape recording; slideshows and video films, selected according to the objectives of the topics. Use of these tools should always be followed by discussion.

Flipcharts are often used for brainstorming, recording and reviewing key points from learners and responding to queries. Sheets from flipcharts can also be displayed like posters following the discussion (Gough 1997). The advantages of using flip charts is that they allow different coloured marking pens to be used (coloured chalk is difficult to read), and the notes need not be erased during or after class (Lowman 1984).

Audiotape and videotape cassettes have many of the advantages of motion pictures, although television screen sizes severely limit the number of students to whom they can be shown effectively. Modern video projectors are a decided improvement over standard monitors. Cassettes have the advantage of allowing the instructor to show desired segments easily (Lowman 1984).

4.5 Discussion

4.5.1 Utility of Discussion

4.5.1.1 Processing an Activity

All the above activities need to be processed to capitalise the significant happenings in the here-and-now interactions of the group. Processing can be done by asking questions for self-reflection and discussion in the large group. Processing questions help the group to reflect on the thoughts, feelings and meaning of their experience that helps them to transfer their learning to their real lives (Delucia-Waack 2006). Lowman (1984) described the utility of the discussion method as follows:

4.5.1.2 Processing Content

Though not effective for presenting the content per se, discussion does aid its mastery by encouraging participants to actively process what they learn, assimilate and integrate through reading or in class. Asking participants to think and a few to speak out loud encourages all participants to think more fully about the content. Discussion is useful for emphasising the connections between new and old knowledge. Participants can also be asked to compare and contrast different concepts.

4.5.1.3 Stimulating Thinking Skills

Discussion is most useful to teach the process of learning that is thinking. Participants learn to approach a problem or topic rationally, monitor their own thinking processes, and question their implicit assumptions. Thinking is also stimulated in those who merely listen to their classmates and consider what they might have said themselves.

4.5.1.4 Awareness of Attitudes

Discussion is particularly good at revealing participants' attitudes. Whether they participate in the discussion or not, participants become more aware of their own attitudes and values, by comparing them with the values and attitudes expressed by others. Exposure to different views can lead some participants to question or even change their implicit assumptions.

4.5.1.5 Participant Involvement

In addition to clarifying content, teaching rational thinking and highlighting affective judgements, discussion is particularly effective at increasing participant involvement in class. However, a facilitator who lets participants talk on and on with little control or direction will soon lose the group's attention.

4.5.2 Techniques of Leading a Discussion

4.5.2.1 Asking Questions

Asking questions is an important technique for discussion and facilitating reflections. Motivation to learn is increased because participants want to work for a facilitator who values their ideas and encourages them to be independent. A facilitator, who by discussion asks for participants' opinions, communicates that he or she cares about their responses to the topic (Lowman 1984). It is important to emphasise that there is no wrong answer to these questions. According to Smith and Delahaye (1987), the participants need to be clear at all times why they are doing what they are doing. Asking questions helps to check reactions and understanding.

The ORID method: The ORID method developed by the Institute of Cultural Affairs (1991a) recommends questions for processing the activity in the following order:

1. O: Objective focus on what they saw/heard (getting the facts),
2. R: Reflection on what feelings were aroused (emotions, feelings, associations),
3. I: How one interprets it (values, meaning, purpose) and
4. D: Decision on what one wants to therefore do (future resolves).

For the experiential PEG work the questions may be adapted as follows:

- What did they do/see/hear?
- How did they feel? If they liked it, why? If there was any discomfort, why?
- What did they learn about self and others?
- Can you make any future resolves for yourself?

Dos: Do's according to Smith and Delahaye (1987):

- Include questions in your session plan.
- Use easy questions at the start of the session (to get the group used to answering questions successfully) and for the shy or quiet person (to encourage participation).
- Distribute your questions equally among the trainees.
- Use a direct question for the inattentive person.
- Rephrase your question if a trainee does not understand it. Try to avoid the temptation to answer the question yourself. You can rephrase a question with simpler words, relating it more directly to an idea the trainee already understands, expanding it with some explanation, or breaking it down into component stages or questions that can be answered sequentially. Alternatively, you could redirect the question to another participant.

Do's according to the Lions Quest (no date) *Skills for Adolescence* Manuals:

- Ask the question and direct participants to think about or write their ideas rather than raise their hands. After a few seconds, call for responses.
- Address the question to the group, not to a specific student. Allow time for all participants to think before calling on someone to share.
- Some of the things participants say will be surprisingly insightful; others will seem frivolous. But when participants express an idea that is important to them, take them seriously. Otherwise they may not feel comfortable sharing.
- Accept multiple answers where appropriate, but correct misinformation.
- Draw shy participants out by occasionally calling on them by name. They still have the right to pass, but showing special interest in them builds self-confidence.

Don'ts: Don'ts according to Smith and Delahaye (1987):

- Don't question the group in a regular order (for example from right to left around the room).
- Don't use long, involved questions. Don't use leading questions. These you can often identify because they can start or end in "don't you?"
- Don't overuse yes/no questions. These give limited response variety and have a 50/50 chance of being answered correctly. You can effectively use a yes/no question to get a "sleeper" involved initially. Then you can ask the sleeper to justify his or her answer.
- Don't use ambiguous questions. These are questions that are open to different interpretations. They usually generate confusion and/or argument.

Don'ts according to the Lions Quest (No date) *Skills for Adolescence* Manuals:

- Do not accept rudeness or inappropriate responses.
- Avoid using more "air time" than participants, during a discussion.
- If you stop discussions after only one student has responded, participants get the impression there was one right answer to the question.

4.5.2.2 Probing

According to Rees (1998), probing helps in the following ways:

- Find the root of an issue or problem.
- Enlighten other group members.
- Explore a concern or idea that may otherwise be overlooked.
- Encourage group members to explore issues in greater depth and to value their own thinking process.
- Open the group up to more honest sharing of information and concerns.
- Increase creativity and open-mindedness.

4.5.2.3 Redirecting Questions and Comments

Provide frequent opportunities for participants to ask questions for clarification. Redirecting invites group members to respond to questions or comments that were directed to the facilitator. The technique encourages dialogue among participants and draws attention away from you. It encourages group members to come up with their own solutions and thoughts as much as possible (Rees 1998).

4.5.2.4 Referencing Back

Referencing back is the technique of referring back to something one of the group members said earlier for the purposes of enhancing the discussion and tying group members' ideas to one another. This encourages members to acknowledge and build on one another's ideas. It demonstrates that you are listening to everyone and giving credit to people for his or her comments (Rees 1998).

4.6 Programme Planning

One needs to make a commitment to praxis in planning and conducting a PEG programme that involves moving between preparation and planning, conducting the programme, evaluative reflection on the programme, and back again to fresh preparations and replanning. Thus, planning such a programme is not a one-time activity, but an ongoing process. In spite of a good plan, the facilitator should have the skill to change the plan at the last minute, depending upon the group processes and the emerging needs.

4.6.1 Components of a Programme Plan

A programme plan for PEG work should include the following components:

- Background for planning
- Composition of the group and its baseline assessment

- Objectives
- Topics and schedule
- Planning the opening session
- Planning topicwise sessions
- Planning the closing session
- Organisational plan.

4.6.2 Background for Planning

The group should be homogenous with reference to age and life situations. Decide on the following factors as the background for planning a PEG programme:

- Age group of children in a life situation
- Relevant theme
- Theoretical/conceptual framework of the theme.

4.6.3 Baseline Assessment of Needs and Expectations

A brief questionnaire may be prepared to obtain the baseline assessment of the needs as well as expectations of the group with reference to the theme. It may include questions related to:

- Developmental tasks of the age group
- Gender-related needs
- Socio-economic class-related needs
- Protection needs of their life situation
- Setting in which they are coming together: schools, colleges, hospitals, health centres, workplaces, clubs and associations, institutions, voluntary organisations and housing societies
- What psychosocial skill modules they have already been trained for and current level of these skills
- Expectations from the programme.

This questionnaire may be administered before the programme starts or in the opening session of the programme.

4.6.4 Objectives

The objectives of the PEG programme may be identified based upon the baseline assessment of the participants and the total time available for the programme. Objectives normally refer to an intended and pre-specified outcome of a planned programme of teaching and it is expressed in terms of what it is hoped the student will learn (Eraut 1989). These should include (either within the objective or in an associated set of assessment criteria) a description of the kind of performances by which achievement will be judged (Toohey 1999). Leaving aside technical considerations such as clarity, the justification of an objective is based on two kinds of argument – feasibility and desirability (Bloom et al., cited from Eraut 1989). Feasibility arguments are normally based on evidence from practice. Desirability arguments are of two main kinds: evidence of expressed preferences and arguments from basic values – the former concerns who thinks an objective is desirable, the latter concerns why it should be thought desirable (Eraut 1989).

4.6.5 Topics and Schedule

The topics may be selected depending on the theme and the objectives. The sequence of the topics may be organised so that the group progresses in learning the skills through logical steps.

The schedule may include the time allocation for the opening session, topicwise sessions and the closing session. The duration of each topicwise session may be planned depending on the age group: half an hour for preschoolage children, 1 hour for middle childhood and 1½–2 hours for adolescents and parents. One or more sessions may be planned per day, depending upon the organisation in which the programme is being conducted. When more than one session is planned in a day, at least a 10-minute break should be planned between sessions.

4.6.6 Planning the Opening Session

The opening session may be planned to include the following essentials:

- Welcome to the group
- Introduction of the facilitators and the participants
- Baseline assessment
- Clarification of the objectives
- Confirmation of administrative details
- Methodologies of experiential learning and group process
- Ground rules
- Formation of committees
- Icebreaker for introducing teamwork or the theme.

4.6.6.1 Setting Ground Rules

The group may be involved in setting ground rules for self-behaviour, behaviour with reference to the facilitator and behaviour with reference to other group members. Examples of such ground rules are given below:

Self-behaviour:

- Be punctual about the programme timings, including the breaks.

Behaviour with reference to the facilitator:

- Raise a hand to speak.
- Ask questions for clarity.
- Attempt to respond to questions asked.

Behaviour with reference to other group members:

- Do not talk among yourselves.
- Listen to others sensitively.
- Do not dominate the discussion.
- Support issues/concerns of others.
- Criticise the opinion, not the person.
- Do not make fun of others.
- Point out if someone is getting distracted.
- Give positive feedback to others.
- Motivate others as learners.
- Invite the quiet ones to talk.
- Care about success of others.
- Use strength of others as learners.
- Maintain confidentiality of personal sharing.
- Be creative in response to problems.
- Help the group reach a decision.

4.6.6.2 Formation of Committees

The following committees may be formed among the participants, for their active participation in the planning and conducting of the sessions:

Committee for monitoring of ground rules: monitors the implementation of ground rules and the group process.

Venue committee: maintains the sitting arrangement every day and switch-off the lights and fans after the session is over.

Maintenance of the black/whiteboard: keeps the black/whiteboard clean and assists the resource person with writing on it.

Creative use of the flannel boards: coordinates use of the flannel boards for display by the facilitator and the participants.

Use of the audio-visual equipment: assists the facilitator with use of the audio-visual equipment.

Timekeeper: maintains the time factor with reference to the starting and ending times and breaks.

Coordination of preparation of daily summaries: allocates the task of preparation of daily summaries and their presentations, beginning of the next day.

The objectives, method/procedure, tool and questions for processing the ice-breaker and the estimated time should be planned.

4.6.7 Planning Topicwise Sessions

4.6.7.1 Topicwise Plan

Each topicwise session may be planned to include the following based on the baseline assessment and the objectives:

- Topic
- Theoretical/conceptual framework of the topic
- Objectives
- Plan for posters
- Schedule

The topicwise schedule may be planned as follows:

Introduction:

- Summary/recapitulation of the previous session/sharing of home-work done
- Linking to and introduction to the topic
- Initial sharing on the topic.

Activities:

The activities may be sequenced as follows:

1. Activity for initiating the topic
2. Activity to provide a sensitising experience
3. Activity to practice self-exploration with reference to the new skills.

Plan for each activity may include the following:

- Objectives
- Method/procedure
- Tool
- Questions for processing the activity
- Estimated time.

Conclusion:

- Discussion on integration and application of new skills
- Self-assessment

- Homework activity for application of new skills
- Writing reflections in the diary.

At the end of each session, the participants may be asked to carry out their self-assessment in their diary with reference to their baseline assessment of needs and expectations, by writing down the following in their diary and/or verbally sharing with others:

- What was a new learning for you in this session?
- What did you like the best in this session and why?
- Which activity was most effective?
- How did you feel during and after the session and why?
- What will you do to practice what you have learnt?

4.6.7.2 Estimation of Time

The approximate time taken by each type of activity is given in the chart below:

Type of method and its processing	Approximate time to be planned
• Lecturette	15 minutes
• Pairing and sharing	5–10 minutes
• Small group activities and presentation to the large group	45–60 minutes
• Role-plays and simulations	45–60 min
• Rounds and brainstorming	30 minutes
• Workshops	2 hours
• Self-reflection and expression	10 minutes
• Diary keeping	5–10 minutes
Type of tool and its processing	Approximate time to be planned
• Use of case studies	30–45 minutes
• Story telling	15 minutes
• Games and exercises	15 minutes
• Energisers	15 minutes
• Use of audio-visual aids	Depends

4.6.8 Planning the Closing Session

The closing session should be planned to include the following:

- Summarising
- Overall self-assessment
- Programme review

The overall self-assessment can be carried out with the help of a questionnaire similar to the baseline assessment to see the impact of the programme.

The programme review questionnaire may include review of the following aspects of the programme:

- Review of the objectives and their fulfilment
- Review of the methodology and the schedule
- Review of the sessions, activities, methods and tools
- Review of the facilitators
- Review of implementation of the ground rules, the group process and participation
- Suggestions for future programmes

The written review can be kept anonymous and followed by an oral discussion.

4.6.9 Organisational Plan

The organisational plan may include planning of the venue, equipment and stationery, use of flannel board and budget.

4.6.9.1 Venue

The venue should be spacious enough for a circular or semi-circular arrangement of chairs, so that everyone can see each other and have adequate space for small group and role-play sessions in the centre.

4.6.9.2 Equipment and Stationery

The equipment to be arranged includes a black/white board and chalks; a couple of flannel boards and pins; computer and projector for slideshow, video cassette player and television, as found necessary. The stationery necessary includes chart papers, flip chart board and sketch pens, cello tape and scissors; transparencies and pens; index cards, markers and so on. The participants should be asked to bring a diary/notebook and pen for themselves.

4.6.9.3 Use of Flannel Boards

One flannel board should be planned by the organisers to display the programme schedule, relevant poems, quotations, fact sheets, news and so on. Another flannel board may be used for participants to express themselves in terms of satisfaction with the programme, output of the small group activities, relevant poems, quotations and so on.

4.6.9.4 Budget

The budget may include items such as rent for the venue and the equipment, stationery, transportation and honorarium for the facilitators, their meals, communication and photocopy charges. The participants' expenses such as their transportation and meals may either be budgeted, or they may be asked to pay for themselves, and/or they may be charged a fee to meet the expenses related to the organisation of the programme.

Note

This chapter is adapted from a chapter on "Methodology of Participatory Training Programmes" in *Methodology of Progressive Social Work Education*, authored by Murli Desai and published by Rawat Publishers in 2004.

References

Corey, G. (2008). *Theory and Practice of Group Counselling* (7th ed.). South Melbourne, VIC: Brooks/Cole.

Covey, S. R. (1997). *The 7 Habits of Highly Effective People*. London: Simon and Schuster.

DeLucia-Waack, J. L. (2006). *Leading Psychoeducational Groups for Children and Adolescents*. Thousand Oaks, CA: Sage.

Elkins, D. P. (1983). *Teaching People to Love Themselves. A Leader's Handbook of Theory and Technique for Self Esteem and Affirmation Training*. Princeton, NJ: Growth Associates.

Eraut, M. (1989). Selecting and justifying objectives. In M. Eraut (Ed.) *The International Encyclopaedia of Educational Methodology* (pp. 338–341). Oxford: Pergamon Press.

Gough, J. (1997). *Developing Learning Materials*. Hyderabad: Orient Longman.

Institute of Cultural Affairs. (1991a). *An Introduction to Discussion Method*. Mumbai: Institute of Cultural Affairs.

Institute of Cultural Affairs. (1991b). *The Workshop Method*. Mumbai: Institute of Cultural Affairs.

Johnson, D. W. (1986). *Reaching Out: Interpersonal Effectiveness and Self-Actualisation*. Upper Saddle River, NJ: Prentice-Hall.

Johnson, D. W. and Johnson, F. P. (2009). *Joining Together: Group Theory and Group Skills* (10th ed.). Columbus, OH: Pearson.

Khavari, K. A. and Khavari, S. W. (1989). *Creating a Successful Family*. London: Sterling Publishers.

Kirst-Ashman, K. K. and Hull, G. H., Jr. (2009). *Understanding Generalist Practice* (5th ed.). Belmont, CA: Brooks/Cole.

Kroehnert, G. (1995). *Basic Training for Trainers: A Handbook for New Trainers*. New York, NY: McGraw Hill Book Co.

Lions Quest Skills . . . (No date). Lions Quest Skills for Adolescence Programme. Mumbai: Lions Quest in India Foundation.

Lowman, J. (1984). *Mastering the Techniques of Teaching*. New Delhi: Prentice Hall.

A Manual for . . . (1998). *A Manual for Participatory Training Methods in Development*. New Delhi: Society for Participatory Research in Asia.

Rees, F. (1998). *The Facilitator Excellence Handbook: Helping People Work Creatively and Productively Together*. San Francisco, CA: Jossey-Bass Pfeiffer.

Smith, B. J. and Delahaye, B. L. (1987). *How To Be an Effective Trainer: Skills for Managers and New Trainers*. New York, NY: Wiley.

Spinks, T. and Clements, P. (1999). *Facilitating Learning: A Sourcebook of Activities*. New Delhi: Viva Books Private Limited.

Staley, J. (1982). *People in Development: A Trainer's Manual for Groups*. Bangalore: SEARCH.

Thompson, C. L. and Henderson, D. A. (2007). *Counseling Children*. Belmont, CA: Thomson/Brooks/Cole.

Tillman, D. (2000). *Living Values Activities for Children Ages 8–14*. New Delhi: Sterling Publishers.

Toohey, S. (1999). *Designing Courses for Higher Education*. Buckingham: Open University Press.

UNICEF. (2000). *Involving People, Evolving Behaviour*. New York, NY: UNICEF.

Williams, S., Seed, J. and Mwau, A. (1994). *The Oxfam Gender Training Manual*. Oxford: Oxfam.

Chapter 5
Enrichment of Self-Awareness

5.1 Concepts of Self-Awareness

Self-awareness is awareness of who we are and how we think, feel, communicate and behave. Such awareness is necessary for congruence among our thinking, feeling, speaking and behaviour. It leads to genuineness, which is important for promotion of positive mental health and prevention of negativities and mental diseases. Genuineness also means that one continues to be oneself and conveys a sense of honesty to others and makes them feel that we are someone they can trust (Hull and Kirst-Ashman 2004).

According to Bayne et al. (1994), self-awareness helps us to

- Be clearer with other people;
- Have more information on which to base decisions;
- Be more ourselves; and
- Detect signs of stress earlier.

Following are the techniques used in Gestalt therapy for stimulating self-awareness:

- Use of first person language, for example I feel, I am and so on.
- Acceptance of responsibility for the way we are and for what we do.
- Expression of feelings here and now.
- Shedding one's defence mechanisms.
- Unlocking one's potential (Morgan et al. 1993).

One way to increase self-awareness is to explore the Johari Window model in which there are four categories of self: open, blind, hidden and unknown.

The open self: This represents all the information about us that we and other people know.

M. Desai, *A Rights-Based Preventative Approach for Psychosocial Well-Being in Childhood*, Children's Well-Being: Indicators and Research 3,
DOI 10.1007/978-90-481-9066-9_5,

The blind self: This is the part of us that others can see but we cannot. To understand this self, we need to be willing to accept feedback and be more aware of our impact on others.

The hidden self: This comprises of our secrets that we do not want others to know.

The unknown self: This represents what is outside of conscious awareness, unknown to us and to others (Ford 2006).

The open self requires genuineness or congruence between thinking, speaking and behaviour. Self-awareness helps us to move towards expansion of the open self by minimising the blind and the hidden self.

5.2 Self-Identity

5.2.1 Concepts of Self-Identity

Erikson (1963, cited by Lesser and Pope 2007) described identity as providing the ability to experience one's self as something that has continuity and sameness and to act accordingly. Self-identity provides a boundary that facilitates separation of understanding of self from others. A highly closed self-identity can lead to indifference to others and a very open self-identity can lead to enmeshment with others. A healthy self-identity has a sense of separation from others and is yet connected with others.

Marcia (1980, cited by Shaffer 2005) developed a classification of four identity statuses:

- Identity diffusion: Identity status characterising individuals who are not questioning who they are and have not yet committed themselves to an identity.
- Foreclosure: Identity status characterising individuals who have prematurely committed themselves to occupations or ideologies without really thinking about these commitments.
- Moratorium: Identity status characterising individuals who are currently experiencing an identity crisis and are actively exploring identity positions in which to invest themselves.
- Identity achievement: Identity status characterising individuals who have carefully considered identity issues and have made firm commitments to them.

Sue and Sue (2003, cited by Lesser and Pope 2007) offer a tripartite model, which provides an integrated conceptual framework for the individual, group and universal dimensions of identity.

1. On the universal level are the shared experiences of humanity, such as birth, death and language.
2. The group-level identity.
3. The individual-level identity.

5.2.2 Individual-Level Self-Identity

The individual-level identity includes the uniqueness of each person by nature of their genetic endowment and non-shared experiences. It refers to the distinctive combination of personality characteristics and social style by which one defines oneself and by which one is recognised by others. According to Bean (1992), people with a high sense of uniqueness:

- Feel there is something special about themselves.
- Feel they know things or can do things that no one else knows or can do.
- Are able to express themselves in their own unique way.
- Feel creative and imaginative and have opportunities to safely express their creativity.
- Feel respect for themselves.
- Are able to enjoy feeling different or unusual.

People from individualist cultures value their individual-level identity more than their group-level identity.

Personality types form an important aspect of individual-level self-identity. According to Jung (cited by Hergenhahn and Olson 2003), the psyche could take two general orientations or attitudes: introversion, which is inward towards the subjective world, and extroversion, which is outward towards the external environment. He then identified four functions of thought pertaining to how a person perceives the world and deals with information and experience: sensing, thinking, feeling and intuiting. By combining the two attitudes and four functions, Jung described eight personality types: thinking extrovert, feeling extrovert, sensing extrovert, intuiting extrovert, thinking introvert, feeling introvert, sensing introvert and intuiting introvert.

5.2.3 Group-Level Self-Identity

The group-level identity includes similarities individuals share by age, gender, education, occupation, disability/ability, sexual orientation and marital status; and race, ethnicity, socio-economic status, geographical location and culture domains of their family identity over which one has no control (adapted from Grotevant 1998). Group identity provides values and connectiveness. According to Bean (1992), people with a high sense of connectiveness

- Feel they are a part of something and feel good about it.
- Feel related in important ways to specific people, places or things that are thought well of by others.
- Feel connected to a past or heritage.
- Feel something important belongs to them and that they are important to others.

People from collectivist cultures value their group-level identity more than their individual-level identity.

5.2.4 Activities

Activity 1: I am . . .
This activity is useful as an icebreaker on the topic.

Procedure:

1. Ask the participants to think of the meaning of their name.
2. Each participant expresses this meaning with the large group through a drawing or acting.
3. Each participant shares the following about their name:
   - Who gave them this name and why?
   - Does the name indicate the race/religion/region of the person?
   - Do they have a pet/nick name, given by whom and why?
   - Were there any humourous events linked to their name?
4. Ask questions and lead the discussion for processing the activity.
5. Discuss the importance of one's name for individual-level as well as group-level self-identity.

Estimated time: Depends on number of participants

Activity 2: My unique palm-print

Procedure:

1. Give an A4 size paper to each child.
2. Each child dips their left palm in a plate of coloured water and makes an imprint on the paper.
3. Each child looks for another child whose imprint matches with his/her own.
4. Discuss the fact and importance of uniqueness of each of us.

This activity can also be used for children's thumbprints.

Estimated time: 30 minutes

Activity 3: Symbol for me

Procedure:

1. Give an index card to each participant.
2. Each participant identifies a symbol that would best describe themselves and draws their symbol on the index card.
3. Each participant may think of a name they would like if they could change their name and write that name on the symbol.
4. Each participant shares their symbol and the new name with the large group, with the rationale.

5. Each participant pins up the card on their dress for the first session of the workshop.
6. In subsequent sessions, the participants may be asked to recall everyone's symbols as a mid-course energiser.
7. Ask questions and lead the discussion for processing the activity.

Estimated time: 30 minutes

Activity 4: My unique self

Procedure:

1. Give a full size paper to each child and form pairs of children.
2. Each pair draws each other's silhouette by making the partner sleep on the floor or stand in front of his/her paper after placing it on the wall. Each child writes one's name at the top of one's drawing
3. Give each child the following Exercise on My Unique Self, which they complete and pin on their drawing:

   (1) I like to...
   (2) I laugh when..
   (3) My favourite food is...
   (4) My favourite movie is..
   (5) My favourite song is...
   (6) My favourite television show is...
   (7) My favourite book is...
   (8) My favourite character is...
   (9) My favourite subject in school is..
   (10) My favourite game is...
   (11) My favourite animal is..
   (12) I do not like to...

4. Share the unique self with the partner and/or display in the hall.
5. Ask questions and lead the discussion for processing the activity.
6. Discussion may be conducted on the importance of uniqueness in all of us.

Estimated time: 45 minutes

Activity 5: My personality type

Procedure:

1. Circulate the following self-exploration of extrovert–introvert personality type (adapted from O'Connell et al. 2005) to the participants.
2. Participants to read the statements and tic mark the boxes that are true for them. Then add up the marked boxes and decide on their personality type.

Self-exploration of extrovert–introvert personality type

Extroverts		*Introverts*	
Volunteers opinions		Does not express opinion unless asked	
Enjoy social events		Enjoy prefer peaceful and quiet atmosphere	
Enjoy working in teams		Enjoy working alone	
Need some social contact each day to feel good		Need some private time each day to feel good	
Have many friends and casual acquaintances		Have few intimate friends	
Total			

3. The participants then share their personality type with their partner.
4. Ask questions and lead the discussion for processing the activity.

Estimated time: 15 minutes

Activity 6: Who I identify with

Procedure:

1. Give the following identity sheet to each participant to fill in the blanks:
   I am .... year old male/female, studying/working in ....
   My family belongs to the .... race/ethnicity.
   They originated from .... region and their mother tongue is .... They follow the .... religion.
   They belong to the .... socio-economic class.
2. Give a group identity chart to each participant to tic mark to what extent they feel identified with persons having the same characteristics as their own with reference to the following attributes:

	To a large extent	*To some extent*	*Hardly/not at all*
Age			
Sex			
Education			
Occupation			
Race/ethnicity			
Region/mother tongue			
Religion			
Socio-economic class			

3. The participants then share their identity sheet and the group identity chart with their partner.
4. Ask questions and lead the discussion for processing the activity.
5. Discuss the importance of being connected.

Estimated time: 15 minutes

5.3 Self-Esteem

5.3.1 Concepts of Self-Esteem

Self-identity is what we think of ourselves and self-esteem is how we feel about ourselves (Ford 2006). Self-esteem is based on a self-identity and comprises of self-acceptance, self-worth, self-love, self-confidence and assertiveness.

5.3.2 Self-Acceptance

According to Branden (1995), in self-acceptance, people choose to value and respect themselves as they are. They are willing to experience and accept their thoughts, their feelings and their behaviour as an expression of their true self. Even when they do something wrong, they have compassion for themselves. They become their own best friend. Self-acceptance helps one be honest and open about oneself and facilitates acceptance of limitations of others.

5.3.3 Self-Worth

Humphreys (2002) noted that self-worth is a sense of being worthy, worthy of giving and receiving love, unique, individual, possessing vast potential and giftedness. Each person needs to identify one's strengths, actual and potential and find oneself worthy.

5.3.4 Self-Love

Where there is self-acceptance and a sense of self-worth, there are positive feelings about self or self-love. According to Fromm (1956), it is a widespread belief that it is sinful to love oneself because self-love is selfishness. However, the ability to love oneself is necessary to be able to love others. Instead of leading to arrogance or conceit, self-love makes us more humble.

5.3.5 Self-Confidence

Self-acceptance, self-worth and self-love leads to self-confidence, that is a belief in ourselves and our capabilities. Persons with high level of self-confidence have clear goals and enjoy working hard to reach their goals. They are not afraid of making mistakes as with every mistake they learn something new. Their self-confidence leads to others' trust in them and in their capabilities. People who lack self-confidence focus on their limitations and ignore their strengths, and feel victimised by the society. They doubt their capacity as how they feel about themselves depends upon how others feel about them. It makes them dependent on others. It leads to self-pity or a life full of regrets that they could have done something differently than the way we did (Finley 1998).

Ellis (2002) suggests the following steps for developing self-confidence:

1. Be determined that no matter what it takes or how hard it is, I am going to work towards a goal.
2. Acquire knowledge of what not to do – stop whining about the adversities that are encountered; and what to do – change my thinking, feelings and behaviour to cope with adversities.
3. Act on determination and knowledge.
4. Keep steadily and persistently determining and acting to change.

5.3.6 Assertiveness

Persons with low self-confidence tend to be passive or aggressive and those with high self-confidence tend to be assertive. Ford (2006) noted the following differences among them:

Chart 5.1 Comparison of Passive, Aggressive and Assertive Behaviours

Passive behaviour	Aggressive behaviour	Assertive behaviour
• Self-denying	• Self-enhancing at others' expense	• Self-enhancing with respect to others
• Allowing others to take decisions for self	• Taking decisions for others	• Taking decisions for oneself
• Not expressive, not responding to obvious provocation	• Expressing through insults, sarcasm, labels, putdowns or hostile statements and actions	• Expressing oneself in an honest and appropriate manner
• Violates one's own right to be treated with respect	• Violates others' right to be treated with respect	• Stands up for one's rights (and rights of others)

According to Alberti and Emmons (1998), assertiveness is a positive self-affirmation, which also values the other people in our life. It contributes both to our personal life satisfaction and to the quality of our relationships with others in following ways:

- To act in one's own best interests refers to the ability to make one's own decisions, to take initiative in starting conversations and organising activities, to trust one's own judgment, to set goals and work to achieve them, to ask help from others, to participate socially.
- To stand up for ourselves includes such behaviours as saying no, setting limits on time and energy, responding to criticism or put-downs or anger, expressing or supporting or defending an opinion.
- To exercise personal rights relates to competency as a citizen, as a consumer, as a member of an organisation or school or work group, as a participant in public events to express opinions, to work for change, to respond to violations of one's own rights or those of others.
- To not deny the rights of others is to accomplish the above personal expressions without unfair criticism of others, without hurtful behaviour towards others, without name-calling, without intimidation, without manipulation, without controlling others.

5.3.7 High Self-Esteem

People with high self-esteem are very close to the full expression of their unique presence and self-worth by feeling of being loveable and capable. According to Berne and Savary (1990), high self-esteem is a capacity to see oneself as valuable and competent, loving and lovable, having certain unique talents and a worthwhile personality to share in relationship with others. People with high self-esteem have a realistic awareness of one' self and of one's rights. They accept their limitations and are not ashamed of them. Because people with healthy self-esteem are usually self-confident, they are able to build healthy relationships, see themselves as successful and act towards others in non-threatening ways.

Humphreys (2002) suggests the following indicators of high self-esteem:

- Loving and caring for oneself.
- Owning and taking responsibility for one's thoughts, feelings, communication and behaviour.
- Being honest and open about oneself.
- Owning mistakes and failures, seeing them as opportunities for further learning and realising that these do not take away one's capacities.

Elkins (1979) suggested the following ways to accept and love oneself:

- Celebrate yourself.
- Rejoice in yourself, with yourself.
- Be happy that you are you!
- You have been given a great gift. It is yourself! It is a privilege to be you. Only you are you. No one else can be you.
- Thank the world that you are here to be you in it.

- Thank God that you are made as you are. Love all of you, fully, completely and deliciously.
- Smile and say to you, I'm glad, I'm me!

5.3.8 Low Self-Esteem

Humphreys (2002) note that people who face a threat to their expression of their self-worth, have a low self-esteem which either leads to passiveness or aggressiveness. Low self-esteem, negative self-image and a poor self-concept hinder the ability to build relationships, to feel unthreatened, to feel successful, to experience kinship with the world, to express their assertiveness, to deal with fear and other strong emotions and to share their own love with others (Berne and Savary 1990).

5.3.9 Activities

Activity 7: Acceptance of my limitations

Procedure:

1. Ask each participant to reflect and write about anyone of their limitations, whether they can change this limitation or not and whether this limitation may actually be strength.
2. The participants share their reflections with their partners.
3. Ask questions and lead the discussion for processing the activity.
4. Discussion can focus on accepting our limitations that we cannot change and finding strengths in them.

Estimated time: 20 minutes

Activity 8: When I do not like myself, I am ...

Procedure:

1. Give the checklist for indicators of lack of self-love (prepared from the behaviour traits identified by Matthews (1988) as evidence of poor self-image) to each participant to respond to:
   Codes: To a great extent – 1, To some extent – 2, Not at all – 3
2. Ask questions and lead the discussion for processing the activity.
3. The discussion can focus on how lack of self-acceptance leads to negativities about self and others.

Estimated time: 15 minutes

Activity 9: I can ...

Procedure:

No.	*Behaviour trait*	*The extent to which present in me*
1	Jealousy	
2	Negative talk about ourselves	
3	Experiencing chronic guilt	
4	Failure to give compliments	
5	Non-acceptance of compliments	
6	Not taking our own needs into account	
7	Not asking for what we want	
8	Failure to give affection	
9	Inability to receive and enjoy affection	
10	Criticism of others	
11	Comparison of ourselves with others	
12	Constant poor health	

1. Ask each participant to complete the following sentences and share with the large group:

    (1) I can..
    (2) I am good at..

2. Invite other participants to add to and celebrate everyone's strengths.
3. Ask questions and lead the discussion for processing the activity.

Estimated time: 30 minutes

Activity 10: Introduction of the chief guest

Procedure:

1. Place an empty chair in front of the participants.
2. Each participant comes forth and introduces themselves as though they are sitting on the empty chair as the chief guest for a programme, in the third person.
3. All the participants applaud after the introduction like they would for a chief guest.
4. Ask questions and lead the discussion for processing the activity.
5. Discussion can be conducted along the following points:

    - Is self-love necessary to love others? When we have high self-esteem, we have less criticism and jealousy of others.

- How is self-esteem different from selfishness? Selfishness is being insensitive to other persons' needs, aiming at achievement in life at the cost of others, being arrogant or conceited or self-centred.

Estimated time: 30–45 minutes

Activity 11: My self-esteem tree

Procedure:

1. Ask each participant to make their personal self-esteem tree as follows:

   (1) List strengths as roots.
   (2) List actions as branches.
   (3) List goals as fruits for children and adolescents.
   (4) List achievements as fruits for adults.
   (5) On the trunk, write whom this self-esteem tree belongs to.

2. Each participant shares their self-esteem tree with the large group.
3. Celebrate everyone's self-esteem, after their sharing.
4. Ask questions and lead the discussion for processing the activity.
5. The discussion can focus on the following:

   - Why are our strengths the roots? What happens to a tree without the roots?
   - Why are our actions the branches? What happens to a tree without branches?
   - Can our roots/strengths increase as time goes? How?

Estimated time: 45 minutes

Activity 12: Characteristics of self-confident persons

Procedure:

1. Ask participants to think of self-confident persons, who they may have come across in their lives.
2. The participants write the names of these persons in their diary and identify the qualities that they think are related to these persons' self-confidence and share them with the large group.
3. Compile these qualities on the board/chart for everyone to see.
4. Ask questions and lead the discussion for processing the activity.

Estimated time: 30 minutes

Activity 13: Steps for developing self-confidence to reach a goal

Procedure:

1. Distribute maze sheets, selected according to the age groups of the participants.
2. The participants find out the way to reach the goal in 2 minutes.
3. Discuss the process through which they have worked on the activity.
4. Discuss if the following steps helped them to reach the goal:

- Self-responsibility
- Determination
- Gaining knowledge
- Action to be undertaken
- Persisting in that action

Chart 5.2 Summary of Self-Identity and Self-Esteem

Self-identity

Individual-level self-identity for uniqueness	*Group-level self-identity for connectiveness*
• Feel there is something special about themselves • Feel they know things or can do things that no one else knows or can do • Are able to express themselves in their own unique way • Feel creative and imaginative and have opportunities to safely express their creativity • Feel respect for themselves • Are able to enjoy feeling different or unusual	• Feel they are a part of something and feel good about it • Feel related in important ways to specific people, places or things that are thought well by others • Feel connected to a past or heritage • Feel something important belongs to them and that they are important to others

↓

Self-esteem

Self-acceptance	Self-worth	Self-love	Self-confidence	Assertiveness
• Valuing and respecting oneself as one is • Being honest and open about oneself • Facilitates acceptance of limitations of others	A sense of being: • Worthy of giving and receiving love • Unique • Individual • Possessing vast potential and giftedness	• Positive feelings about self • Makes us more humble • Necessary to be able to love others	• Belief in oneself and one's capabilities • Clarity of goals • Not being afraid of making mistakes • Leads to others' trust in them and in their capabilities	• Self-enhancing with respect to others • Taking decisions for oneself • Expressing oneself in an honest and appropriate manner • Stands up for one's rights (and rights of others)

5. Ask them to identify one goal from their self-esteem tree and reflect on how they will use the above steps to reach the goal and share with their partner.
6. Ask questions and lead the discussion for processing the activity.

Estimated time: 30 minutes

Activity 14: Role play on assertive behaviour

Procedure:

1. Identify the following situations where assertiveness is required:
   - Making career decisions
   - Saying no to a friend who wants you to try taking drugs
   - Sharing an opinion different than that of the parents
   - Asking a friend's help when you fall down and sprain an ankle
   - Returning to the store a merchandise that has defects
   - Responding to a false allegation by the teacher
2. For the first situation, role-play passive behaviour and aggressive behaviour. Invite one or more volunteers to role-play assertive behaviour.
3. Discuss characteristics of passive and aggressive behaviour and their disadvantages and discuss the characteristics of assertive behaviour and its advantages.
4. Form small groups for other situations listed above and ask them to prepare a role-play on assertive behavior in that situation and present to the large group.
5. Ask questions and lead the discussion for processing the activity.

Estimated time: 45 minutes

References

Alberti, R. and Emmons, M. (1998). *Complete Guide to Assertive Living*. Mumbai: Jaico Publishing House.

Bayne, R., Horton, I., Merry, T. and Noyes, E. (1994). *The Counsellor's Handbook: A Practical A-Z Guide to Professional and Clinical Practice*. London: Chapman and Hall.

Bean, R. (1992). *The Four Conditions of Self-Esteem: A New Approach for Elementary and Middle Schools*. Santa Cruz, CA: ETR Associates.

Berne, P. H. and Savary, L. M. (1990). *Building Self-Esteem in Children*. New York, NY: Better Yourself Books.

Branden, N. (1995). *The Six Pillars of Self-Esteem*. NEW York, NY: Bantam Doubleday Dell Publishing Group.

Elkins, D. P. (1979). Introduction. In D. P. Elkins (Ed.) *Self Concept Sourcebook Ideas and Activities for Building Self Esteem* (pp. 1–3). Princeton, NJ: Growth Associates.

Ellis, A. (2002). *Make Yourself Happy and Remarkably Less Disturbable*. Mumbai: Jaico Publishing House.

Finley, G. (1998). *The Secret of Letting Go*. Delhi: Pustak Mahal.

Ford, L. (2006). *Human Relations: A Game Plan for Improving Personal Adjustment* (4th ed.). Upper Saddle River, NJ: Prentice Hall.

Fromm, E. (1956). *The Art of Loving*. London: George Allen and Unwin.

Grotevant, H. D. (1998). Adolescent development in family context. In N. Eisenberg (Ed.) *Handbook of Child Psychology: Social, Emotional and Personality Development*. New York, NY: Wiley.

Hergenhahn, B. R. and Olson, M. H. (2003). *An Introduction to Theories of Personality* (6th ed.). Upper Saddle River, NJ: Prentice Hall.

Hull, G. H. and Kirst-Ashman, K. K. (2004). *The Generalist Model of Human Service Practice*. Singapore: Thomson.

Humphreys, T. (2002). *Self-Esteem: The Key to Your Child's Future*. Dublin: Newleaf.

Lesser, J. G. and Pope, D. S. (2007). *Human Behavior and the Social Environment: Theory and Practice*. Boston, MA: Pearson Allyn and Bacon.

Matthews, A. (1988). *Being Happy! A Handbook to Greater Confidence and Security*. Singapore: Media Masters.

Morgan, C. T., King, R. A., Weisz, J. R. and Schopler, J. (1993). *Introduction to Psychology*. New Delhi: Tata McGraw Hill.

O'Connell, A., O'Connel, V. and Kuntz, L. A. (2005). *Choice and Change: The Psychology of Personal Growth and Interpersonal Relationships*. Upper Saddle River, NJ: Prentice Hall.

Shaffer, D. R. (2005). *Social and Personality Development* (5th ed.). Belmont, CA: Thomson/Wadsworth.

Chapter 6
Enrichment of Proactive Thinking Skills

6.1 Concepts of Proactive Thinking Skills

Our mind is like an iceberg, while we are more aware of our outer or conscious mind, the part with the greater impact is the hidden part. All of our conscious thoughts, as we grow up, contribute to the building of our subconscious mind (Matthews 1988). Thinking affects our emotions, decisions, communication, behaviour and actions.

6.1.1 Reactive Thinking

In order to avoid facing issues of fear, guilt, failure, emotional pain or embarrassment, or when others try to evaluate or control us, we react to protect our ego through the use of "deceptions", excuses and avoidance of the truth (Defense Mechanisms no date). When we think in this way, we focus our efforts on the weaknesses of other people (and ours), the problems in their (and our) environment and circumstances over which we have no control. The negative energy, generated by that focus, causes neglect in areas we could do something about (Covey 1997). Reactive thinking patterns are comprise of irrational, rigid, protective and negative thinking. Such thinking patterns need to be replaced with proactive thinking skills, which are possible with high self-esteem.

6.1.2 Proactive Thinking

Proactive thinking is a product of one's conscious choice, based on values, rather than a product of one's conditions that is based on feelings. Proactive people use their freedom to choose their response to the stimulus. They focus their efforts on things they can do something about (Covey 1997). Proactive thinking skills include the skills of rational and critical, flexible, realistic and creative, self-responsible and positive thinking skills.

Proactive thinking requires affirming self-talk that reminds one about the realistic factors that are in our favour (Nelson-Jones 1999). An affirmation is a positive

M. Desai, *A Rights-Based Preventative Approach for Psychosocial Well-Being in Childhood*, Children's Well-Being: Indicators and Research 3,
DOI 10.1007/978-90-481-9066-9_6, © Springer Science+Business Media B.V. 2010

thought that we repeat to ourselves. For example, "I can handle this situation". Using affirmations allow us to select quality thoughts and implant them into our subconscious so that we can feel better and perform better. Our words affect how we think and how we feel. What we think affects what we say and how we think. Hence our words can have a positive effect on our thinking and feeling (Matthews 1988).

6.2 Reframing Irrational Thinking with Rational and Critical Thinking Skills

6.2.1 Irrational Thinking

Over-generalisation, emotional reasoning, mind reading and so on are examples of irrational thinking.

Over-generalisation: Over-generalisation is comprised of thinking in terms of never, always, everybody, nobody and so on. In such thinking, a single negative event or lack of ability becomes proof of general failure on our part (Atkinson 1992). The over-generalised statements need to be reframed with factual accuracy. Thoughts such as "My father is always shouting at me" can be reframed rationally as "My father shouts at me when I tell a lie".

Emotional reasoning: Emotional reasoning is an irrational thinking pattern when we think something must be true because we "feel" it so strongly, ignoring or discounting the evidence to the contrary (Lesser and Pope 2007). Emotional reasoning such as "I feel something terrible has happened" can be reframed rationally as "I will not worry about something that I do not know anything about".

Mind reading: Mind reading is an irrational thinking pattern when we believe we know what others are thinking, failing to consider other more likely possibilities (Lesser and Pope 2007). Mind reading such as "I know my neighbour does not like me as he never says hello to me" can be reframed rationally as "My neighbour seems to be a reserved person, I will try to say hello to her if she does not mind."

Hamilton (2007, p. 151) lists primacy effect, false consensus bias, confirmation bias and fundamental attribution error, that may lead to cognitive misperceptions as follows below.

Primacy effect: Paying greater attention to the first information we get about a person or situation than to information that comes later.

False consensus bias: Assuming that other people perceive and interpret things the same way we do.

Confirmation bias: Noticing and remembering information and events that support the beliefs we already have about something, while simultaneously failing to notice or remember information or events to the contrary.

Fundamental Attribution Error: Assuming other people's behaviour is a result of their personality, while failing to acknowledge potential situational influences.

6.2.2 Rational and Critical Thinking Skills

Irrational thinking patterns need to be replaced by rational thinking skills. Rational thinking uses a critical thinking approach which is making a judgment about information with the use of relevant criteria. Critical thinkers can distinguish between:

- Reliable and unreliable information.
- Facts and opinions.
- Definite and indefinite conclusions (Langrehr 2001).

According to Brookfield (1987), following are components of critical thinking:

- Simply because a practice or structure has existed for a long time does not mean that it is the most appropriate for all time, or even for this moment.
- Just because an idea is accepted by everyone else does not mean that we have to believe in its innate truth without first checking its correspondence with reality as we experience it.
- Awareness that practices, structures, and actions are never context-free. Awareness of how context shapes what one considers normal and natural ways of thinking and living. Critical thinkers realise that in other contexts entirely different norms are considered normal.
- Capacity to imagine and explore alternatives to existing ways of thinking and living. Critical thinkers realise that alternatives to supposed fixed belief systems, habitual behaviours, and entrenched social structures always exist, so they become sceptical of claims to universal truth or to ultimate explanations.

Gibbs and Gambrill (1999) have identified the following attitudes as related to critical thinking:

- Believe in and respect human rights and the dignity and intrinsic worth of all human beings.
- Respect the truth above self-respect.
- Respect opinions that differ from one's own.
- Seek reasons for beliefs and claims.
- Rely on sound evidence.
- Remain relevant to the main point.
- Seek alternatives.
- Seek clarity.

Brookfield (1987) suggested the following characteristics of critical thinkers:

Clarity: Act in ways that are perceived clearly by observers.

Consistency: Act in consistent ways. They do not change their behaviour or responses to similar situations in ways that appear unjustified, irrational, or capricious.

Openness: Honest and willing to account for their actions, to admit to frustrations and anxieties as well as to successes and pleasures, and to admit to dilemmas and ambiguities they are facing.

Communicativeness: Able to explain the reasons for their actions in terms that are understood clearly. They are able to use illustrative examples, metaphors, and analogies in discussing what they hope to achieve by acting in certain ways.

Specificity: Exhibit external, specific behaviours that allow for interpretative imitation. Observers can perceive particular actions, responses, and behaviours that they can try out, in appropriately adapted ways, in their own contexts.

6.2.3 Activities

Activity 1: Reframing irrational thinking with rational thinking skills

Procedure:

1. Divide the participants into small groups to discuss the following types of irrational thinking patterns:
   (1) Over-generalisation
   (2) Emotional reasoning
   (3) Mind reading.
2. Each small group may discuss the following questions for the respective type of irrational thinking and present them to the large group:
   (1) What are other examples of such thinking?
   (2) What is unrealistic in such thinking?
   (3) What makes us think this way?
   (4) What are the implications of this type of thinking?
   (5) How can such thinking be reframed in a rational manner?
3. Ask questions and lead the discussion for processing the activity.

Estimated time: 30 minutes

Activity 2: Critical review of mass media

Procedure:

1. Divide the participants into small groups to critically review the following media: (1) newspapers, (2) magazines, (3) hoardings, (4) radio programmes, (5) TV

serials, (6) TV advertisements and (7) movies with reference to the following questions:

- Is the message clear and consistent?
- How does this medium deal with reliable versus unreliable information, facts versus opinions, or definite versus indefinite conclusions?
- Who benefits from what they portray?
- What effects does it have on the common person?
- How can this medium promote rational and critical thinking?

2. The small groups share their discussion with the large group.
3. Ask questions and lead the discussion for processing the activity.

Time: 45 minutes

Activity 3: Identification of the subjective "Normal"

Procedure:

1. Divide the participants into small groups to discuss the concept of "normal" with reference to topics such as (a) dressing, (b) eating, (c) wedding ceremonies and (d) dancing through the following questions:

    (1) What is the normal way in my culture?
    (2) Is it normal because it is biological/god-given? Or is it normal because the majority does it? Or is it normal because it is being done for a long time?
    (3) What is my attitude to those who do not use these "normal" ways?
    (4) Is "normal" same in all cultures? Do different cultures have different norms?

2. The small groups share their discussion with the large group.
3. Ask questions and lead the discussion for processing the activity.

Time: 45 minutes

6.3 Reframing Rigid Thinking with Flexible and Creative Thinking Skills

6.3.1 Rigid Thinking

We often tend to make rigid rules about how to live our lives (Hay 2004). Examples of rigid thinking patterns are "should and must" statements, inflexible approach and "all or nothing" type of thinking.

"Should and Must" statements: We have precise fixed ideas of how we or others should behave and we overestimate how bad it is when these expectations are not met (Lesser and Pope 2007). Should and must thoughts such as "My wife

should cook like my mother" can be reframed with "My wife has different talents than the ones my mother had."

Inflexible approach: Very often we get used to thinking and behaving in a particular way and cannot be flexible about it. Moreover, when we plan or expect something and it does not move that way, because of others, we get very upset. Such inflexibility creates an enormous amount of inner stress and is often irritating and insensitive to other people (Carlson 1997). When we have an inflexible approach, we tend to have low frustration tolerance and awfulise our problem out of proportion. We believe that we cannot stand a situation, which we demand must not occur (Dryden 1994). The inflexible approach in thoughts such as "I have planned the day perfectly so I will not accept any changes" can be reframed with flexibility as "I have planned the day perfectly but I am ready for changes as demanded by the situation".

"All or Nothing" type of thinking: We often tend to do "all or nothing" type of thinking when we think in terms of black and white, ignoring shades of grey. If we cannot get total control/do something perfectly/have exactly what we want, we see it as a total failure or not worth bothering. By setting all or nothing standards we diminish our ability to change or adapt to a situation; we also discount small steps achieved towards a goal (Atkinson 1992). "All or nothing" type of thinking such as "I want a first rank or else I will leave studies" can be reframed as "I will study hard for a good result".

Rigid thinking patterns need to be replaced with realistic, flexible and creative thinking skills.

6.3.2 Flexible and Creative Thinking Skills

When we are flexible, we are more relaxed and save the energy that goes in getting upset. Our flexibility makes the persons around us also relaxed (Carlson 1997). Flexibility comes with creativity.

Creative thinking is generally considered to be involved with the creation or generation of ideas, processes, experiences or objects. Creativity is a way of thinking that leads to something new and different. According to Csikszentmihalyi (1996), most of the things that are interesting, important and human are the result of creativity. Each of us is born with two contradictory sets of procedure: a conservative tendency, made up of instincts for self-preservation, self-aggrandisement and saving energy; and an expansive tendency made up of instincts for exploring, for enjoying novelty and risk – the curiosity that leads to creativity belongs to this set. If too few opportunities for curiosity are available, if too many obstacles are placed in the way of risk and exploration, the motivation to engage in creative behaviour is easily extinguished. When we are creative, we feel that we are living more fully than during the rest of our life. Our perceptions are fresh and judgements insightful (Csikszentmihalyi 1996).

According to Epstein (2000), it is a myth to believe that creativity is rare and only the highly intelligent people are creative. Everyone can learn to be more creative.

Creativity in thinking includes cognitive flexibility. Not knowing, that is the humility to admit that we do not know, is one key that opens the door to creativity. It helps not to react out of past habits but deal with each situation in a creative and appropriate manner (Carlson and Bailey 1997). According to Langrehr (2001), some characteristics of creative thinkers are:

- Risk taking,
- Curiosity,
- Lack of inhibition,
- Non-conforming attitude and
- Fantasising/daydreaming attitude.

The strategies for developing creative thinking are adapted below from Langrehr (2001):

- Combine ideas of what exists.
- Reverse thinking of what exists.
- Eliminate the unnecessary from what exists.
- Think of the alternatives to what exists.
- Elaborate or extend what exists.

6.3.3 Activities

Activity 4: Story on accepting reality and flexibility

Procedure:

1. Share the following story of "Four Bears without Hair" with the participants and conduct a discussion.

   Once upon a time, four hairless bears, named Denial, Herd, Arrogant and Adaptable lived together, enjoying the warm climate. When the climate started getting cold, Denial denied that there was going to be any problem. Herd felt that what would happen to others will happen to him. Arrogant said that he will fight with the climate and make it change. All three of them perished in the cold wave. Adaptable grew hair to face the cold and survived.

2. Ask questions and lead the discussion for processing the activity.

Activity 5: Reframing rigid thinking patterns with flexible and creative thinking skills

Procedure:

1. Divide the participants into small groups to discuss the following types of rigid thinking patterns:

(1) Inflexible approach
(2) "All or nothing" type of thinking
(3) "Should and must" statements

2. Each small group discusses the following questions for the respective type of rigid thinking and presents them to the large group:

   (1) What are the other examples of such thinking?
   (2) What is unrealistic in such thinking?
   (3) What makes us think this way?
   (4) What are the implications of this type of thinking?
   (5) How can such thinking be reframed in a realistic, flexible and creative manner?

3. Ask questions and lead the discussion for processing the activity.

Estimated time: 45 minutes

Activity 6: Alternate use of a common item

Procedure:

1. Divide the participants into three small groups to discuss the alternate use of a common item. Examples of common items are pencil, table, chair, handkerchief and so on.
2. The small groups may write down as many different uses of the item as the members can think of and share with the large group.
3. Ask questions and lead the discussion for processing the activity.

Time: 25 minutes

Activity 7: Creative strategies by small groups

Procedure:

1. Divide the participants into three small groups, to discuss creative strategies for a task each, depending upon their age group and life situation. Examples of the tasks are

   - Develop new hairstyles to beat the heat
   - Develop new ways of walking to skip potholes on the road
   - Develop new ways of greeting someone
   - Develop new ways of posing for your group photo
   - Rearranging the classroom
   - Rearranging the public garden
   - Planning a sports centre

   Alternatively, the same task may be given to all the small groups and the outcome compared for examining the range of creative ideas possible for one task.

2. The small groups share their creative strategies with the large group.
3. Ask questions and lead the discussion for processing the activity.

Time: 30–45 minutes

6.4 Reframing Protective Thinking with Self-Responsibility

Passive and aggressive protectivity, distorting the truth and rationalisation are thinking patterns that tend to protect the ego which need to be replaced with taking self-responsibility.

6.4.1 Passive Protectivity

Persons with passive personalities tend to passively protect their ego in following ways:

- *Compliance*: Giving in to the wishes of another to avoid confrontation.
- *Escapism*: Withdrawing to escape from reality.
- *Fantasy*: Using fantasy or daydreaming to escape from reality into a fictitious world a world of success or pleasure.
- *Silence*: Using silence to protect oneself from talking about the problem.
- *Crying*: Self-pity or feeling sorry for ourselves when others have not been fair to us
- *Introjection*: Assuming responsibility for events outside their realistic control.
- *Regression*: The reverting back to an earlier stage of immaturity.
- *Repression*: The involuntary exclusion of unwanted thoughts or feelings from the individual's consciousness.
- *Suppression*: The voluntary exclusion of unwanted thoughts from the individual's consciousness (Defense Mechanisms no date).

Passive reactivity such as "I am the most humiliated person in the world" can be reframed as "I did not like that my sister left the room when I was still talking to her and I will tell her so".

Self-defeating thinking is a combination of negative thinking and passive reactivity. According to Ford (2006), self-defeating behaviour is often rooted in negative beliefs and expectations. It can take forms of self-handicapping, passive self-defeat, high-anxiety avoidance, fear of change and learned helplessness as discussed below.

Self-handicapping: When people fear failure or the inability to sustain success, they create an impediment, or handicap, that makes success less likely. Then if they do fail, they can blame it on the external impediment or handicap rather than some internal flaw. If they succeed, they feel they have done it in spite of the obstacle.

High-anxiety avoidance: The amount of anxiety generated by the possibility of failure or success greatly influences a person's willingness to try. It may seem safer to not make decisions rather than risk doing or saying the wrong thing.

Fear of change: Underlying many of these styles of self-defeating behaviour may be the fear of change itself even when the change is for the better. Many people become so attached to their particular way of being that they even mourn the loss of unhealthy patterns.

Learned helplessness: Many patterns of self-defeating behaviour are the results of past experiences that make people feel as though they have little control over aversive situations. Attributes of learned helplessness are:

- Passivity becomes characteristic behaviour.
- Fatigue and isolation may accelerate feelings of helplessness.
- A feeling of lack of control in one situation is generalised to other situations.

Resistance to change: Following are some beliefs that Hay (2004, p. 52) lists which limit our ideas and make us resist change:

- It is not done.
- It is not right.
- Men/Women do not do that.
- My family never did that.
- It is too much work.
- It is too far.
- It will take too long.

We also resist change by giving our power to others:

- God does not approve.
- This is not the right environment.
- I do not have the right tools.
- My doctor does not want me to.
- I cannot get time off work.
- They have to change first.
- They do not understand.
- I do not want to hurt them (Hay 2004, pp. 52–53).

Following are delaying tactics that we use for resisting change:

- I will do it later.
- I cannot think right now.
- I do not have the time right now.

- It would take too much time away from my work.
- I have too many other things to do.
- I will think about it tomorrow.
- The time is not right.
- It's too late/too soon (Hay 2004, p. 54).

6.4.2 Aggressive Protectivity

Persons with aggressive personalities tend to aggressively protect their ego in following ways:

- *Arguing*: Bringing up a controversy to sidetrack the other individual.
- *Questioning*: The means of firing questions at the potential intruder to keep him/her from bringing up threatening issue in life.
- *Sarcasm*: Making a joke out of a grave or hurtful situation.
- *Defiance*: Daring others to prove that we are wrong.
- *Anger*: Using anger (voice tone, cursing, facial expressions, body jesters, aggression, violence) to control the situation.
- *Threatening*: Using aggression to avoid facing an issue (Defense Mechanisms, no date).

Angered reactivity such as "What do you think of yourself?" can be reframed as "You are free to think the way you want to, but I do not think that way."

Blaming others is also aggressive reactivity where we lay the judgment for our problems upon someone else through the following types of thinking:

- *Judgmentalism*: Placing others on a lower spiritual level to cover one's own spiritual inadequacies.
- *Justification*: Trying to balance our wrong with the wrong of others.
- *Manipulation*: Trying to indirectly blame someone else for our difficulty, then trying to get the other person to straighten up.
- *Projection*: Attributing our own feelings or thoughts to someone else and often passing judgment on the other person (Defense Mechanisms no date).

Blaming others takes an enormous amount of mental energy. It is a drag-me-down mindset that creates stress and disease. It makes us feel powerless over our own life because our happiness is contingent on the actions and behaviours of others, which we cannot control (Carlson 1997). Blaming others by thoughts such as "He first started by being sarcastic with me, I had to give it back to him. Let him change first then I will change." can be reframed as "Even if someone starts the fight first, I need to control my anger and not fight with anyone."

6.4.3 Distorting the Truth

Distortion is the changing of the shape of a reality to make it more acceptable through the following protective mechanisms:

- *Displacement*: The transferring of a strong emotion from its precipitated object to a safer or more acceptable substitute.
- *Denial*: A blatant lie to cover one's back.
- *Minimising*: An attempt to make the problem smaller than it really is.
- *Reaction formation*: When one does exactly the opposite of what one desires to do (Defense Mechanisms no date).

Distortion of truth needs to be reframed by accepting the truth of one's thoughts, feelings, communication and behaviour.

6.4.4 Rationalisation

Rationalisation is a way to avoid facing responsibility through use of logic through the following protective mechanisms:

- *Analysing*: An attempt to explain the cause for our failure, believing that that may resolve the issue. Explaining the problem in minute detail, thinking that that may resolve the problem.
- *Intellectualisation*: The avoidance of unconscious conflicts by the excessive use of an intellectual guise of words, thoughts, or debate.
- *Excuse*: The use of logic that may appear to be acceptable to avoid an issue (Defense Mechanisms no date).

Rationalisating thoughts such as "I come late to work because I have my family responsibilities" can be reframed with self-responsibility as "I come late because I do not plan my time well".

6.4.5 Self-Responsibility

Self-responsibility is taking responsibility for one's thinking, feelings and behaviour (Covey 1997). According to Branden (1995), self-responsibility is accepting that we are responsible for our choices, actions and for achieving our dreams. The quality of our communications, the level of consciousness we bring to our work and relationships and how we prioritise our time are also our responsibility. Thus, we are responsible for raising our self-esteem and for our personal happiness. The experience of self-responsibility is very empowering; it places our life back in our own hands.

Avoiding self-responsibility victimises us with regard to our lives, leaving us helpless. We give power to everyone else except ourselves. When we are frustrated, we look for someone to blame (Branden 1988). Refusing to accept personal responsibility means that we look towards others to rescue us and be overly dependent on them (Dryden 1994). When other persons contribute to our problem, it is we who must rise to the occasion and take responsibility for our own happiness. When we stop blaming others, we regain our sense of personal power (Carlson 1997).

6.4.6 Activities

Activity 8: Celebrity interview

Procedure:

1. Ask for a pair of volunteers to come centre stage. Ask one of them to conduct an interview with the other, who is supposed to be a celebrity in the field of politics or movies.
2. The questions that the first person asks the other person centre around reasons for the second person's recent failure in the respective field, such as a politician being voted out in the recent election, or a movie star's movie turning out to be a flop.
3. The rest of the participants may observe and identify the protective thinking patterns used by the celebrity with reference to:

   - Blaming others
   - Distorting the truth
   - Rationalisation

4. Ask questions and lead the discussion for processing the activity.

Estimated time: 15–20 minutes

Activity 9: Breaking the barricade of protective thinking

Procedure:

1. Arrange a barricade of four chairs in a circle, with labels of the four categories of protective thinking: passive protectivity, aggressive protectivity, distorting the truth and rationalisation.
2. Sit in the centre of the barricade.
3. Volunteers approach you and ask a discomforting question such as why are you late, or why they failed in the exam or why they are angry and so on.
4. Choose any of the chairs from around to protect yourself and role-play that protective pattern.

5. Remove the chairs and then display the card of self-responsibility and role-play self-responsibility.
6. Ask questions and lead the discussion for processing the activity.

Estimated time: 30 minutes

Activity 10: From resistance to acceptance of change

Procedure:

1. Form pairs of participants.
2. Allocate the statements on resistance to change to the pairs and ask them to reframe them for accepting change.
3. Ask questions and lead the discussion for processing the activity.

Estimated time: 20 minutes

6.5 Reframing Negative Thinking with Positive Thinking Skills

6.5.1 Negative Thinking

Negative thinking is to see negativity in oneself and in others, and in one's past, present and future. According to Atkinson (1992), all of us have negative thought patterns at some time, but some people get trapped in a negative way of thinking which limits their ability to act or to change. Everyone faces problems in life. However, we often deny our problem by thinking:

- There is nothing wrong with me.
- I cannot do anything about this problem.
- It was alright last time.
- If I ignore it, the problem will go away (Hay 2004).

Negative thinking patterns comprise of mental filter/selective abstractions, ignoring the positive, catastrophising, labelling, fortune telling and so on, which needs to be reframed with positive thinking skills.

Mental filter/selective abstraction: We pay undue attention to negative details instead of seeing the whole picture (Lesser and Pope 2007). It is similar to ignoring the positive, when we ignore the nice things that happen to us and concentrate on what is not happening or what went wrong (Atkinson 1992).

Catastrophising: When things do not go the way we want them to, we jump to the worst conclusion. A minor upset gets defined as a crisis (Atkinson 1992). This is commonly known as making a mountain out of a mole.

Labelling: Lesser and Pope (2007) identify labelling that is putting a fixed global label on ourselves or others without considering that the evidence might more reasonably lead to a less disastrous conclusion.

Fortune telling: We are so convinced that things will turn out badly that we act as though they already have done so. The future is a fact we have predicted and we intend to make sure it happens (Atkinson 1992).

Negative thoughts about ourselves: We have the following types of ideas about ourselves that we use as limitations or resistance to changing: we are too old/young/fat/thin/short/tall/strong/weak/dumb/smart/poor/worthless and so on (Hay 2004, p. 53).

6.5.2 Positive Thinking Skills

Positive thinking is to see positivity in oneself and in others, and in one's past, present and future. Positive thinking about oneself leads to self-esteem. Positive thinking about others leads to unconditional warmth and love. Positive self-talk also includes countering negative self-talk. Positive thinking does not deny problems; problems in positive thinking are seen as opportunities to learn (Matthews 1988). Such thinking is very essential for positive emotions and action (Carlson and Bailey 1997).

Gratitude for what we have is the core of positive thinking. We all have many persons in our life to be grateful to, for example our family members, friends, our teachers, our neighbours and so on. We need to set zero expectations for what we receive as others do not owe us anything. Thinking that we are entitled to more than we have, leads to feeling deprived and resentful. We need to view every moment and everything that we receive as gifts to appreciate and be grateful for (Stevens 1998). Gratitude makes you and the receiver both happy. Lack of gratitude or complaining brings little to rejoice about (Hay 1996).

The following gratitude prayer is adapted from Louise Hay (1996):

I am grateful for myself and for my body.
I am grateful for my ability to see, hear, feel and taste and touch.
I am grateful for my talents and abilities.
I am grateful for all of nature.
I am grateful for my family, friends, work and income.
I am grateful for my past experiences for I know that they were part of my soul's growth.
I am grateful for today and I am grateful for the tomorrows to come.

Gawain (1996) notes that it is relatively easy to feel gratitude when good things are happening and life is going the way we want it to. Even then we often take things for granted. According to him, a much greater challenge is to get in touch with gratitude when we are going through a difficult time. Gratitude would be the last thing that occurs to us at such a moment. However, after going through a difficult time, in retrospect we often see that there was something important and necessary about that experience. An important lesson was learned, our wisdom deepened and so on. Sometimes we are confronted with a necessary change that we must make within ourselves and/or in our lives (Gawain 1996).

Concentration in whatever activity we may be engaged in, or remaining in the present moment, helps in developing positive thinking. Present is the most important moment of our life. By being positive in the present, we can lay a good foundation for a positive future (Gupta 2002).

6.5.3 Activities

Activity 11: Positive affirmations

Procedure:

1. Ask participants to stop talking, close their eyes and take a deep breath.
2. Initiate the following positive self-talk/affirmations:

   - I like my uniqueness.
   - I am a loveable person.
   - I am my best friend.
   - Others are loveable persons.
   - I have many capabilities.
   - Others have many capabilities.
   - My thoughts, feelings, decisions, communication, behaviour and happiness are in my control.
   - I must give today's activities my best.
   - I am going to enjoy what I do today.
   - I have a problem but it can be solved.
   - I am going to learn from this problem.
   - It is okay if I make a mistake, I will learn from it.
   - Whatever happens, happens for the good.

3. The participants add to these positive affirmations mentally.
4. Ask questions and lead the discussion for processing the activity.

Estimated time: 15 minutes

Activity 12: Awareness of negative thinking patterns

Procedure:

1. Form small groups and allocate the following types of negative thinking patterns to them:

   (1) Mental filter/selective abstractions
   (2) Ignoring the positive
   (3) Catastrophising
   (4) Fortune telling
   (5) Labelling

2. Each small group may discuss the following questions for the respective type of negative thinking pattern and present them to the large group:

   (1) What are the examples of such thinking?
   (2) What is unrealistic about such thinking?
   (3) What makes us think this way?
   (4) What are the implications of this type of thinking?
   (5) How can such thinking be reframed?

3. Ask questions and lead the discussion for processing the activity.

Estimated time: 30 minutes

Activity 13: Story of positive thinking

Procedure:

1. Share the following story of "Whatever Happens, Happens for the Good" with the participants.

> One day a king was standing in the balcony of his palace. It was a windy and cool evening. As the wind started getting wilder, the king went to the door to get back into his chamber. Just then a strong wind blew. The doors to the chamber shut with a loud bang. As the king had placed his hand on the door to get in, his finger got caught between the two doors and was cut. Hearing his cries, the guards and the king's wise prime minister arrived on the scene immediately. Seeing that the king's finger was cut, the guards said some sympathetic words but the prime minister said, "Whatever happens, happens for the good." Hearing these unconsoling words, the king lost his temper. He said, "Guards, go and put him in prison." So the prime minister was imprisoned. The king appointed a new prime minister.
>
> A few days later, the king and some staff went on a hunting trip. In the jungle, some dacoits caught the king as they were looking for a prefect man to be sacrificed in the name of their goddess. When they examined the king, they saw that his finger was missing. So they set him free. The king reached back to his palace. He asked the guards to free and fetch the imprisoned prime minister. The king said to him, "You were right. Whatever happens, happens for the good. I was saved due to my missing finger. You are free now. Now hold your post as usual." The prime minister smiled, bowed low and said, "Yes, Your Majesty, whatever happens, happens for the good." (Tiny Tot 2002).

2. Ask questions and lead the discussion for processing the activity.

Estimated time: 15 minutes

Activity 14: Positive thinking about the past

Procedure:

1. Ask participants to form pairs to share the following about their childhood/adolescence:

   - Share one happy memory.
   - Share one sad memory.
   - Think of the positive outcomes of the sad event, with the help of their partner.

2. The pairs to volunteer to share their thoughts with the large group, only if they feel comfortable doing so.
3. It is important that the group is sensitive while listening to sad memories and does not invalidate any negative feelings associated with the memories.
4. Ask questions and lead the discussion for processing the activity.

Estimated time: 30 minutes

Activity 15: Gratitude prayer

Procedure:

1. Ask participants to write what they are grateful about with reference to the following aspects in their diary:

    (1) About their body.
    (2) About their talents and abilities.
    (3) About my family and friends.
    (4) About education and teachers.

Chart 6.1 Summary of Reframing Reactive Thinking with Proactive Thinking Skills

Reframing irrational thinking with rational thinking skills		Reframing rigid thinking with realistic, flexible and creative thinking skills	
Reframe irrational thinking	*With rational thinking skills*	*Reframe rigid thinking*	*With realistic, flexible and creative thinking skills*
• Over-generalisation • Emotional reasoning • Mind reading • Biases/cognitive misperceptions	Value: • Clarity • Reasoning • Evidence • Specificity • Consistency • Contextualisation of what is "normal" • Alternatives to "normal"	• "Should and must" statements • Inflexible approach • "All or nothing" type of thinking	• Accepting reality • Flexibility • Creative thinking skills
Reframing protective thinking with self-responsibility		Reframing negative thinking with positive thinking skills	
Reframe protective thinking	*With self-responsibility*	*Reframe negative thinking*	*With positive thinking skills*
• Passive protectivity • Aggressive protectivity • Distorting the truth • Rationalisation	• Take responsibility for one's thinking, feelings, behaviour and choices • Place our life back in our own hands	• Mental filter/selective abstractions • Ignoring the positive • Catastrophising • Labelling • Fortune telling	Acknowledgement and gratitude for the positive in: • Oneself • Others • One's past • One's present • One's future

(5) About work, colleagues and income.
(6) About nature.

2. Ask a volunteer to say a gratitude prayer.
3. Ask questions and lead the discussion for processing the activity.

Estimated time: 15 minutes

Activity 16: Expression of gratitude

Procedure:

1. Ask each participant to make a list of three persons who have contributed/are contributing to their lives.
2. Participants to decide how they will express their gratitude to all the three persons.
3. Participants to write a letter to express their gratitude to one of these persons.
4. Ask questions and lead the discussion for processing the activity.

Estimated time: 30 minutes

References

Atkinson, J. (1992). *Better Time Management*. New Delhi: Harper Collins Publishers.
Branden, N. (1988). *How to Raise Your Self-Esteem*. New York, NY: Bantam Books.
Branden, N. (1995). *The Six Pillars of Self-Esteem*. New York, NY: Bantam Doubleday Dell Publishing Group.
Brookfield, S. D. (1987). *Developing Critical Thinkers: Challenging Adults to Explore Alternative Ways of Thinking and Acting*. San Francisco, CA: Jossey-Bass Publishers.
Carlson, R. (1997). *Don't Sweat the Small Stuff. . .and It's all Small Stuff: Simple Ways to Keep the Little Things from Overtaking Your Life*. London: Hodder and Stoughton.
Carlson, R. and Bailey, J. (1997). *Slowing Down to the Speed of Life: How to Create a More Peaceful Simpler Life from the Inside Out*. New York, NY: Harper Collins Publishers.
Covey, S. R. (1997). *The 7 Habits of Highly Effective People*. London: Simon and Schuster.
Csikszentmihalyi, M. (1996). *Creativity: Flow and the Psychology of Discovery and Invention*. New York, NY: Harper Collins Publishers.
Defense Mechanisms. (No date). *Defense Mechanisms*. www.wholeperson-counseling.org/ndoc/defenses.html. Accessed 8 May 2005.
Dryden, W. (1994). *10 Steps to Positive Living*. New Delhi: Orient Paperbacks.
Epstein, R. (2000). *The Big Book of Creativity Games: Quick, Fun Activities for Jumpstarting Innovation*. New Delhi: Tata McGraw Hill.
Ford, L. (2006). *Human Relations: A Game Plan for Improving Personal Adjustment* (4th ed.). Upper Saddle River, NJ: Prentice Hall.
Gawain, S. (1996). Being grateful during life's challenges. In Hay, L. L. and Friends (Eds.) *Gratitude: A Way of Life* (pp. 85–88). New Delhi: Hay House India.
Gibbs, L. and Gambrill, E. (1999). *Critical Thinking for Social Workers: Exercises for the Helping Profession*. Thousand Oaks, CA: Pine Forge Press.
Gupta, M. K. (2002). *How to Control Anger – The Deadly Enemy*. New Delhi: Pustak Mahal.
Hamilton, V. M. (2007). *Human Relations: The Art and Science of Building Effective Relationships*. Upper Saddle River, NJ: Pearson Prentice Hall.

Hay, L. L. (1996). Gratitude prayer. In Hay, L. L. and Friends (Eds.) *Gratitude: A Way of Life* (pp. 311–312). New Delhi: Hay House India.
Hay, L. L. (2004). *You Can Heal Your Life*. New York, NY: Hay House, Inc.
Langrehr, J. (2001). *Become a Better Thinker*. Bangalore: Mastermind Books.
Lesser, J. G. and Pope, D. S. (2007). *Human Behavior and the Social Environment: Theory and Practice*. Boston, MA: Pearson Allyn and Bacon.
Matthews, A. (1988). *Being Happy! A Handbook to Greater Confidence and Security*. Singapore: Media Masters.
Nelson-Jones, R. (1999). *Creating Happy Relationships*. London: Continuum.
Stevens, T. G. (1998). *You Can Choose To Be Happy*. Counselling and Psychological Services at California State University.
Tiny Tot (2002). *Tiny Tot Best of Moral Stories*. Delhi: Tiny Tot Publications.

Chapter 7
Enrichment of Emotional Intelligence

7.1 Concepts of Emotional Intelligence

7.1.1 Emotions

According to Plutchik (1982, cited by Kalat and Shiota 2007), an emotion is an inferred complex sequence of reactions to a stimulus including cognitive evaluations, subjective changes, autonomic and neural arousal, impulses to action and behaviour designed to have an effect upon the stimulus that initiated the complex sequence. Kalat and Shiota (2007) identify the following key points of this definition:

1. Every emotion includes three aspects: cognition, feeling and action.
2. Emotions are functional – that is useful.
3. Every emotion is a reaction to a situation whereas mood or affect is a general long-lasting disposition not dependent on any single event.
4. Emotion is inferred, not observed. You feel your own emotions but infer others'.

Koprowska (2005) describes the purpose of emotion as survival. The good feeling we experience in relation to food, companionship and sexual relationships, motivate us to keep healthy, stay safely with others and reproduce the species. Anger helps us to protect ourselves through fighting; fear protects us through running away and so on.

7.1.2 Emotional Intelligence

Salovey and Mayer (1990, cited by Compton 2005) proposed the following five characteristics of emotional intelligence:

1. Recognising and expressing one's emotions
2. Ability to manage/regulate one's emotions

M. Desai, *A Rights-Based Preventative Approach for Psychosocial Well-Being in Childhood*, Children's Well-Being: Indicators and Research 3,
DOI 10.1007/978-90-481-9066-9_7, © Springer Science+Business Media B.V. 2010

3. Using emotions to motivate oneself to reach goals and remain focused
4. Recognising emotions in others and being empathic
5. Ability to create and maintain effective interpersonal relationships

7.1.3 Linkage Between Thinking and Emotions

Every feeling we experience is the outcome of a thought and leads to some action. Hepworth et al. (2006) note that the dynamic interaction among cognitions, emotions and behaviours influence social functioning. Cognitive-behavioural therapy (CBT) explores the relationship between thoughts and subsequent feelings and behaviour (McInnis-Dittrich 2002). Its founder, Albert Ellis (cited from Ellis 1999) described the sequence of events that ultimately lead to our experiencing feelings:

- "G" is our Goal that we assume will bring us happiness.
- "A" refers to an Activating event.
- "B" refers to Beliefs or thinking or interpretation about the Activating event. People differ with regard to their feelings associated with events solely due to the fact that they have different interpretations.
- "C" refers to the Consequences that follow the Activating Event and the Beliefs or the Consequent emotion, which may be positive or negative. When the activating event hinders the fulfilment of our goal, the consequent emotion will be negative, depending upon our belief system.
- "D" is Disputing the irrational beliefs that make us feel the negative emotions and making them rational.

Fischer and Bidell (1998) suggest negative and positive emotions as superordinate categories of emotions. These flow from negative and positive thinking, respectively, and emotions within each category are intercorrelated. CBT is based on the assumption that both cognitive and behavioural responses to events and situations are learned. Through a process of relearning, people can change their emotional and behavioural response to situations (McInnis-Dittrich 2002).

7.2 Emotional Awareness and Expression

7.2.1 Awareness and Expression of Emotions in Self

It is important that we recognise the emotion that we may be experiencing at a given point of time and identify the reason for the same. Second, the emotion and its rationale need to be expressed in the I-language conveying self-responsibility (West and Turner 2006). According to Johnson (1986), the following are difficulties that arise when feelings are not recognised, accepted and expressed constructively:

- Suppressing and denying feelings can create relationship problems.
- Suppressing and denying feelings can interfere with the constructive diagnosis and resolution of relationship problems.
- Denying feelings can result in selective perception.
- Suppressing feelings can bias judgments.

7.2.2 Awareness of Emotions in Others/Empathy

Besides being aware of our own emotions it is also important to empathise with others' emotions. Empathy is the capacity to understand the feelings and views of another person (Shebib 2003, p. 73). Kadushin and Kadushin (1997) noted that empathy is the expression of placing of credence on what the other feels and experiences. By being empathic, we share the emotions of another person – excitement, sadness, joy, exhilaration and so on. We particularly need to understand the needs of others that may be different from ours. In doing so, we are able to achieve a subjective understanding of what the other person is experiencing. According to Cartledge and Milburn (1995), others' feelings can be inferred from their verbal communication, for example tone of voice, words and timing and from their non-verbal behaviour, for example facial expressions, posture and gestures. Following inference of other's feelings and emotions, we can help others identify their true feelings, help air them, clarify their exact feelings, and so on.

Ford (2006) proposes the following classification of people by the combination of the two levels of emotional awareness:

1. People who experience others' emotions but ignore their own.
2. People who easily step into their own feelings and increase them and ignore others'.
3. People who downplay their own as well as others' emotions through overintellectualisation.
4. People who can experience others' as well as their own emotions. This approach is necessary for emotional intelligence.

7.2.3 Activities

Activity 1: Understanding one's feelings and emotions

This activity is useful as an icebreaker on emotions.

Procedure:

1. Show the chart of "How do you feel today?" and ask participants to identify their feeling/emotion of the day and express its rationale in the I-language.
2. Alternately ask the participants to draw their own faces expressing their emotions and share it with the large group with the rationale in the I-language.
3. Ask questions and lead the discussion for processing the activity.

Estimated time: 20–30 minutes

Activity 2: Dumb Charade on Awareness and Expression of Emotions

Procedure:

1. Make a number of chits with one feeling/emotion written on each, fold them and ask the participants to take turns to pick one and act the emotion through body language.
2. The rest of the participants observe and try to infer the feeling/emotion that is being acted out.
3. The acting participant then shares one situation when he/she experiences that emotion.
4. Ask questions and lead the discussion for processing the activity.
5. Discussion can focus on the importance of recognition, expression, verbalisation and inference of emotions.

Estimated time: 30 minutes

Activity 3: Assessment of Emotional Awareness

Procedure:

1. Ask each participant to reflect whether they are aware of their own and/or others' emotions with reference to the following classification:
   - People who experience others' emotions but ignore their own.
   - People who experience their own feelings and increase them and ignore others'.
   - People who downplay their own as well as others' emotions through overintellectualisation.
   - People who can experience others' as well as their own emotions.
2. Ask questions and lead the discussion for processing the activity.

Estimated time: 15 minutes

7.3 Regulating Negative Emotions

7.3.1 Concept of Regulating Negative Emotions

7.3.1.1 Messages of Negative Emotions

The negative emotions are essential and beneficial as they signal the need for change and problem-solving, and provide motivation (Webster-Stratton 1999). Cornelius and Faire (2006, p. 130) note that each emotion delivers a message:

- Anger: I need change; I need to communicate this.
- Resentment: I need to take charge of my feelings; I need to take responsibility for changing the situation.

- Hurt: I need to restore empathy; I need to be healed.
- Guilt: I need to make amends; I will do things differently next time.
- Fear: I need to take care; I need support; I need more facts, I need to slow down.

We need to work on these messages before expressing them to the persons concerned.

7.3.1.2 Types of Negative Emotions

According to Bayne et al. (1994), anger, sadness and fear are three kinds of basic negative emotions and there are subordinate emotions within each. Healthy negative emotions are essential and lead to action to resolve a problem. Unhealthy negative emotions narrow an individual's momentary thought–action repertoire (Fredrickson and Levenson 1998, cited from Fredrickson 2000) that prevents us from taking any constructive action.

7.3.1.3 Effects of Negative Emotions

Negative emotions lead to stress, biological changes and changes in behaviour and relationships.

Stress: Events that create negative emotions are stressful (Kalat and Shiota 2007). Stress is experienced when the demands of a situation tax or exceed a person's resources and some type of harm or loss is anticipated (Lazarus 1966, cited from Rice 2000). It is also caused by wanting more of something that we cannot have, or having more of something that we do not want (Carlson and Bailey 1997). Stressors are stressful events or situations, chronic stressors are those, which are long-term and not resolved quickly and acute stressors are those that are short-term and require immediate response (Hamilton 2007). Modern life tends to present people with many long-term non-life threatening stressors (Kalat and Shiota 2007).

Biological effects of negative emotions: Whenever we experience negative emotions, the nerves of the brain and the nervous system get activated which leads to many biological changes. Gupta (2002) lists the following biological changes that take place in order to provide the increased energy to face the impending threat:

- Blood pressure is increased and blood vessels are dilated.
- Digestion is shut down, and blood is diverted from stomach towards skeleton muscles to provide them energy.
- Sweating increases and skin resistance decreases.
- Blood is diverted away from the skin because peripheral blood vessels are constricted.
- The activity of the immune system gets withdrawn for the time being.

As a result of these biological changes, frequent episodes of emotional problems can bring about the following problems in the body:

- Migraine and headache
- Digestive disorders, ulcers

- Heart problems
- Muscular tightness, backache and spondylitis (Gupta 2002).

Effects on behaviour and relationships: Emotional problems have major effects on behaviour as these destroy the reasoning capacity and intellect for the time being. Bonds of friendship and love, which may have been developed over years, can easily be destroyed (Gupta 2002).

7.3.1.4 Regulating Negative Emotions

Negative emotions can be regulated by

- Accepting reality
- Letting go and forgiveness

Accepting reality: We need to expect reality of life even if it is different from our expectations. We need to be comfortable with imperfection. When we let go our expectations, when we accept life as it is, we are free (Carlson 1997). Dryden's (1994) recommendations of ways to accept reality are as follows:

- Learn to accept self and others as they are;
- Acknowledge that the situation does exist;
- Tragedies can and do happen to all of us;
- Unfairness does exist in this world;
- Rate the tragedy/unfairness on a realistic scale of badness;
- Acknowledge that we dislike it;
- Develop a high frustration tolerance, change the "I can't stand it" attitude to "I don't like it but I can stand it" attitude and
- Decide to take constructive action to try and change the situation.

When we accept that life is not fair, it makes us feel compassion for others and ourselves. That will help us spend our energy in loving-kindness to improve the situation for others and ourselves (Carlson 1997). Stevens (1998) suggests that it is important to replace the "fairness" doctrine with the "happiness" doctrine. Expecting justice with reference to a calculation of what we have given with reference to what we receive, generally have little correspondence to outside reality. However, psychological justice does prevail in the sense of lack of real intimacy and love in the life of those who harm others. They are punished by their own anger and negative beliefs, which torment them with conflict, anger and anxiety.

Letting go and forgiveness: When someone has hurt us, we do not have to be the one who punishes them (Brahm 2005). It is better to let go of the heavy load of past resentments, not just for the sake of others, but also for our sake. Learning to forgive people, who hurt us, is the best way to stop feeling victimised. The moment we stop blaming others, we are in a position to take some action to improve things (Matthews 1988). Forgiveness is a powerful tool to let go of the pain, making peace with your past and getting on with your life. It helps you heal yourself by replacing anger with understanding. Rather than thinking of the person who hurt you as bad, you may begin to see that person as someone who was weak, sick, needy or ignorant and direct good wishes towards the person (Ford 2006). It implies giving love, understanding and acceptance where there has been hate, resentment and disharmony. It means changing the attitude of disappointment by cancelling expectations and allowing an attitude of unconditional love to flow out to the person who disappointed us. It is a willingness to take responsibility for oneself and to allow others to take responsibility for themselves (Stauffer 1998). The process of forgiving can be carried out mentally as well as by writing about it (Ford 2006). Brahm recommends positive forgiveness which includes appreciating the good in the other person and tackling the root problem, which result in positive changes in the other person.

7.3.2 Anger

Anger is a natural, healthy, non-evil human emotion and, despite our best efforts to minimise its influence in our lives, all of us experience it from time to time, whether we express it or not (Alberti and Emmons 1998). Stevens (1998) noted that anger is caused by our fear, helplessness, or inability to mentally cope with some situation. Anger can overcome anxiety and fear and encourage us to take actions we would never take otherwise. Such actions can be highly constructive or destructive, depending on the circumstances (Johnson 1986). Feeling exasperated, frustrated, provoked, sore, annoyed and fed-up are healthy and need to be regulated. Feeling disgust, furious, bitter or seething is unhealthy, and need to be prevented. If we have a persistent problem with anger, it is unhealthy as then we either have important underlying issues that we have not resolved or we are using emotional coping methods that are ineffective (Stevens 1998).

According to Gupta (2002), we should not repress anger. Repressed anger is more harmful than expressed anger because the former is pushed into our subconscious or unconscious mind, from where it subtly affects our mental functioning and behaviour. In Brahm's (2005) opinion, anger is our frustrated expectation based on our "should" beliefs. In order to express anger, we have to justify it to ourselves first. So we reconstruct the "crime" committed by the other person against us like a mental trial, we as the judge, without allowing the other person to defend him/her. Then we feel okay at being angry with them. In a fair trial, it is important to pause and let the other person defend him/her.

7.3.2.1 Regulating Anger

Alberti and Emmons (1998) and Stevens (1998) provide the following steps for minimising anger in a particular situation:

- Identify the real issue that is causing the anger.
- Increase your empathy; consider the possibility that the other person may be having a really bad day. Try to understand the issue from the other person's point of view.

- Assume the best intentions; even the most hostile people are usually not trying to hurt others. They primarily want to protect or defend themselves.
- Be tolerant of the infinite variety of human beings.
- Holding on to anger, to punish the other person, is self-destructive, it only hurts ourselves. It has negative effects on the body and our life.
- If you want to change the other person's behaviour, rewards are more effective than punishments.
- Work towards resolution of problems with others in our life, not "victory". The best way to eliminate an enemy is to make him/her our friend.
- Forgive, let go of your need to blame somebody for everything that goes wrong in life.

The following chart shows the healthy response to certain anger-provoking situations adapted from Gupta (2002):

Chart 7.1 Healthy Response to Anger-Provoking Situations

Anger-provoking situations	Healthy response
• When someone does not agree with us and criticises us	• Remain calm and do not give any clarification. Truth does not depend upon people's opinion about us
• When people do not behave according to our expectations	• Everyone is unique and need not think and behave same as us
• When someone or something becomes an obstacle in the path to meet our desires	• Take all obstacles in our path as opportunities to grow and learn
• When people do not stand by the commitments and promises they make to us	• Accept the reality that the world is a mixture of good and bad people

Alberti and Emmons (1998) make the following recommendations for dealing with anger:

- Make some assertive verbal expression of concern.
- "Schedule" time for working things out. If you are able to do so spontaneously, fine; if not, arrange a time with the other person to deal with the issue later.
- State your feelings assertively.
- Accept responsibility for your feelings. You got angry at what happened; the other person did not "make" you angry.
- Stick to specifics and to the present situation. Avoid generalising. Do not dig up the entire history of the relationship!
- Work towards resolution of the problem.

7.3.2.2 Coping with Someone Else's Anger

What do we do when someone is furious and directing their full hostility at us? When a person is angry with us, we should not indulge in logical arguments because he/she cannot appreciate our logic in an emotional state. Do not get angry with the angry person as that would harm both of you (Gupta 2002). Alberti and Emmons (1998) recommend the following steps to deal with someone else's anger:

- Allow the angry person to vent the strong feelings.
- Respond only with acknowledgement and acceptance of the other person's feelings at first, for example "I can see that you're really upset about this."
- Take a deep breath, and try to stay as calm as possible.
- Offer to discuss a solution later giving the person time to cool off, for example "I think we both need some time to think about this. I'd like to talk with you about it in an hour/tomorrow/next week."
- Admit when you are wrong, even in the face of insult.
- Assert yourself about the way the angry person is reacting.
- Make a short statement to bring the encounter to an end.
- Follow the conflict resolution approach.

7.3.3 Hurt

Hurt is pain caused by perceived injustice in a relationship in which we are deeply involved. The extent of hurt depends upon the significance we attach to the relationship. We need to understand why we get hurt so that we can avoid getting hurt (Ford 2006). When we are hurt, "why", "how could it be" and similar self-pitying responses crowd the mind, which do not lead to the resolution of the problem, but only keep us running in circles (TT Ranganathan Clinical Research Foundation no date). If we confront the person who has hurt us, they will most likely get defensive, not be able to hear us and even find something to blame us for. This keeps the cycle of blame–resentment–defensiveness–transgression going (Carlson and Bailey 1997). Some of us carry a huge burden of hurts of the distant past. Pulled down by the sheer weight of negative feelings, we cannot relate to the present (TT Ranganathan Clinical Research Foundation no date).

Left to itself, hurt heals over a period of time. However, people often do not allow the hurt to be healed and hang on to it for the following reasons (Carlson and Bailey 1997):

- *To avoid repetition of the past*: People mistakenly believe that refusing to forgive another will help them avoid repeating the past. They often say that if they forgive others they will get hurt again.
- *To avoid condoning the behaviour*: People believe that if they forgive the other person, they are in some way condoning what was done.
- *To motivate change*: People hold on to grudges because they think that the anger gives them energy to change things in the future.

7.3.4 Sadness

Sadness is the emotional reaction to a sense of loss (Kalat and Shiota 2007). Sadness includes feeling discouraged, unhappy, low, bruised, disappointed, hurt, ashamed, upset, guilty and gloomy. If we lose something or someone, it is natural to feel sad, and it may make us do something constructive about it. However, if loss leads to the feelings of being depressed, defeated, devastated, empty, worthless, hopeless, crushed and battered, it is unhealthy and need to be prevented, as it makes us feel helpless and stops us from being constructive (Dryden 1994).

Brahm (2005) notes that when tragedies occur in our life, we go through the following thoughts:

- It is not our fault so we wonder why this happened to me.
- We feel stuck with it, as even our near and dear ones cannot take it away.
- Its pain fills our whole life.
- When we continue to feel sad about it, our sadness brings more sadness to us and to our near and dear ones.

Brahm (2005) recommends the following to deal with sadness:

- Overcoming sadness is the work that we have to do for ourselves.
- We need to believe that "this too will pass" and take nothing for granted.
- We need to welcome tragedies as fertilisers for life.

7.3.5 Fear and Anxiety

Fear and anxiety are similar experiences, characterised by feelings of danger and a sense of being threatened. We experience fear when the danger is directed towards a specific object or event. It is a response to a perceived danger, either to oneself or to a loved one, and it subsides quickly when the threat is gone. A moderate amount of fear of real dangers leads to intelligent precautions. However, excessive fear is unhealthy as it becomes a barrier in undertaking safe action and making use of opportunities (Kalat and Shiota 2007). Brahm (2005) noted that experiencing fear is finding faults with the future. So staying in the present and being open to the uncertainty of the future releases us from the prison of fear.

The following statements listed by Hay (2004) show how fear of the future can be a barrier to behaviour:

- I might fail.
- They might reject me.
- I might get hurt.
- It might cost me money.
- Who knows where I might end up?
- I may lose my freedom.
- I might lose my friends.

For many young people, anxiety or nervousness is normatively associated with developmental transitions. Children experience anxiety when separating from their parents or when entering school for the first time. Adolescents experience anxiety when moving from school to college (Rose and Fatout 2003).

7.3.6 Activities

Activity 4: Regulating negative emotions

Procedure:

1. Divide the participants into five small groups to discuss the following four questions for (a) anger, (b) hurt, (c) sadness, (d) fear and (e) anxiety:

   (1) What situations make me feel this emotion?
   (2) How do I express this emotion?
   (3) What effect my expression has on me, on the other person, our relationship and the situation?
   (4) What thoughts make me feel this emotion? Is my thinking realistic? Can I reframe my thinking to prevent this emotion?
   (5) How can I express this emotion more constructively?

2. The small groups can prepare role-plays on expressing the negative emotions constructively and present to the large group.
3. Ask questions and lead the discussion for processing the activity.

Estimated time: 60 minutes

Activity 5: Reflections on Forgiving and Letting Go

Procedure:

1. Ask the participants to close their eyes and remember experiencing hurt by someone and feel the emotions it aroused in them.
2. The participants ask the following question to themselves:

   (1) Who has hurt me and how?
   (2) How long have I carried the hurt?
   (3) Has it helped the other person change?
   (4) Who is suffering from the hurt?
   (5) Can I replace hurt with understanding of the other person?
   (6) Can I leave the responsibility of change to that person?
   (7) Can I wish good for that person without any expectations?
   (8) Can I forgive that person and let go the hurt?

3. Ask them to share their thoughts with their partner if they feel comfortable doing so. The partners may help each other understand the person who hurt, wish him/her good and mentally forgive the person and throw away the negativity from their present life. Those who are not comfortable sharing, may carry out the process by themselves.
4. Ask questions and lead the discussion for processing the activity.

Estimated time: 30 minutes

7.4 Enrichment of Positive Emotions

7.4.1 Concepts of Enrichment of Positive Emotions

According to Fredrickson and Levenson (1998, cited from Fredrickson 2000), positive emotions that broaden an individual's momentary thought–action repertoire, which in turn can build that individual's enduring personal resources, resources that also served the ancestral function of promoting survival. By broadening the momentary thought–action repertoire, positive emotions loosen the hold that negative emotions gain on an individual's mind and body by undoing the narrowed psychological and physiological preparation for specific action. Love, joy and happiness are the main types of positive emotions.

Positive emotions can be enriched by:

- Positive thinking, that is acknowledgement and gratitude for the positive in oneself and others and in one's past, present and future.
- Tools of smile, humour and laughter.

7.4.2 Love

7.4.2.1 Capacity to Love

According to Erich Fromm (1956), most people see the problem of love primarily as that of *being loved* rather than that of *loving*, of one's capacity to love. Most people also have the attitude that the problem of love is the problem of an *object*, not the problem of a *faculty*. People think that to love is simple, but that to find the right object to love – or to be loved by – is difficult. However, according to Fromm, love is not primarily a relationship to a specific person; it is an attitude, an orientation of character, which determines the relatedness of a person to the world as a whole, not towards one object of love. When we put more efforts on being a loving person, which is something in our control, we will anyway receive more love, and love is its own reward (Carlson 1997).

Peck (1985) defined love as the will to extend one's self for the purpose of nurturing one's own or another's spiritual growth. True love is a committed thoughtful decision. It is total commitment to the security, satisfaction and well-being of another person whose development and growth towards his/her greatest potential matters to us more than our own. Love's sole intention is the good of another. It does not count the cost or expect a return.

7.4.2.2 Unconditional Love

Unconditional love is allowing people to be where they are and loving them anyway (Matthews 1988). Unconditional love not only means acceptance, care, affirmation and the absence of comparison, but also encouragement of behaviour that builds competence while keeping behaviour and person separate. Problematic behaviours, whether they be of a minor or serious nature, need to be confronted and responsibility has to be demanded but without threatening the relationship with the perpetrators of the problematic behaviour (Humphreys 2002). Some people are frustrating to spend time with as they are self-centred, have lots of needs, are very demanding and are unreasonable in their attitudes. Yet, if we can love them, they may feel our love, and it may bring out the best in them. Our love can transform people and make them more lovable (Keith 2001).

7.4.3 Joy and Happiness

When we feel an intense pleasure in response to a particular event, the emotion we feel is joy (Kalat and Shiota 2007). Happiness is the sense of contentment or general satisfaction with life. Since every emotion is a reaction to a situation whereas mood or affect is a general long-lasting disposition not dependent on any single event, happiness is more a mood than an emotion (Kalat and Shiota 2007).

Happiness is born from the internal workings of our own minds. No other person or external condition can make us happy or unhappy. We should not become overly attached to any one particular goal, person, event or external condition. We need to replace the external control with internal control. We control our own happiness by our thoughts and actions. We need to overcome our greatest fear and learn that we can be happy in any situation (Stevens 1998). We cannot choose our external circumstances, but we can always choose how to respond to them. Regardless of what is going on around us, we need to make the best of what is in our control, and take the rest as it occurs. Every difficulty in life presents us with an opportunity to turn inward and invoke our strengths. We need to look beyond the event and form the habit to put it to good use (Epictetus 2003).

Dalai Lama and Cutler (1998) say that happy people are sociable, flexible, creative, loving, forgiving and are able to tolerate life's daily frustration more easily than unhappy people. They demonstrate a certain quality of openness and a willingness to reach out to help others. Unhappy people are more self-focused and often socially withdrawn, brooding and even antagonistic.

7.4.4 Smile, Humour and Laughter

Joy and happiness can be expressed through smile and laughter which, in turn, leads to more happiness for us and the people around us.

7.4.4.1 Smile

Nierenberg and Calero (1975, cited by Lewis 2000) described three very common smiles, the simple, the upper, and the broad, indicating increasing levels of joy:

- *Simple smile*: This is when the teeth are not exposed. We generally wear the simple smile when we are watching something interesting or pleasant but are not physically involved in the action. We smile to ourselves.
- *Upper smile*: This smile exposes the upper set of teeth. It is a friendly smile, usually when we greet someone. It is accompanied by eye contact.
- *Broad smile*: This smile exposes both sets of teeth, and is usually accompanied by laughter, often without eye contact.

7.4.4.2 Humour and Laughter

Humour and laughter can be effective self-care tools that provide quality of perception, which enables us to experience joy even when faced with adversity (Wooten 1996).

Humour gives us a different perspective on our problems and, with an attitude of detachment; we feel a sense of self-protection and control in our environment. An ability to laugh at our situation or problem gives us a feeling of superiority and power. Humour and laughter can foster a positive and hopeful attitude. We are less likely to succumb to feelings of depression and helplessness if we are able to laugh at what is troubling us. Laughter provides an opportunity for the release of uncomfortable emotions, which if held inside, may create biochemical changes that are harmful to the body (Wooten 1996).

According to Loomans and Kolberg (2002, p. 20), positively used, humour and laughter have many benefits. Its physical benefits are enhanced immune system functioning, acting as an internal massage and regulating blood pressure. It enhances self-esteem, creative/critical thinking skills, communication skills, coping skills and enthusiasm, confidence, optimism, joy and openness. Its social benefits are it builds of a sense of team and reduces conflict. All these benefits result in reduced stress and feeling good. They note that humour can also heal, affirm, uplift, inspire and give joy to the other person through merriment or through wordplay.

Smith (2009) notes that the sound of roaring laughter is far more contagious than any cough, sniffle, or sneeze. When laughter is shared, it binds people together and increases happiness and intimacy. In addition to the domino effect of joy and amusement, laughter also triggers healthy physical changes in the body. Humour and laughter strengthen our immune system, boost our energy, diminish pain, and protect us from the damaging effects of stress. Best of all, this priceless medicine is fun, free and easy to use.

7.4.5 Activities

Activity 6: Qualities of loveable persons

Procedure:

1. Ask the participants to list five persons they love and five they can never love and the characteristics of the loveable persons and the unlovable persons.

2. When each shares the characteristics with the large group, put them on the board.
3. Ask questions and lead the discussion for processing the activity.

Estimated time: 20 minutes

Activity 7: Is it possible to love others unconditionally?

Procedure:

1. Ask the participants to think of three persons whom they love and the expectations they have from each of them.
2. Ask if they would still love them even if the expectations are not met.
3. Ask questions and lead the discussion for processing the activity.
4. The discussion can focus on how to separate the behaviour from the person.

Estimated time: 20 minutes

Activity 8: Sharing joy

Procedure:

1. Ask the following questions and write the responses on the board:

   (1) When do we feel joy?
   (2) How do we express joy?
   (3) What effect our expression has on us, the other person and our relationship?

2. Participants form pairs to share any joyous event from their life with each other.
3. Ask questions and lead the discussion for processing the activity.

Estimated time: 15 minutes

Activity 9: Who is in charge of my happiness?

Procedure:

1. Participants to form two groups:

   (1) Those who depend on others for their happiness and
   (2) Those who are in charge of their own happiness.

2. The first group to discuss what others should do that would make them happy. The second group to discuss what they do to make themselves happy.
3. Each group to share their discussion with the large group.
4. Discussion can focus on how being in charge of one's own happiness makes one happier than when one depends on others for happiness.

Estimated time: 20 minutes

Activity 10: Prescription for happiness

Procedure:

1. Create a Happiness Pharmacy, which provides the following medicine:

   - Develop connected self-identity
   - Develop unique self-identity
   - Increase self-esteem
   - Be assertive
   - Be proactive
   - Use rational and critical thinking
   - Use realistic and flexible thinking
   - Use creative thinking
   - Take self-responsibility
   - Feel gratitude for what you have
   - Express gratitude to others
   - Make positive affirmations
   - Be aware of emotions in self
   - Express emotions
   - Regulate negative emotions
   - Ask for forgiveness
   - Give forgiveness and let go
   - Practice unconditional love
   - Enhance joy and happiness
   - Use humour
   - Use smile
   - Use laughter

2. Ask for two volunteers to role-play on being a sad patient and a happiness doctor. The sad patient presents his/her sadness problem to the doctor for a prescription to cure his/her sadness. Depending on the problem, the doctor prescribes a happiness medication from the Happiness Pharmacy.
3. Ask questions and lead the discussion for processing the activity.
4. Participants form pairs and practice being the sad patient and the happiness doctor alternately.
5. Ask questions and lead the discussion for processing the activity.

Estimated time: 60 minutes

Activity 11: Homework of Smiling at the Mirror

Procedure:

1. Give a homework activity to the participants, they should look at a mirror and smile at themselves.
2. The next day, ask questions and lead the discussion for processing the activity.

3. The discussion can focus on the importance of smiling at self for self-esteem and happiness.

Estimated time: 15 minutes

Activity 12: Laughter club

Procedure:

1. Ask participants to form pairs to share an event with each other when they laughed heartily.
2. Ask volunteers to make the whole group laugh.
3. Ask questions and lead the discussion for processing the activity.

Estimated time: 30 minutes

References

Alberti, R. and Emmons, M. (1998). *Complete Guide to Assertive Living*. Mumbai: Jaico Publishing House.
Bayne, R., Horton, I., Merry, T. and Noyes, E. (1994). *The Counsellor's Handbook: A Practical A-Z Guide to Professional and Clinical Practice*. London: Chapman and Hall.
Brahm, A. (2005). *Who Ordered this Truckload of Dung?: Inspiring Stories for Welcoming Life's Difficulties*. Boston, MA: Wisdom Publications.
Carlson, R. (1997). *Don't Sweat the Small Stuff. . .and It's All Small Stuff: Simple Ways to Keep the Little Things from Overtaking Your Life*. London: Hodder and Stoughton.
Carlson, R. and Bailey, J. (1997). *Slowing Down to the Speed of Life: How to Create a More Peaceful Simpler Life from the Inside Out*. New York, NY: Harper Collins Publishers.
Cartledge, G. and Milburn, J. F. (1995). *Teaching Social Skills to Children: Innovative Approaches* (2nd ed.). New York, NY: Pergamon.
Compton, W. C. (2005). *An Introduction to Positive Psychology*. Australia: Thomson/Wadsworth.
Cornelius, H. and Faire, S. (2006). *Everyone Can Win: Responding to Conflict Constructively*. Australia: Simon and Schuster.
Dalai Lama and Cutler, H. C. (1998). *The Art of Happiness: A Handbook for Living*. London: Coronet Books.
Dryden, W. (1994). *10 Steps to Positive Living*. New Delhi: Orient Paperbacks.
Ellis, A. (1999). *Make Yourself Happy and Remarkably Less Disturbable*. Mumbai: Jaico Publishing House.
Epictetus. (2003). *The Art of Living*. New Delhi: The India Today Group.
Fischer, K. W. and Bidell, T. R. (1998). Dynamic Development of Psychological Structures in Action and Thought. In R. M. Lerner (Ed.) *Handbook of Childhood Psychology* (pp. 467–561). New York, NY: John Wiley and Sons.
Ford, L. (2006). *Human Relations: A Game Plan for Improving Personal Adjustment* (4th ed.). Upper Saddle River, NJ: Prentice Hall.
Fredrickson, B. L. (2000). Cultivating positive emotions to optimize health and well-being. *Prevention and Treatment*, 3, Article 0001a.
Fromm, E. (1956). *The Art of Loving*. London: George Allen and Unwin.
Gupta, M. K. (2002). *How to Control Anger – The Deadly Enemy*. New Delhi: Pustak Mahal.
Hamilton, V. M. (2007). *Human Relations: The Art and Science of Building Effective Relationships*. Upper Saddle River, NJ: Pearson Prentice Hall.
Hay, L. L. (2004). *You Can Heal Your Life*. New York, NY: Hay House, Inc.

Hepworth, D. H., Rooney, R. H., Rooney, G. D., Strom-Gottfried, K. and Larson, J. A. (2006). *Direct Social Work Practice: Theory and Skills* (7th Ed.). Belmont, NY: Thomson Higher Education.

Humphreys, T. (2002). *Self-Esteem: The Key to Your Child's Future*. Dublin: Newleaf.

Johnson, D. W. (1986). *Reaching Out: Interpersonal Effectiveness and Self-Actualisation*, Upper Saddle River, NJ: Prentice-Hall.

Kadushin, A. and Kadushin, G. (1997). *The Social Work Interview: A Guide for Human Service Professionals* (4th ed.). New York, NY: Columbia University Press.

Kalat, J. W. and Shiota, M. N. (2007). *Emotion*. Australia: Thomson Wadsworth.

Keith, K. M. (2001). *Anyway: The Paradoxical Commandments: Finding Personal Meaning in a Crazy World*. London: Hodder and Stoughton.

Koprowska, J. (2005). *Communication and Interpersonal Skills in Social Work*. Exeter: Learning Matters.

Lewis, H. (2000). *Body Language: A Guide for Professionals*. New Delhi: Response Books.

Loomans, D. and Kolberg, K. (2002). *The Laughing Classroom: Everyone's Guide to Teaching with Humor and Play*. Novato, CA: New World Library.

Matthews, A. (1988). *Being Happy! A Handbook to Greater Confidence and Security*. Singapore: Media Masters.

McInnis-Dittrich, K. (2002). *Social Work with Elders: A Biopsychosocial Approach to Assessment and Intervention*. Boston, MA: Allyn and Bacon.

Peck, M. S. (1985). *The Road Less Traveled*. New York, NY: Simon and Schuster.

Rice, V. H. (Ed.) (2000). *Handbook of Stress Coping and Health Implications for Nursing Research, Theory and Practice*. Thousand Oaks, CA: Sage Publications.

Rose, S. R. and Fatout, M. F. (2003). *Social Work Practice with Children and Adolescents*. Boston, MA: Allyn and Bacon.

Shebib, B. (2003). *Choices: Counseling Skills for Social Workers and Other Professionals*. New York, NY: Allyn and Bacon.

Smith, M. (2009). *Laughter Is the Best Medicine*. http://www.helpguide.org/life/humor_laughter_health.htm#authors. Accessed 13 June 2009.

Stauffer, E. R. (1988). *Unconditional Love and Forgiveness*. Whittier, CA: Triangle Publishers.

Stevens, T. G. (1998). *You Can Choose To Be Happy*. Counselling and Psychological Services at California State University.

TT Ranganathan Clinical Research Foundation. (No date). *I Feel Hurt . . .How Do I Get Over It?* Madras: TT Ranganathan Clinical Research Foundation.

Webster-Stratton, C. (1999). *How to Promote Children's Social and Emotional Competence*. London: P. Chapman; Thousand Oaks, CA: Sage Publications.

West, R. and Turner, L. H. (2006). *Understanding Interpersonal Communication: Making Choices in Changing Times*. Australia: Thomson.

Wooten, P. (1996). Humor: An antidote for stress. *Holistic Nursing Practice*, 10(2), 49–55.

Chapter 8
Enrichment of Interpersonal Relationship Skills

8.1 Concepts of Interpersonal Relationship Skills

The evolution and the survival of our species are intimately intertwined with our ability to initiate, develop and stabilise our relationships with other people. All members of our society are highly interdependent and therefore need to be skilled in building and maintaining relationships with each other (Johnson 1986). An interpersonal relationship is a relationship based on personal interaction rather than on any legal or structural basis (Schvaneveldt 1966), for example relationships between family members, friends, neighbours and colleagues. Interpersonal skills require enhanced self-identity and self-esteem, proactive, rational, realistic, flexible, creative and positive thinking skills and emotional intelligence.

Interpersonal relationship skills are comprised of

- Interdependence in relationships
- Positive perception of others
- Positive feelings for others
- Win–win goals in relationships
- Collaborative conflict management skills
- Interpersonal communication skills

8.2 Interdependence in Relationships

Interdependent social interactions can create synergy in relationships, which can lead to new energy or new alternatives in life (Covey 1997). Interdependence can be achieved through a semi-open boundary between two individuals, which is defined by cohesion and maintained by adaptability.

8.2.1 Cohesion

Cohesion is defined as the emotional bonding that two persons have towards one another. There are four levels of cohesion, ranging from disengaged (very low), to separated (low to moderate), to connected (moderate to high), to enmeshed (very

M. Desai, *A Rights-Based Preventative Approach for Psychosocial Well-Being in Childhood*, Children's Well-Being: Indicators and Research 3,
DOI 10.1007/978-90-481-9066-9_8, © Springer Science+Business Media B.V. 2010

high). It is hypothesised that the central levels of cohesion (separated and connected) make for optimal family functioning. The extreme levels (disengaged and enmeshed) are generally seen as problematic (Olson 1988).

8.2.2 Adaptability

Adaptability in interpersonal relationships is the ability of two persons to change in response to one another and move towards a state of homeostasis. The four levels of adaptability range from rigid (very low), to structured (low to moderate), to flexible (moderate to high), to chaotic (very high). It is hypothesised that the central levels of adaptability (structured and flexible) are more conducive to relationships with the extremes (rigid and chaotic) being the most problematic (Olson 1988).

8.2.3 Activities

Activity 1: Assessment of cohesion and adaptability in interpersonal relationships

Procedure:

1. Give the following chart on assessment of cohesion and adaptability in interpersonal relationships to each participant to reflect and respond.

Relationships with	Cohesion Our relationship is • Non-existent (disengaged) – 1 • Good (separated) – 2 • Very good (connected) – 3 • Cannot live without each other (enmeshed) – 4	Adaptability Our interaction is • Rigid – 1 • Structured – 2 • Flexible – 3 • Chaotic – 4
Parents		
Spouse		
Children		
Siblings		
Grandparents		
Cousins		
Aunts and uncles		
Friends		

2. Ask questions and lead the discussion for processing the activity.
3. The discussion can focus on the need for semi-open self-boundary, separated but connected cohesion, and structured and flexible adaptability in interpersonal relationships.

Estimated time: 15 minutes

8.3 Positive Perception of Others

For enrichment of interpersonal relationships, we need to perceive others as equal, recognise their strengths, accept and respect them, and if there are differences, celebrate them.

8.3.1 Egalitarian Perception

Cornelius and Faire (2006) noted that we all operate in a variety of power relationships, such as male–female, parent–child, teacher–student, employer–employee. According to them, those in power can play the role of a persecutor or a rescuer. The persecutors use coercive power or aggression to silence opposition whereas the rescuers use manipulative power by offering unwelcome or uninvited help. Both need victims, those who either are genuine victims or play the role of victims. These relationships are based on perception of inherent physical and mental incapability, based on sex, age and class of individuals and/or groups. These power relationships justify role stereotypes, hierarchy, intolerance and discrimination and, thereby, justify violence. An egalitarian approach values equity and equality, non-hierarchy, non-discrimination, and non-prejudicial approach to all human beings.

8.3.2 Recognition of Strengths

According to Saleeby (2006), every individual, group, family and community has strengths that are assets, resources, wisdom and knowledge. Trauma and abuse, illness and struggle may be injurious, but they may also be sources of challenge and opportunity. The strengths-based approach implies the following:

- Recognising uniqueness and strengths in everyone and respecting their self-esteem
- Understanding and accepting the limitations of others
- Celebrating differences with others

Everyone has strengths and limitations and nobody is perfect. However, we tend to find more faults in others than in ourselves as we judge ourselves by our intentions and others by their behaviour (Covey 1997). We need to try to recognise strengths instead of faults in people around us, as follows (Skills for School Success 1993):

Chart 8.1 Recognition of Strengths in Faults

Recognition of faults	*Recognition of strengths*
Rudeness	Being straightforward
Bossiness	Leadership
Sissyness	Gentleness
Nosy behaviour	Curiosity
Stubbornness	Determination
Anger	Standing up for beliefs
Laziness	Being able to relax
Disorganisation	Comfortable

In the strengths-based approach, it is also important that we communicate our appreciation to the other person with words such as *I appreciate your thoughtfulness, it is very nice of you, I like what you did, I trust your determination.*

8.3.3 Acceptance and Respect

Acceptance is a non-judgmental attitude, manifested by behaving in a manner that shows respect and concern for others, regardless of behaviour. It means giving others freedom to be themselves, to express themselves freely (adapted from Kadushin and Kadushin 1997). Respect to others is shown as follows:

- Respect them as equals
- Respect their right to have their own opinions
- Respect their decisions
- Respect their values and experience (Cornelius and Faire 2006)

8.3.4 Celebration of Differences

A relationship, by definition, has to be between two different people who will have physical, mental, emotional and other differences. Most of the time, we are so convinced that ours is the best way of living that we cannot accept people who are living differently than us. So we often expect others to be exactly like ourselves or we become indifferent to those who are different. Some of us ridicule those who are different than us. Some of us can tolerate differences. What is needed for synergy is a celebration of our differences. We need to see differences as an advantage for creating new alternatives in life, without necessarily having to agree with them (Covey 1998).

8.3.5 Activities

Activity 2: Reflections on recognition of strengths in faults

Procedure:

1. Ask the participants to select one person with whom they are disengaged and identify their negative characteristics that bother them and write down in their diary.
2. Participants to reflect if they can see strengths in those negative characteristics.
3. Participants to also identify strengths of the same person (for example, a person may have a short temper, but may be a very diligent and sincere worker).
4. Ask questions and lead the discussion for processing the activity.

Estimated time: 30 minutes

Activity 3: Game of guess whose strengths?

Procedure:

1. Ask one participant to go out of the room.
2. The rest of the participants decide on the "it", a participant in the large group whose identity has to be guessed by the participant who went out.
3. When the person is called back, he or she asks the participants for clues about strengths of this person to identify him/her.
4. Play a couple of rounds of this game.
5. Ask questions and lead the discussion for processing the activity.
6. The discussion may focus on do they remember everyone's strengths.

Estimated time: 15 minutes

Activity 4: Story of blind men's description of an elephant

Procedure:

1. Narrate the following story of blind men's description of an elephant:

    Six blind men were asked to describe an elephant.
    The first blind man, who was touching the elephant's trunk, said it was like a tree branch.
    The second blind man, who touched its tusk, said it was like a pipe.
    The third blind man, who touched its leg, said it was like a pillar.
    The fourth blind man, who touched its tail, said it was like a rope.
    The fifth blind man, who touched its ear, said it was like a hand-fan.
    The sixth blind man, who touched its belly, said it was like a wall.
    They started fighting over who is right, until a wise person made them realise that they were all right and wrong as the whole elephant is made of all these aspects.

2. Discuss the following points:

    - The complete reality is made of different dimensions, and all are equally necessary.

- When we have differences, it is futile to argue that only we are right, as in a way everyone is right.
- Only by welcoming differences we can see the total picture.

Estimated time: 15 minutes

8.4 Positive Feelings for Others

For enrichment of interpersonal relationships, our feelings for others should comprise of warmth, humility and empathy that can be expressed by verbal and body language.

8.4.1 Warmth

According to Shebib (2003, pp. 72–73), warmth is an expression of non-possessive caring. It is demonstrated by showing sincere interest in the comfort of the other person. Kirst-Ashman and Hull (2009) noted that displaying warmth involves genuinely conveying a feeling of interest, concern, well-being and affection to another individual. It is a vehicle for acceptance. Alberti and Emmons (1998) have observed that positive, caring feelings are more difficult for many people to express than assertiveness. Embarrassment, fear of rejection or ridicule, the idea that reason is superior to emotion are excuses for not expressing warmth, caring and love spontaneously. Warmth can be expressed by eyes, smile, touch and words.

8.4.2 Humility

According to Stauffer (1988), humility opens our mind to perceive accurately the needs of others as they see them and to desire to meet those needs when it is practical to do so. Without humility, the needs of others, as they see them, are blocked from our mind. The one who practices humility develops the ability to listen, to hear the needs of others. The one who is humble also sees value in others. The humble person not only senses the sometimes unexpressed needs of others but also relates to the one in need in an appropriate manner.

8.4.3 Empathy

Empathy is the capacity to understand the feelings and views of another person. Its practice makes one other-centred. Sympathy merely mirrors another person's trouble; empathy discovers the causes of the trouble with the searchlight of insight (Peterson 1961). An empathic attitude is characterised by one's willingness to learn about the world of another and begins with suspending judgement (Shebib 2003, p. 73). Kadushin and Kadushin (1997) noted that empathy is the expression of placing of credence on what the other feels and experiences. By being empathic, we share the emotions of another person – excitement, sadness, joy, exhilaration and so on. We particularly need to understand needs of others that may be different from ours. In doing so, we are able to achieve a subjective understanding of what the other person is experiencing.

According to Cartledge and Milburn (1995), empathy leads to acceptance or appreciation of the individuality and dignity of persons. It provides accessibility, a pre-condition for the emergence of relationships that are free of constraining obligation and conformity.

8.4.4 Activities

Activity 5: Story of the stork and the fox

Procedure:

1. Share the story of the stork and the fox to discuss how it is necessary to recognise individual needs

> A fox and a stork were fast friends. Once the fox invited the stork for lunch. She prepared a delicious soup. When the stork arrived for lunch, he was very hungry. The fox soon served two dishes of steaming soup. But the fox had served the soup in flat dishes. The fox lapped up the soup quickly but the poor stork could not taste the soup. His long, thin beak could not taste a single drop of the soup.
>
> After the lunch, the stork invited the fox for dinner to his own house. The fox was delighted. She started thinking about all the delicious dishes the stork would serve. As soon as the sun set, the fox dressed up and arrived at the stork's doorstep. She could smell the tasty soup being prepared in the kitchen. Soon the stork welcomed the fox in. The soup was served in a narrow and long mouthed jar. The stork quickly dipped his beak into the jar and drank up the soup. Alas! All that the fox could do was smell the soup. The narrow mouth of the jar did not let her get at the soup in the jar (Tiny Tot 2002).

2. Ask volunteers to rewrite the story with the stork and fox behaving with humility, empathy and warmth and share with the large group.
3. Ask questions and lead the discussion for processing the activity.

Estimated time: 30 minutes

Activity 6: Warm greetings

Procedure:

1. Make participants stand in a circle.
2. Each participant warmly greets the person on his/her left side, one at a time so that everybody enjoys the warmth.
3. Ask questions and lead the discussion for processing the activity.

Estimated time: Depends on the number of participants

Activity 7: Blindfolded walk with partners

Procedure:

1. Make pairs of participants.
2. One partner in each pair blindfolds the other and guides the blindfolded partner for a brief walk for 5 minutes outside the hall and back.
3. Ask questions and lead the discussion for processing the activity.
4. The discussion can focus on use of warmth, humility and empathy by the guide for the blindfolded person and experience of humility and empathy by the blindfolded person for the blind persons.

Estimated time: 30 minutes

8.5 Win–Win Goals in Relationships

8.5.1 Concepts

Covey (1997) has laid down four goals in a relationship, depending upon whether we want to win or lose and whether we want the other person to win or lose as discussed below.

8.5.1.1 Goal of Win–Lose

Persons with low self-esteem and aggressiveness want to win and others to lose all the time in the following ways:

- Use other people for their own selfish purposes.
- Try to get ahead at the expense of others.
- Insist on getting their way without being concerned about the feelings of others.
- Become jealous when something good happens to others.

When two win–lose persons get together, it ends in a lose–lose outcome. Both of them lose as is evident in wars or in revenge.

8.5.1.2 Goal of Lose–Win

Persons with low self-esteem and passiveness want to lose and others to win all the time in the following ways:

- In a doormat approach, they set low expectations and compromise their standards.
- It can lead to an abusive relationship.

8.5.1.3 Goal of Win–Win

Persons with high self-esteem and assertiveness want them and others, both to win all the time in the following ways:

- It does not eliminate the differences in perspectives; it eliminates the negative energy normally focused on the differences.
- It creates a positive and cooperative energy focused on thoroughly understanding the issues and resolving them in a mutually beneficial way.
- It is a belief in the third alternative, neither "your" way nor "my" way, but a better way.
- This approach creates synergy, which produces solutions better than the originally proposed approaches.

8.5.2 Activity

Activity 8: Win–win goals in relationships

Procedure:

1. Participants to reflect on their goals in their main relationships and identify the relationships for which they have the following goals:

Relationships with	• I win and you lose – 1 • I lose and you win – 2 • I lose and you lose – 3 • I win and you win – 4
Parents	
Spouse	
Children	
Siblings	
Grandparents	
Cousins	
Aunts and uncles	
Friends	

2. Ask questions and lead the discussion for processing the activity.

Estimated time: 30 minutes

8.6 Collaborative Conflict Management Skills

Interpersonal conflict is the interaction of persons who perceive incompatible goals and interference from each other in achieving those goals (Folger et al. 2001, cited by West and Turner 2006). Conditions of scarcity create competitive zero-sum structure whereby gains for one party result in losses for other members. Such a structure produces behaviours of confrontations, threats, promises and appeasement (Zimmerman 2001).

8.6.1 Types of Interpersonal Conflict

According to West and Turner (2006), the various types of conflict are image conflicts, content conflicts, value conflicts and relational conflicts:

- Image conflicts concern self-presentation.
- Content conflicts revolve around an issue, public or personal.
- Value conflicts are content conflicts in which the content is a question of right or wrong.
- Relational conflicts focus on issues concerning the relationship between two people.

Kilmann and Thomas (1975), cited by Galvin et al. (2008), have developed a model to demonstrate that conflict style consists of two partially competing goals, concern for others (or cooperativeness) and concern for self (or assertiveness) as follows.

Cooperativeness	*Assertiveness*	*Conflict style*
Low	Low	Avoiding
Low	High	Competition
High	Low	Accommodation
Moderate	Moderate	Compromise
High	High	Collaboration

8.6.2 Self-Fulfilling Prophecy in Conflicts

According to Johnson (1986), in conflict situations, there are often perceptual distortions about our own and the other person's behaviour, motivations and position. When selective perception or distortions in perception operate, it is very easy to fall into a trap where we see only the hostile feelings of the other person and fail to see the positive feelings. This can very easily result in a self-fulfilling prophecy in the following manner:

1. We assume that the other's feelings are entirely hostile;
2. We take defensive action by either attacking the other person before he or she can attack us or cutting off contact with the other person;
3. Our action intensifies the other person's hostility and decreases his or her positive feelings towards us; and
4. Our original, but false, assumption is confirmed. Self-fulfilling prophecies are very common in conflict situations, and whenever we become involved in a conflict we should be careful not to fall into these traps.

8.6.3 Collaborative Conflict Management Skills

When there is a conflict in a relationship, do not try to "get your way" or "get back at" the other person or "turn the other cheek". The important thing is to affirm the self-worth of both people involved (Alberti and Emmons 1998). The collaborative conflict management skills include attitude adjustment, reducing defensiveness in others, understanding the other person's perception of the conflict for win–win goals.

8.6.3.1 Attitude Adjustment

According to Ford (2006), attitude adjustment in conflict management includes the following:

- Let go of the need to be right.
- Do not offer resistance.
- Acknowledge the other person's position.
- Offer your point of view.
- Agree to disagree.
- Realise that the other person has important reasons.

8.6.3.2 Reducing Defensiveness in Others

Conflict gets aggravated with defensiveness spiral when one negative comment tends to be reciprocated, then each provokes another, getting worse as we go along, creating a downward spiral that is very difficult to turn around (Wilmot 1987, cited by Hamilton 2007). Hamilton (2007) discusses the following techniques for reducing defensiveness in self and others:

- Replace evaluation or judgemental communication with non-judgemental description.
- Replace certainty or closed-mindedness with provisionalism or open-mindedness.
- Replace control or making decisions for other people with working collaboratively and in a problem-focused manner.

- Replace manipulative strategy with spontaneity.
- Replace neutrality or lack of concern with empathy.
- Replace superiority with equality.

8.6.3.3 Understanding the Other Person's Perception of the Conflict

Resolving conflicts constructively requires that we understand the other person's thoughts, feelings and needs. To achieve such understanding, we need to use good listening skills and try to view the conflict from the other person's point of view. Different people have different perspectives. No two people will see a conflict in exactly the same way. Each person will interpret the same event differently. To resolve a conflict constructively, we need to keep in mind both our own perspective and the perspective of the other person (Johnson 1986).

Role-playing is an easy way to increase our understanding of another person's perspective. By trying to present the other person's position and feelings as if we were the other person, we can gain insight into the other person's perspective. For example, when two friends are having a conflict, they need to try presenting each other's position as if they were the other friend. The more involved we get in arguing each other's positions, the more we will understand how the conflict appears from the other person's perspective, and therefore the more we will be able to find solutions that are mutually acceptable (Johnson 1986).

8.6.3.4 Steps for Collaborative Conflict Management

The following steps are recommended for collaborative conflict management:

(1) Find appropriate time and place to discuss the conflict. Take a deep breath to physically relax.
(2) Begin with an attitude of respect for and acceptance of each other.
(3) Only if we are sincerely appreciative of each other, when things go well, do we have the right to criticise each other.
(4) Identify the real issue of the conflict and determine to solve the conflict.
(5) Focus on one issue at a time, decide what is of the uppermost concern and discuss it.
(6) Own one's opinions, feeling and action and not transfer to or label the other.
(7) Ask and express one's expectations of the other and reasons for disappointment.
(8) Ask questions instead of making personal attacks or counter-attacks.
(9) Understand the other's views with a non-judgmental attitude and be sensitive to each other's needs and perceptions, by imagining oneself in the other's role.
(10) Maintain a here-and-now orientation.
(11) Be specific and realistic about expectations from each other.

(12) Emphasise points of agreement as a foundation for discussion of points of argument.
(13) Put forth one's suggestions to solve the conflict and to discuss the pros and cons of each suggestion.
(14) Develop goals, which are basically compatible. If they both want to preserve the relationship more than to win, they have a better chance.
(15) Seek solutions rather than deciding who is to blame.
(16) Work towards a win–win outcome.
(17) Make a commitment to implement the solution and take responsibility for its consequences.
(18) If one has made a mistake, admit it and if one has hurt the other, apologise. Apologies disarm the other person.
(19) If conflict resolution is not possible, agree to disagree.
(20) Learn from the experience.

8.6.3.5 Agreement to End the Conflict

According to Johnson (1986), a conflict ends when two persons reach an agreement. All parties need to be satisfied with the agreement and committed to abide by it. The agreement should specify the following:

1. The joint position being adopted.
2. The ways in which the two will act differently in the future.
3. The ways in which cooperation will be restored if one person slips and acts inappropriately.
4. The times the two will meet to discuss the relationship and to see if further steps can be taken to improve cooperation with each other.

It is important that both the persons understand which actions trigger anger and resentment in the other. Criticism, put-downs, sarcasm, belittling and other actions often trigger a conflict. If the two understand what not to do as well as what to do, the conflict will be resolved more easily.

8.6.4 Activities

Activity 9: Story on futility of verbal aggression

Procedure:

1. Share the story of the two goats to discuss the futility of verbal aggression

> Once a white goat and a black goat were crossing a river from the opposite banks. They were on a narrow bridge across the river. Only one person or animal could walk on it at one time. As the two goats met at the middle, the black goat said, "Hey! Why are you blocking my path? Go back and let me go on my way."

The white goat grew angry and said, "How dare you order me? I'll not step back. Why don't you go back?" Soon the argument heated up. The two goats locked horns in anger. As they were fighting on the narrow bridge, they lost their balance and fell into the swift flowing river and both of them drowned (Tiny Tot 2002).

2. Ask questions and lead the discussion for processing the activity.

Estimated time: 15 minutes

Activity 10: Role reversal to understand the other perspective

Procedure:

1. Identify a controversial topic for debate and divide the participants into two groups, one to argue in favour of the topic and the other against it. Examples of the topic are should euthanasia or mercy killing be permitted, should child labour be banned, should women work.
2. In the next step, ask the groups to reverse their stands, the one which argued in favour of it should now argue against it and vice versa.
   This activity can also be carried out through role-plays, with following examples:

   - In a mixed sex group, men and women may be asked to reverse their sex roles and present a role-play.
   - In a family situation, the traditional parents and children/adolescents' roles may be reversed.
   - In a work situation, employers and employees' roles may be reversed.

3. Ask questions and lead the discussion for processing the activity.

Estimated time: 45 minutes

Activity 11: Role-plays on collaborative method to manage conflict

Procedure:

1. Form small groups, and give each small group a chit of a conflictual situation, depending on their age group and life situation. Examples of these situations are conflict over the boundary wall/use of the common area between two neighbours, conflict between two classmates competing for the first rank, marital conflict, parent–adolescent conflict and siblings fighting over parental property.
2. Small groups prepare role-plays on collaborative conflict management skills and present to the large group.
3. Ask questions and lead the discussion for processing the activity.

Estimated time: 45 minutes

Activity 12: Reflection of personal conflict

Procedure:

1. Ask the participants to select one of their relationships that is conflictual.
2. Participants reflect on the following questions:

   - If they had made any prior attempts to resolve the conflicts. If yes, which kind of approach they had tried?
   - What prevented the conflict from getting resolved?
   - How will you overcome those difficulties now?

3. Participants write a plan of rebuilding that relationship in their diaries.
4. Ask questions and lead the discussion for processing the activity.

Estimated time: 15 minutes

References

Alberti, R. and Emmons, M. (1998). *Complete Guide to Assertive Living*. Mumbai: Jaico Publishing House.

Cartledge, G. and Milburn, J. F. (1995). *Teaching Social Skills to Children: Innovative Approaches* (2nd ed.). New York, NY: Pergamon.

Cornelius, H. and Faire, S. (2006). *Everyone Can Win: Responding to Conflict Constructively*. Australia: Simon and Schuster.

Covey, S. R. (1997). *The 7 Habits of Highly Effective People*. London: Simon and Schuster.

Covey, S. (1998). *The 7 Habits of Highly Effective Teens*. London: Simon and Schuster.

Ford, L. (2006). *Human Relations: A Game Plan for Improving Personal Adjustment* (4th ed.). Upper Saddle River, NJ: Prentice Hall.

Galvin, K. M., Bylund, C. L. and Brommel, B. J. (2008). *Family Communication: Cohesion and Change* (7th ed.). Boston, MA: Pearson.

Hamilton, V. M. (2007). *Human Relations: The Art and Science of Building Effective Relationships*. Upper Saddle River, NJ: Pearson Prentice Hall.

Johnson, D. W. (1986). *Reaching Out: Interpersonal Effectiveness and Self-Actualisation*. Upper Saddle River, NJ: Prentice Hall.

Kadushin, A. and Kadushin, G. (1997). *The Social Work Interview: A Guide for Human Service Professionals* (4th ed.). New York, NY: Columbia University Press.

Kirst-Ashman, K. K. and Hull, G. H., Jr. (2009). *Understanding Generalist Practice* (5th ed.). Belmont, CA: Brooks/Cole.

Olson, D. H. (1988). *Family Perspectives in Child and Youth Services*. New York, NY: The Haworth Press.

Peterson, W. A. (1961). *The New Book of the Art of Living*. New York, NY: Simon and Schuster.

Saleeby, D. (2006). Introduction: Power in the people. In D. Saleeby (Ed.) *The Strengths Perspective in Social Work Practice* (4th ed., pp. 1–24). Boston, MA: Pearson.

Schvaneveldt, J. D. (1966). The international framework in the study of the family. In F. I. Nye and F. M. Berardo (Eds.) *Emerging Conceptual Frameworks in Family Analysis* (pp. 70–129). New York, NY: The Macmillan Co.

Shebib, B. (2003). *Choices: Counseling Skills for Social Workers and Other Professionals*. New York, NY: Allyn and Bacon.

Skills for School Success. (1993). *Working with Others*. Fairfax Station, VA: The Parent Institute.

Stauffer, E. R. (1988). *Unconditional Love and Forgiveness*. Whittier, CA: Triangle Publishers.

Tiny Tot. (2002). *Tiny Tot – Best of Moral Stories*. Delhi: Tiny Tot Publications.
West, R. and Turner, L. H. (2006). *Understanding Interpersonal Communication: Making Choices in Changing Times*. Southbank, VIC: Thomson.
Zimmerman, S. L. (2001). *Family Policy: Constructed Solutions to Family Problems*. London: Sage Publications.

Chapter 9
Enrichment of Interpersonal Communication Skills

9.1 Concepts of Interpersonal Communication Skills

A relationship is formed whenever reciprocal information processing occurs, that is when two or more individuals mutually take account of one another's verbal or non-verbal activities. Thus, interpersonal communication is the means, through which relationships of all types are initiated, develop, grow and deteriorate (Ruben 1988). In short, it is a necessity for our development as social beings (Tubbs and Moss 1980).

9.1.1 Interpersonal Communication

Communication involves

- The person who generates a message (sender),
- The message (verbal or non-verbal),
- The channel through which the message is transmitted, and
- The person who receives the message (receiver) (Tubbs and Moss 1980).

At any given point of time, a person or a communicator may be the sender and receiver, because when one is speaking, one is simultaneously observing the behaviour of the other person and reacting to it. This is also true of the other person. We constantly give and receive feedback that may be verbal or non-verbal. The channels of interpersonal communication are the sensory organs. We simultaneously make use of information from a number of different channels. We convey and receive messages through speech/hearing, eyes, body and touch (Tubbs and Moss 1980).

Communication is said to be effective when the sender's intended message corresponds closely with the receiver's perceived message. Technical or semantic barriers prevent effective communication. Technical interference refers to either a speech impediment on the part of the sender or the factors that cause the receiver to perceive distortion in the intended information. In semantic interference, the

---

Chapter 9 has been written by Murli Desai and Sheetal Goel.

M. Desai, *A Rights-Based Preventative Approach for Psychosocial Well-Being in Childhood*, Children's Well-Being: Indicators and Research 3,
DOI 10.1007/978-90-481-9066-9_9,

receiver does not attribute the same meaning to the message that the sender does (Tubbs and Moss 1980).

9.1.2 Interpersonal Communication Skills

According to Johnson (1986), some skills in sending messages for effective communication include the following:

1. Clearly "own" your messages by using the first person singular pronouns: "I", "my".
2. Make your messages complete and specific.
3. Make your verbal and non-verbal messages congruent.
4. Make the message appropriate to the receiver's frame of reference.
5. Ask for feedback concerning the way your messages are being received.

The interpersonal communication skills are comprised of

- Verbal communication skills
- Body language skills
- Listening skills
- Feedback skills

9.2 Verbal Communication Skills

9.2.1 Verbal Communication and Context

Verbal messages comprise of the language or words we use. A word is merely a symbol of the object it represents. Meanings are not inherent in words. It is human beings who assign meanings to words. As experiences of human beings change, meanings change. People can have similar meanings only to the extent they have had similar experiences. Meanings can have denotations and connotations. Denotations refer to primary associations a word has for most members of a given linguistic community. Connotations refer to other secondary associations a word has for one or more members (Tubbs and Moss 1980).

According to Donn (2000), communication happens in the psychological, relational, situational, environmental and cultural context as given here in:

Psychological context, which is who we are, and what we bring to the interaction. Our needs, desires, values, personality and so on, all form the psychological context.

Relational context, which concerns our relations to the other person.

Situational context deals with the psychosocial "where" we are communicating.

Environmental context deals with the physical "where" we are communicating. Furniture, location, noise level, temperature, season, time of day, all are examples of factors in the environmental context.

Cultural context includes all the learned behaviours and rules that affect the interaction.

The collectivistic cultures use high-context communication that relies more heavily on attention to contextual details and less on explicit language to transmit its message. Messages are conveyed subtly to save the listener from embarrassment as high value is placed on "saving face". On the other hand, the individualistic cultures use low-context communication that relies on clear, concrete and explicit language. They favour instrumental communication that is task-oriented and focuses on achieving the speaker's goal. The collectivistic cultures, on the other hand, favour affective communication that is person-oriented, and focuses on building and maintaining good relations between the communicators (Hamilton 2007, pp. 294–297).

Hamilton (2007, pp. 296–297) identifies another cultural variation that can be seen with reference to the quantity of words considered appropriate by a culture: elaborate, exacting and succinct communication styles.

- The elaborate communication style uses many words to convey its message and is very colourful and expressive.
- The succinct communication style is understated language that says very little and relies on the listener to understand the unspoken meaning, similar to the high-context language. Silence is highly valued in these cultures and those who talk a lot may be suspected of being dishonest.
- The exacting communication style is clear and specific language that states the facts, no more, similar to the low-context communication.

9.2.2 Open Communication Skills

We often use judgemental, controlling, superior and certain communication patterns that are aggressive and used to protect one's ego. Open communication is non-judgmental, permissive, spontaneous, empathic, equal and provisional. Such communication is essential for the fulfilment of goals of the individual and the relationship. It is a way of communicating where each person experiences openness, intimacy and understanding with the other and where what is discussed is relevant and appropriate to each other's personal growth and the development of the relationship (Humphreys 2002). Open type of communication is compared in the chart below with the protective type by Humphreys:

Protective communication	Open communication
Judgmental (criticising, name-calling, blaming, cross-examining)	Non-judgmental
Controlling (directing, commanding, ordering, warning, threatening, punishing, moralising)	Permissive
Strategic (sulking, manipulation, hidden agenda)	Spontaneous
Neutral (ignoring, dismissing, excusing)	Empathic
Superior (advising, recommending)	Equal
Certain (persuading, arguing)	Provisional

Open communication requires the use of non-discriminatory language. Our language may tend to reflect our biases or stereotypes on the basis of gender, ethnicity, disability or age, either intentionally or accidentally. This should be avoided and replaced with non-discriminatory language. Consider some of the following examples:

- It is a common practice to talk in terms of male specific words in the generic sense almost denying the existence of the female species. Instead it is preferable to use terms like "human beings", "humankind", "women and men", "persons", "individuals" and so on, instead of the term "men".
- An ethnic group should not be trivialised by describing it with words such as "culturally backward".
- A family situation should not be denigrated with words such as "broken family".
- It is advisable to describe the situation of people instead of using words that label them. Some examples are given below:

Avoid	*Prefer*
Servant	Domestic worker
Aged	Elderly/older persons
Delinquent	Child in conflict with law
Disabled	Person with disability
Illegitimate	Born out of wedlock
Divorcee	Person after divorce
Prostitute	Woman in prostitution

9.2.3 Activities

Activity 1: Game of passing the message
This activity is useful as an icebreaker on the topic.

Procedure:

1. Prepare a chit with a sentence not exceeding 10–12 words and ask the participants to sit in a circle.
2. A volunteer picks up a chit, reads it in his/her mind and whispers it to the person seated on his/her right.
3. This person on the right then whispers it to the person on his/her right. This goes on till the last person in the circle.
5. Participants should not repeat the sentence twice.
6. The last person speaks aloud the sentence that he/she has heard from the partner.
7. The volunteer who picked up the chit shares the original sentence aloud.
8. Ask questions and lead the discussion for processing the activity.

In a large group, two simultaneous groups can be made for the same game as follows:

(1) By size: One large and one small group
(2) By type of message: One short and simple statement and one long and complicated statement

(3) By language: One in the language familiar to the group and one in a new language
(4) By subject: One on a familiar topic and one on an irrelevant topic.

Estimated time: 30 minutes

Activity 2: Saying the same but Not meaning the same

Procedure:

1. Divide the participants into four small groups and ask them to share experiences wherein they have had communication gaps because of usage of words that have implied different meanings for different persons for the following reasons:
   (1) One word has different meanings depending on people's life experiences or variations.
   (2) One word has more than one meaning in the same language.
   (3) One word has different meanings in different dialects of the same language.
   (4) One word has different meanings in different languages.
2. Ask questions and lead the discussion for processing the activity.

Estimated time: 20–30 minutes

Activity 3: Role-plays on passive, aggressive and assertive communication

Procedure:

1. Identify a situation and demonstrate passive and aggressive communication patterns as follows:

	Passive communication	*Aggressive communication*
Verbal language		
	Ambiguous and negative	Authoritarian and commanding
	Self blame	Lectures and moralises
	Feels worthless	Blames and accuses
	Apologetic	Uses criticism, sarcasm or ridicule
	Wants sympathy	Hostile
		Name-calling
		Threatening
		Confrontational
		I win, you lose approach
		Magnifies disagreements and plays down agreement
		States one's opinion as fact
		Insists on 'rightness' and won't discuss options
		Dismisses other people's ideas/opinions/values as worthless
Voice	Soft or not at all	Loud and shouting

	Passive communication	*Aggressive communication*
Body language		
Timing and place	No sensitivity to convenience of others	No sensitivity to convenience of others
Facial expression	No expressions Makes faces	Frowns
Eye contact	No eye contact, looks down	Glaring look
Posture	Cringes, physically makes oneself small, fidgets	Intimidating towering over others Finger pointing

	Assertive communication
Verbal language	
	Organised Straightforward and positive Persistent Solution-oriented Treats people with respect instead of taunting and negative statements Makes self-responsible "I" statements rather than using the passive voice Expresses facts, supported by evidence Links feelings to the analysis of the facts
Voice	Clear and modulated instead of soft and ambiguous
Body language	
Timing and place	Sensitive to time (when to talk) and place (where to talk)
Facial expression	Pleasant, conveys a smile and not a frown
Eye contact	Eye contact conveys attention to the person spoken to
Posture	Stands up straight and relaxed

2. Ask questions and lead the discussion for processing the activity.
3. The discussion can focus on

- Advantages of passive communication that confrontation is avoided.
- Disadvantages of passive communication that a passive person is not respected or taken seriously and suffers stress.
- Advantages of aggressive communication that a narrow victory is achieved.
- Disadvantages of aggressive communication that the aggressive person is disliked or feared by people and loses in the long run.

4. Ask for volunteers to demonstrate assertive communication skills as follows:
5. Ask questions and lead the discussion for processing the activity.
6. The discussion can focus on

- Advantage of assertive communication is that a solution is achieved with mutual respect.
- Disadvantages of assertive communication are none.

Estimated time: 20–30 minutes

Activity 4: Role-plays on open communication

Procedure:

1. Divide the participants into small groups and ask them to discuss the following types of verbal communication:
   (1) Judgmental versus non-judgmental language
   (2) Permissive versus controlling language
   (3) Spontaneous versus strategic language
   (4) Empathic versus neutral language
   (5) Equal versus superior language
   (6) Provisional versus certain language
   (7) Discriminatory versus non-discriminatory language.
2. Each group may prepare role-plays on their topic and present to the large group.
3. Ask questions and lead the discussion for processing the activity.

Estimated time: 60 minutes

9.3 Body Language Skills

9.3.1 Concepts of Body Language

Lewis (2000) defines body language as the communication of personal feelings, emotions, attitudes and thoughts through body movements – gestures, postures, facial expressions, walking styles, positions and distance – either consciously or involuntarily, more often subconsciously, and accompanied by the spoken language. He cites Mehrabian's (1971) finding that if the verbal, voice and non-verbal elements are consistent, the message is effective. If the elements are inconsistent, the impact is as follows:

7 percent is verbal (the words or the message),
38 percent is voice (intonation, projection and resonance of the voice) and
55 percent is non-verbal (or body language).

Much of our time is spent in learning to speak and write a language, but much less attention is paid to non-verbal aspects of communication. According to Michelson, Sugai, Wood, and Kazdin (1983), an important part of being a skilled communicator is being able to use non-verbal signals to illustrate or emphasise what is being said.

9.3.2 Functions of Body Language

According to Michelson et al. (1983), non-verbal cues help to provide feedback and information exchange between people in addition to conveying the affect and intensity of the verbal message. Researchers have found that non-verbal communication plays an important role in guiding interactions and in defining relationships among people. Thus, it is easy to understand how deficient non-verbal skills can affect not only the content of what is said, but also the flow of conversation. Lewis (2000) lists the following functions of body language:

- Supplement, repeat, reinforce or even contradict the verbal message
- Substitute for words
- Express emotions
- Regulate interaction
- Indicate status relationships

9.3.3 Difference Between Verbal and Body Language

Hamlin (1988, cited from Lewis 2000) made the following distinctions between use of verbal language and body language:

Chart 9.1 Difference Between Verbal and Body Language

Verbal language	Body language
• Words are on the head level. They are symbols which one has to translate mentally into meaning	• Non-verbal language is at the feeling or gut level, its meaning is absorbed instinctively. We feel its meaning rather than think about it
• Words can be edited and controlled through training. We choose what we wish to express	• Body language – posture, gesture, and movement – is unedited, unconscious, involuntary, and spontaneous. Hence, its message is more truthful and genuine
• Words are specific. As symbols, they call forth the same images for all of us; for instance, "nose" is nose, "window" is window. Words express concrete ideas and facts	• Body language needs interpretation. A person may use only posture and gesture and no words containing certain elements that are coloured by our background and culture. Hence, these need to be interpreted by the observer, according to his/her knowledge.
• Words can be found in abundance. It is convenient to describe and explain things with them, but it is not possible to comprehend the depth of feelings through words alone	• Body language is compact. It expresses feelings in a more economical way, and can be more direct and eloquent than verbal language. It evokes immediate response.
• Words separate. There are differences between foreign languages and one's own. Then, vocabulary and pronunciation define class, level of accomplishment, education, and social status	• Body language can unify because it has, by and large, universally understood meanings.

9.3.4 Non-verbal Cues

The different non-verbal cues as pointed out by Ruben (1988) include paralanguage, appearance, gesture, touch, use of space and use of time, as described below.

9.3.4.1 Paralanguage

Refers to any cues created in the process of verbalising other than the words themselves. For example, sniffs, sneezes, pitch, rate of speech, nasality, accents, pauses and even silence. These help to interpret the content of the verbal message, speaker's educational background, interest in the topic, level of comfort, self-concept, personality, mood and the nationality or region of the country to which the person belongs. For example, on the basis of pitch one can determine whether a particular utterance is a statement or a question, a serious comment or a sarcastic remark.

9.3.4.2 Appearance

We often form our first or initial impressions based on appearances that comprise of face, eyes, physique, dress and adornment. Facial expressions are a rich source of the emotional state of the person. Eye contact serves as a signal of readiness to interact and the absence of such contact whether accidental or intentional reduces the likelihood of such interaction. However, cultural factors like gender and hierarchy strongly govern the rules of eye contact. Dress and adornments like cosmetics, jewellery, eyeglasses, tattoos, hairstyles, footwear or carrying a purse, radio, newspaper, briefcase, credit cards, cell phone and so on are a basis for judgment of gender, age, personality, approachability, financial well-being, class, taste, values and cultural background.

9.3.4.3 Gestures

Movement of the head, body, arms, legs or feet play an important role in communication. They can be used as substitutes or complements for language (for example nodding of head instead of saying yes and so on) and may convey messages with a particular purpose, or those that are incidental or unintended.

9.3.4.4 Touch

Levels of contact and comfort with touching vary according to cultures.

9.3.4.5 Use of Space

Intensity of tactile messages often depends on the well-defined expectations that we have about the invasion of our personal space. Edward Hall (cited in Ruben 1988) has suggested the following categories of use of space:

- For intimate conversations and relations, space between individuals varies between 0 and 18 inches;

- While engaging in casual or personal discussions, the space is 18 inches to 4 feet;
- Informal and business conversations takes place between 4 and 12 feet apart and
- In a public setting, the space between individuals ranges from 12 feet to the limits of visibility.

According to Hall cited in Ruben (1988), fluctuations with each category depend on various factors like the age, gender and culture of the individuals, nature of the relationship, topic of discussion, setting and so on.

9.3.4.6 Use of Time

We often communicate through use of time. For example, keeping up with assignments/appointments on time, promptly replying to letters, phone calls, e-mails and so on. Reaching on time implies the eagerness and discipline of the person while being late may refer that a person is not serious and so on.

9.3.5 Modes of Body Language

John Mole (1999, cited from Lewis 2000) gives graphic descriptions of the four basic modes of body language as below.

Open: These are gestures indicating "open" attitudes, open palms, open arms, open body; face-to-face body direction.
Closed: Into this category fall the most obvious gestures and postures, like crossed arms, crossed legs, body turned away.
Forward: This involves postures that indicate a person is active in the communication process. He/She leans forward, feet firmly planted on the ground; points towards you when he/she actively accepts or rejects a message.
Back: This indicates leaning-back postures, staring at the ceiling, doodling, or cleaning one's glasses, signalling whether the person is passively absorbing or ignoring the message.

One can find combinations of these posture groups in four basic modes, as follows:

Open-forward: The responsive mode that shows active acceptance.
Open-back: The reflective mode that shows interest and receptivity, but no active acceptance.
Closed-back: The fugitive mode that shows an attempt to escape, either physically out the door or mentally into boredom.
Closed-forward: The combative mode that shows active resistance (Mole 1999, cited from Lewis 2000).

9.3.6 Activities

Activity 5: Can actions speak louder than words?

Procedure:

1. Give verbal instructions and ask the participants to follow your gestures.
2. Use gestures that are not congruent with the verbal instructions. For example, ask them to touch their nose but you touch your ear. Most of the participants will follow your gestures rather than your verbal instructions.
3. Alternately or in addition, other demonstrations of body language dominating verbal language may be carried out. For example, saying you are happy to meet someone but without a smile, sitting at a distance while giving condolence to a bereaved colleague.
4. Demonstrate gestures that convey negative perception and feelings to others that should be avoided.
5. Ask volunteers to demonstrate gestures that convey positive perception and feelings to others that need to be promoted.
6. Ask questions and lead the discussion for processing the activity.

Estimated time: 20 minutes

Activity 6: Dumb charade on mode of communication

Procedure:

1. Prepare four chits of:

   (1) Open-forward: The responsive mode of communication;
   (2) Open-back: The reflective mode of communication;
   (3) Closed-back: The fugitive mode of communication and
   (4) Closed-forward: The combative mode of communication.

2. Ask for four volunteers to pick each one and enact the mode of communication, without using any words, while the participants have to guess these modes.
3. Ask questions and lead the discussion for processing the activity.

Estimated time: 60 minutes

9.4 Sensitive Listening Skills

9.4.1 Barriers in Listening

Following are some of the common barriers to listening:

(a) *Selective listening*: Listening and responding to only the part of the conversation that interests us.

(b) *Word listening*: Paying attention to the words but not paying attention to the body language or the feelings behind the words.
(c) *Interrupting*: Saying something else or reacting without letting the person complete one's saying.
(d) *Predicting*: Predicting what the speaker is trying to say or finishing their sentences or putting words in the mouth of the speaker robbing them of the opportunity to express themselves.
(e) *Frozen evaluation or prejudgment*: Blocking in listening due to an earlier assessment of the speaker.
(f) *Passiveness*: Not responding, spacing out, looking away, yawning, fidgeting, looking at one's watch or pretending to be listening, but being caught up in our own thoughts.
(g) *Me too syndrome*: Responding about oneself rather than the person who is talking, projecting one's own biography.
(h) *Being defensive*: Being defensive when the speaker's ideas are different than ours.
(i) *Denial and contradicting*: Denial of the speaker's feelings and insisting on a contradictory opinion.
(j) *Judging and instant advice*: Making judgments and instant advising, conveying that one knows more than the other person.
(k) *Pity*: Expressing pity to the speaker undermining his/her self-esteem.

9.4.2 Sensitive Listening Skills

Covey (1997) points out that one should listen not only with ears, but also with eyes and most importantly with the heart with the intent to understand, not just the words that are spoken, but also the body language that conveys feelings. Gerard Egan (1986, cited in Burnard, 1994) has suggested a simple acronym "SOLER" for the body language that enhances listening skills. The acronym stands for the following:

'*S*': Sit *squarely* in relation to the person you are listening to.
'*O*': Maintain an *open* relaxed position.
'*L*': *Lean* slightly towards the person who is speaking.
'*E*': Maintain reasonable *eye contact.*
'*R*': *Relax* while listening.

Following are some more suggestions to enhance sensitive listening:

(a) *Just listen*: Allow the speaker to complete speaking and listen with interest and an intent to understand. Do not rush or get preoccupied with replying. Often a person reaching out to us may not particularly want answers/solutions to his/her problems, but may simply want to be heard out.

(b) *Observe body language*: Read non-verbal cues and try to understand.
(c) *Express concern*: Ask open-ended questions for more information, opinion and feeling by asking where, who, how and why.
(d) *Express understanding and acceptance*: Restate or interpret the speaker's ideas and feelings in our own words, instead of repeating their exact words. Allow others to have their own opinions even if one does not agree.
(e) *Preserve and promote self-esteem*: Preserve their self-esteem even if we think they have made a mistake. Promote their self-esteem by reminding them of their strengths. Give opinion or suggestions only if asked or ask before giving opinion or suggestions.

9.4.3 Activities

Activity 7: Sharing without sensitive listening

Procedure:

1. Ask the participants to form pairs.
2. In phase one, one of the partners become speakers who share an event in their life with the other partners. The listeners show lack of interest.
3. In phase two, the speakers replay sharing of the same event in their life. The listeners now listen with interest.
4. Ask questions and lead the discussion for processing the difference between the two phases of the activity.

Estimated time: 30 minutes

Activity 8: Sensitive listening

Procedure:

1. Demonstrate problems in listening through a role-play on a situation related to the participants' family, colleagues or friends, for example discussing a career plan with a colleague or any problem with a friend.
2. Ask volunteers to demonstrate sensitive listening skills.
3. Ask questions and lead the discussion for processing the activity.

Estimated time: 30–45 minutes

9.5 Feedback Skills

Giving and receiving positive and negative feedback is an essential aspect of all interpersonal communication and an imperative to be able to grow in our relationships with people.

9.5.1 Negative Feedback Skills

9.5.1.1 Giving Negative Feedback

It is best to give negative feedback when it is invited because then the receptivity is greater, but it is also important to let other people know if their behaviour disturbs or bothers us. However, this is not always an easy thing to do, as people may feel threatened and react defensively. At other times the individual is not aware that he or she is doing something that is bothersome. In this situation, a tactful comment or request can be welcome information. The act of giving negative feedback can be carried out in the form of requesting behaviour change of another person. In most cases, this can be mutually beneficial. The person who makes the request may be able to change an uncomfortable situation and the person of whom change is requested receives necessary feedback (Michelson et al. 1983).

According to Humphreys (2002), we often give negative feedback to the other person indirectly and/or unclearly:

- In indirect but clear expression, the person for whom the request or statement is intended is not directly addressed, for example "Nobody loves me in this house".
- The direct but unclear communication is typified in the "you" messages, which say nothing about the sender of the message, for example "You are always shouting". They also judge or blame the other person, which generally leads the other person to withdraw or attack back.
- Cynicism and sarcasm typify indirect and unclear communication, for example "Looks like I'm not your real son".

We need to learn to express our needs directly and clearly. It requires directly addressing the intended person, "I" language, declaration of how we feel and clear expression of our needs (Humphreys 2002). Cornelius and Faire (2006, pp. 80–83) note that an I-statement tells the other person how we see the situation, without blaming and without demanding that the other person change. They recommend that it includes describing the behaviour, the resulting problem/feelings and the future as follows:

- We need to describe the facts of the behaviour that bothers us and not interpret it with reference to its motive. For example, "Who are you to shout at me . . ." can be reframed as "When you shout at me in front of my friends . . ."
- We have the right to feel the way we do but not blame others for the same. For example, "You humiliate me" can be reframed in an I-statement as "I am hurt."
- Our preferred approach for future can be constructively stated as "I would appreciate you telling me what you do not like after my friends leave" instead of "You better not talk to me in this language".

9.5.1.2 Receiving Negative Feedback

When attacked with criticism, especially personal, most humans get defensive. However, it is to our advantage to turn around the criticism and make it into a useful feedback. According to Ricucci (2001), we can practice handling criticism more effectively as follows:

- Try to remain as calm as possible when sensing an "onset" of criticism. Do not tense up or get bristled before it's delivered. The reason you have to be this calm, is when it is your turn to talk and accept the criticism or answer any questions regarding the criticism, you will look like a rational, cool-headed individual with a good head on your shoulders.
- Try not to cut the person off with excuses or explanations right away. Hear the person out. You may want to start thinking of a couple of comments to back yourself up, but not defensive or excuses.
- It is a good thing to remember to accept the persons' viewpoint and thank them for what they have just told you. Remember that you are the one benefitting from the insight of the criticism.
- If the criticism is based on false assumptions, thank the person for the advice and apologise for conveying something that was not meant to. However, state the facts in the right perspective.

9.5.2 Positive Feedback Skills

9.5.2.1 Giving Positive Feedback

Dryden (1994) noted that we often do not communicate our appreciation to others either because they have not communicated their appreciation to us, or because we feel they already know how good they are, or we are just not used to giving compliments. In any social interaction or relationship, it tremendously helps to communicate to others what we like about, both, them and what they have done. However, it is important that the positive feedback given is genuine, unconditional and without ulterior motives (Humphreys 2002). Brahm (2005) notes that without positive feedback the good qualities in the other person wither and die. It is necessary not only to encourage the good qualities in them, but also to enrich our relationship and create happiness. Alberti and Emmons (1998) recommend expressing positive feedback by a warm, firm and extended handshake, a warm smile and extended eye contact, and/or words such as *I respect you, I understand what you mean, I will be there, count on me, may be you are right, thank you, I appreciate your thoughtfulness, it is very nice of you, I like what you did, I trust you, I'm glad to see you,* and so on.

9.5.2.2 Receiving Positive Feedback

Accepting appreciation is difficult if we are not feeling good about ourselves. Nevertheless, it is an assertive act and mutually enhancing to accept praise from another person (Alberti and Emmons 1998). It could be expressed by words such as "thank you for your kind words" and "it is nice of you to say that".

9.5.3 Activities

Activity 9: Requesting behaviour change

Procedure:

1. Take an example of a situation when the father shouts at the adolescent son for bringing home friends late at night and the son shouts back.
2. Ask for two volunteers to act father and son and demonstrate the skills to request behaviour change with eachother.
3. Ask questions and lead the discussion for processing the activity.

Estimated time: 30 minutes

Activity 10: Communication of I am OK, you are OK

Procedure:

1. Use one or more of the following methods to bring about communication of appreciation among the participants. Every participant has to give a genuine compliment to the other without expecting anything in return.

   (1) Ask participants to stand in a circle. Start by communicating appreciation to the person standing on your right hand side. He/She does the same to the person standing on his/her right hand side and it continues till the circle is complete and you receive the communication of appreciation. The receivers thank but not return a compliment immediately after receiving one (adapted from "I Appreciate: A Validation Exercise" from Elkins 1983, p. 106).
   (2) Give each participant a paper plate on which they should write their name and then have it pinned up on their back. Each participant writes a compliment on the plate of each of the others (adapted from "Have a Hand" from *Energize* 1991).
   (3) Ask the participants to think of people who contribute to our lives significantly, but to whom we do not communicate our appreciation, for example our parents, our teachers, persons who work for us and so on. Ask them to write a note of appreciation to one of them.

2. Ask questions and lead the discussion for processing the activity.

Estimated time: 30–60 minutes (depending on the combination of activities).

References

Alberti, R. and Emmons, M. (1998). *Complete Guide to Assertive Living*. Mumbai: Jaico Publishing House.

Brahm, A. (2005). *Who Ordered This Truckload of Dung? Inspiring Stories for Welcoming Life's Difficulties*. Boston, MA: Wisdom Publications.

Burnard, P. (1994). *Counselling Skills for Health Professionals*. London: Chapmen and Hall.

Cornelius, H. and Faire, S. (2006). *Everyone Can Win: Responding to Conflict Constructively*. Sydney, NSW: Simon and Schuster.

Covey, S. R. (1997). *The 7 Habits of Highly Effective People*. London: Simon and Schuster.

Donn, C. (2000). *Four Principles of Interpersonal Communication*. www.pstcc.cc.tn.us/facstaff/dking/interpr.htm. Accessed 9 June 2004.

Dryden, W. (1994). *10 Steps to Positive Living*. New Delhi: Orient Paperbacks.

Elkins, D. P. (1983). *Teaching People to Love Themselves. A Leader's Handbook of Theory and Technique for Self Esteem and Affirmation Training*. Princeton, NJ: Growth Associates.

Energize. (1991). *Energize*. Granville, NC: Quest International.

Hamilton, V. M. (2007). *Human Relations: The Art and Science of Building Effective Relationships*. Upper Saddle River, NJ: Pearson Prentice Hall.

Humphreys, T. (2002). *Self-Esteem: The Key to Your Child's Future*. Dublin: Newleaf.

Johnson, D. W. (1986). *Reaching Out: Interpersonal Effectiveness and Self-Actualisation*. Englewood Cliffs, NJ: Prentice-Hall.

Lewis, H. (2000). *Body Language: A Guide for Professionals*. New Delhi: Response Books.

Michelson, L., Sugai, D. P., Wood, R. P. and Kazdin, A. E. (1983). *Social Skills Assessment and Training with Children: An Empirically Based Handbook*. New York, NY: Plenum Press.

Ricucci, R. (2001). *Utilizing Constructive Criticism*. www.ga.essortment.com/constructivecri_revy.htm. Accessed 29 June 2005.

Ruben, B. D. (1988). *Communication and Human Behaviour*. New York, NY: MacMillan Publishing Co. Inc.

Tubbs, S. L. and Moss, S. (1980). *Human Communication*. New York, NY: Random House.

Chapter 10
Family Life Education

10.1 Concepts of Family Life Education

10.1.1 Family and Household

The family may be broadly defined as a unit of two or more persons united by ties of marriage, blood, adoption or consensual unions, generally constituting a single household, and interacting and communicating with each other (Desai 1994). Every individual has a family of orientation or family of origin as it is the family he/she is born into. Most individuals also form a family of procreation, mostly by marriage and child bearing but may be also by consensual relationships, reproductive technologies or adoption (Collins et al. 2007). Family and household are, often, used synonymously. However, a household means a residential unit, composed of one or more persons living under the same roof and eating food cooked in a single kitchen (Shah 1973) and may or may not comprise a family.

10.1.2 Family in the Ecological Perspective

The ecological perspective views an individual in the context of his/her family and the family in the context of its environment as these constantly interact with and, therefore, influence one another. The family's immediate environment is comprised of the ethnic/kinship community, neighbourhood, natural environment, work place, school/college, friends, media and so on. The state, corporate sector and the market influence the family indirectly. The macro-system is the larger international eco-political contexts in which these systems are embedded. Diversity in the environment brings variations in family life, which, in turn, explains differences in individual members' well-being to a large extent. Similarly, changes in the environment influence the family life, which affects its individual members (Desai 1994).

M. Desai, *A Rights-Based Preventative Approach for Psychosocial Well-Being in Childhood*, Children's Well-Being: Indicators and Research 3,
DOI 10.1007/978-90-481-9066-9_10, © Springer Science+Business Media B.V. 2010

10.1.3 Types of Families

Families are classified as follows based on the classification of groups by performance given by Johnson and Johnson (2009):

1. *Pseudo-families*: Pseudo-families are families whose members have no interest in one another. Although they talk to one another, they see one another as rivals who must be defeated. As a result, the sum of the whole is less than the sum of the potential of the individual members. The members would be happier staying alone.
2. *Traditional families*: Traditional families are structured in such a way that very little joint work is required. Some members seek a free ride on the efforts of the more conscientious members. The latter may feel exploited and do less or would be happier if staying alone.
3. *Effective families*: An effective family is more than the sum of its parts as the members commit themselves to maximising their own and others' potentials. The characteristics of effective families are positive interdependence, two-way communication, distributed leadership, power based on expertise and constructive resolution of conflicts.

10.1.4 Family Life Education

Family life education (FLE) programmes aim at the achievement of the characteristics of effective families or family well-being. Following are the principles of FLE:

- FLE is relevant to individuals, couples, and families across the life span.
- FLE draws on multidisciplinary knowledge.
- FLE is offered in many venues, including community workshops, video and print media, publications, the Internet and so on.
- FLE is educational rather than therapeutic (adapted from Arcus et al. 1993, cited by Duncan and Goddard 2005).

10.2 Enrichment of Family Dynamics

Family dynamics is comprised of family identity and esteem, composition, family development and family relationships.

10.2.1 Family Identity

10.2.1.1 Group-Level Family Identity

Every family is connected to its immediate environment that is comprised of the ethnic/kinship community, neighbourhood, natural environment, work place, school/college, friends, public services, media and so on (Desai 1994). Family identity is the boundary that separates it from other systems in the environment. It is formed by its composition, ethnic background and financial status. Ethnic background includes race, religion, regional background and mother tongue. Family name is often an indicator of the group-level family identity that provides connectedness to the family.

10.2.1.2 Unique-Level Family Identity

Every family has its own unique character depending on its history.

10.2.2 Family Composition

As a social system, a family is comprised of sub-systems. Each member can be considered a sub-system and its dyad also can be considered a sub-system. The dyadic sub-systems are

- Conjugal sub-systems
- Filial sub-systems
- Fraternal sub-systems
- Grandparent–grandchild sub-systems
- In-law sub-systems
- Consensual sub-systems

The family composition is comprised of its size, age and sex of its members and relationship among them. Families have plurality of composition that varies with class, ethnicity, geographical location and individual choice. The normative or traditional family compositions comprise of joint and nuclear families. The joint family comprises two or more couples and their children, bound together by common movable or immovable property, and may or may not be staying together. Variations in a joint family are lineal joint families, collateral joint families and lineal-cum-collateral joint families. The nuclear family comprises couples and their unmarried children, and is generally financially independent of other families. A variation of an elementary/nuclear family is the supplemented nuclear family, which comprises a nuclear family with single relatives (Kolenda 1987). Leslie and Korman (1984) termed extended families as consanguineous families as they focus on blood relations. They termed nuclear families as conjugal families as conjugal relation is the core of these families.

As marriage and children are considered essential elements of a traditional family, the following comprise alternate family compositions:

- Single-parent families (due to unwed parenthood, death of a spouse, desertion, separation or divorce or migration of a spouse)
- Childless families (due to infertility or out of choice)

- Reconstituted/step-family
- Consensual unions

10.2.3 Family Development

As a family system moves through time, it goes through changes in its composition, as members are added, mature and lost.

10.2.3.1 Stages of Family Development

The development stages in a traditional nuclear family may move through the following stages, with variations in the stages depending on the variations in age and life transitions of family members:

- Young persons getting married
- Young couples bearing and bringing up children
- Middle-aged couples with children forming their own nuclear families
- Old couples with children bearing and bringing up their children

10.2.3.2 Family Developmental Tasks

A family's developmental task is a growth responsibility that arises at a certain stage in the life of a family, determined by the age and developmental needs of the members of the family. Successful achievement of the developmental tasks leads to satisfaction and success with later tasks, while failure leads to unhappiness in the family, disapproval by society and difficulty with later developmental tasks (Duvall 1977).

10.2.3.3 Family Developmental Transitions

Family developmental transitions mean families moving from one developmental stage to another. Examples of family developmental transitions necessary at each stage are adapted as follows from Carter and McGoldrick (2005):

- Moving to the stage of a couple getting married, the family has to (1) make commitment to a new dyadic sub-system (conjugal), (2) realign with the other sub-systems in the family (filial and fraternal) and with friends and (3) make space for the in-law sub-system.
- Moving to the stage of a couple rearing children, the family has to (1) make readjustments in the conjugal sub-system to (2) make space for a new parenting sub-system with their children and (3) make readjustments in their filial system to make space for their parents' grandparental sub-system.
- Moving to the stage of a couple with adolescent children, the family has to (1) make readjustments in their parenting sub-system to allow the adolescent children more independence, (2) refocus on their conjugal sub-system and career

and (3) make readjustments in their filial system accommodating for care giving of and losing ageing parents.
- Moving to the stage of an elderly couple, the family has to (1) make readjustment to a life of a dependent and (2) readjustment to life with losing the spouse and siblings and preparation of death.

10.2.3.4 Family Adaptability

Family developmental transitions require the ability of a family system to adapt to the new demands that create stress with reference to the resources available. Covertly or overtly, the family tries to maintain or restore the balance between demands and resources (Tseng and Hsu 1991). Patterson (1988) has listed different ways in which this can be accomplished by the family system:

- Direct action to reduce the number and/or intensity of demands;
- Direct action to acquire additional resources not already available to the family;
- Maintaining existing resources so that they can be allocated and reallocated to meet changing demands;
- Managing the tension associated with continuing strain on resources; and
- Cognitive appraisal to change the meaning of a situation to make it more manageable.

Tseng and Hsu (1991) also identified promoting changes in family structure and interaction that give the family more strength; and skills for dealing with strain and demands effectively.

The four levels of adaptability range from rigid (very low), to structured (low to moderate), to flexible (moderate to high), to chaotic (very high). It is hypothesised that the central levels of adaptability (structured and flexible) are more conducive to marital and family functioning with the extremes (rigid and chaotic) being the most problematic (Olson 1988). Structured and flexible adaptability therefore facilitates family developmental transitions.

10.2.4 Family Relationships

The following skills of interpersonal relationships can be applied to the family subsystems as well as family as a system for enrichment of family relationships:

Semi-open boundary in relationships

- Cohesion
- Adaptability

Positive perception of others

- Egalitarian perception
- Recognition of strengths
- Acceptance and respect
- Celebration of differences

Positive feelings for others

- Warmth
- Humility
- Empathy

Win-Win goals in relationships
Collaborative conflict management skills
Interpersonal communication skills

- Open communication skills
- Body language skills
- Sensitive listening skills
- Feedback skills.

10.2.5 Family Activities

Family activities include sharing family tasks, having meals together, spending weekends and vacations, and celebrating birthdays and festivals, and decision-making about these. According to Khavari and Khavari (1989), whenever possible, the entire family should read and discuss the ideas and information together. In this way each person is provided with a common background from which to learn the necessary skills and attitudes for improving family life.

10.2.6 Activities

Activity 1: What is a family?

This activity is useful as an icebreaker for the topic.

Procedure:

1. Ask the participants to define family.
2. Lead the discussion along the following points:
   - Does family only mean blood and legal relationship?
   - What about social and emotional relationships?
   - Can unrelated persons staying together be considered a family?

Estimated time: 15 minutes

Activity 2: My family name

Procedure:

1. Ask the participants to think of the meaning of their family name.
2. Each participant expresses this meaning with the large group through a drawing or acting.

3. Each participant shares the following about their family name with their partner:
   - What is the meaning of this family name?
   - What is the history of this family name?
   - Does the family name indicate the race/religion/region of the family?
   - Is any status attached to their family name?
4. Ask questions and lead discussion for processing the activity.
5. Discuss the importance of one's family name for group-level family identity.

Estimated time: 30 minutes

Activity 3: Drawing my family-esteem tree

Procedure:

1. Ask the participants to make their family self-esteem tree as follows:
   (1) List family strengths as roots.
   (2) List family actions as branches.
   (3) List family achievements as fruits.
   (4) On the trunk, write which family this self-esteem tree belongs to.
2. Each participant shares their family self-esteem tree with the large group.
3. Celebrate everyone's family self-esteem, after their sharing.
4. Ask questions and lead discussion for processing the activity.
5. Discussion can focus on need for family members' acceptance, sense of worth and love for the family, confidence about family's capabilities, assertiveness with reference to family rights, and family-level self-responsibility for meeting its needs.

Estimated time: 45 minutes

Activity 4: My family genogram

Procedure:

1. Ask the participants to draw at least a three-generational genogram of their family and share with their partner:
   - Each horizontal line conveys a generation, and generations are joined by vertical lines.
   - They can start with their own generation, including self, siblings and spouses.
   - Their parents' generation can be listed above their own.
   - Their children's generation can be listed below their own.
   - Draw squares for males and circles for females, and place the age of each within. A cross within indicates dead.
   - List siblings/children from the oldest to the youngest, left to right.
   - List husband on the left and wife on the right.
   - Make a circle to include the family members that live together in a household.

2. Ask questions and lead discussion for processing the activity.
3. Discussion can focus on family history, hereditary patterns, characteristics and present composition.

Activity 5: Respecting plurality of household composition

Procedure:

1. Ask the participants to examine their household composition in their family genogram and form six groups according to their present household composition: joint household, nuclear household, single-parent household, childless household, reconstituted/step-family and consensual Union.
2. Each group discusses the reasons and implications of their household type, and shares with the large group.
3. Ask questions and lead discussion for processing the activity.
4. The discussion can focus on the importance of respecting plurality of household composition.

Estimated Time: 45 min

Activity 6: Family adaptability

Procedure:

1. Ask the participants to assess the adaptability of their family in the following situations:

Developmental transitions	The amount of stress created by these transitions: high – 1, medium – 2 low – 3	Family adaptability: rigid – 1, structured – 2 flexible – 3, chaotic – 4
• When there is birth of a child		
• When there is a marriage and addition of a family member		
• When there is a change in the education or occupation of a family member		
• When there is death in the family		

2. Participants share the assessment with their partner.
3. Ask questions and lead discussion for processing the activity.
4. The discussion can focus on how to convert the rigid and chaotic adaptability into structured and flexible.

Estimated time: 20 minutes

Activity 7: Drawing family togetherness

Procedure:

1. Ask the participants to draw a picture of their family, as engaged in the most common activity.
2. Participants list the activities that the family members do together.
3. Participants reflect if they enjoy doing these family activities.
4. Ask questions and lead discussion for processing the activity.
5. Discuss how it is important to together have at least one meal a day, spend weekends and vacations and celebrate birthdays and festivals and so on. The decisions about these also need to be taken together as a family.

Estimated time: 30 minutes

Activity 8: Story on complementarity in family life

Procedure:

1. Share the story of brothers Sonu and Monu

> Once there lived two brothers Sonu and Monu. Sonu was blind while Monu was lame. He could not walk without help. One day Sonu heard that a large fair was being held in the next village. He said to Monu, "Brother, we must go to that fair. We"ll have a lot of fun." "But Sonu, how can we go so far away? You are blind so you can't see the way. I am lame so I can't walk for such a long distance."
>
> Sonu smiled and said, "Don't be disheartened, Monu, I have found a way out. I am blind but I can walk to cover great distances. You cannot walk as you are lame, but you can show me the way to the fair. Now you can sit on my shoulders. You will see the way and tell me which way to go while I'll be your legs to carry you to the fair." So the two friends went to the fair together and enjoyed themselves. (Adapted from Tiny Tot Best of Moral Stories 2002)

2. Ask questions and lead discussion for processing the activity.
3. Discussion may be conducted along the following points:

   - How did Sonu and Monu overcome difficulties together to go to the fair?
   - Complementarity refers to recognising different strengths of individuals in teams and using these to achieve the best possible results in a team effort.

Estimated time: 30 minutes

Activity 9: Family as a team

Procedure:

1. Prepare chits with names of different machines written on them. The examples are oven, bicycle, train engine, airplane, pencil sharpener, mixer/grinder, sewing machine, washing machine and so on.
2. Divide the participants into small groups and ask each small group selects a chit and plan to enact the machine as a group.

3. Each member has a role to play and the enactment shows connections, movements and sounds.
4. Each small group takes turns doing the enactment, which the others try to guess (adapted from "Machines" by Staley 1982).
5. Ask questions and lead discussion for processing the activity.
6. Discussion may focus on application of the activity to family life with reference to importance of complementarity, interdependence, individual accountability, sharing resources, providing mutual support and celebrating joint success.

Estimated time: 30 minutes

Activity 10: Problem-solving in family life

Procedure:

1. Ask the participants (not more than 15) to stand in a circle, close to each other, shoulder to shoulder.
2. Participants randomly grab two other hands of persons not standing next to them. The result is an awkward but hilarious tangle.
3. The participants try to untangle themselves without letting go the hand that they are holding.
4. They jump over some hands, go beneath some hands, turn around with their hands going over others' heads and so on, to untangle themselves.
5. They may end up with a large circle like they started with or some small interconnected circles. Some may not be able to untangle themselves (adapted from "All in Knots" in *Energize* 1991).
6. Ask questions for processing the activity and lead the discussion for application to problem-solving in family life.

Estimated time: 30 minutes

10.3 Democratic Family Structure

10.3.1 Family Structure

Family structure comprises of roles and power, influenced by family ideologies, functional orientation and rules.

10.3.1.1 Family Ideologies

Family ideologies generally comprise of patriarchy, sexism, adultism and ageism. Patriarchy describes a social structure where the actions and ideas of men and boys are dominant over those of women and girls. This circumstance of male dominance is reflected in correlative inequities throughout the society. In the sphere of the family, the father or the eldest male is considered the patriarch or "head of the household" (Wikipedia 2008). There has never been a true matriarchal family in existence.

10.3.1.2 Family Functional Orientation

McIntyre (1966) identified the following three major areas of family functions, which need to be balanced for a democratic family structure:

- The functions of the family for the ethnic community and the larger society (kinship orientation);
- The functions of the family for its unity and joint happiness (familism) and
- The functions of the family for development and well-being of individual family members (individualism).

According to Rogers and Sebald (1962):

- Kinship orientation is the degree to which a family fulfils the role expectations of the kinship reference group. Families have traditionally had a strong kinship orientation that influences family norms and subordinates individual interest.
- Familism is the subordination of individual interest to those of the family group.
- Individualism is the primacy of individual interest.

10.3.1.3 Family Rules

Family rules are formulas or norms for relationships or guides for conduct and interactions in the family in order to maintain family homeostasis (Hepworth et al. 2006). According to Virginia Satir, family rules are usually not consciously known or verbalised by the family members. The family becomes dysfunctional when members do not understand the unwritten rules. Usually such families do not have bad members but bad rules. She would like all family members to understand the rules that govern their emotional interchanges, including freedom to comment, freedom to express what one is seeing or hearing, freedom to agree or disapprove and freedom to ask questions, when one does not understand (Thompson and Henderson 2007).

10.3.1.4 Family Roles

The functions that the family as an institution performs are divided among family members in the form of roles. Roles are culturally defined and are passed on to succeeding generations as correct behaviour (Nye and Berardo 1973). Role expectations are thus learnt from the family of orientation. According to Levy (1949), role differentiation is the distribution of persons among the various positions and activities distinguished in the structure and hence the differential arrangement of the members of the structure. The terms of role differentiation may be age, sex, generation and sometimes economic and political positions. Family roles have implications for locus of power in the family.

10.3.1.5 Power in Family

According to Blood and Wolfe (1960), power is the ability of an individual to influence or control the behaviour of others. In the context of the family, power refers to an act or statement, which indicates an attempt on the part of a family member to control, initiate, change or modify the behaviour or motivation of another member. In patriarchal families, power rests with the oldest man in the family. The egalitarian family implies equal distribution of power between men and women and across age groups. Family power has implication for status in the family. Since men and elderly have more power in patriarchal families, they have a higher status than women and children in these families.

Power leads to abuse of the powerless. The two basic types of family abuse are adult abuse and child abuse. The following factors differentiate family abuse from other types of abuse:

- It occurs within ongoing relationships that are expected to be protective, supportive and nurturing.
- The victim not only wants to escape the violence, but also longs to belong to a family.
- Affection and attention may co-exist with violence and abuse.
- Ongoing family relationships create opportunities for repeated victimisation (American Psychological Association 1996, cited by Mignon et al. 2002).

10.3.1.6 Democratic Family Structure

Democratic family structure requires:

- Egalitarian, gender-aware, child-friendly and elderly friendly ideologies and rules.
- Role flexibility and interchangeability.
- Egalitarian power and status allocation.

10.3.2 Sexism and Rights of Women

10.3.2.1 Sexism

Sexism is a prejudice or discrimination on the grounds of sex, especially against women (Reader's Digest Oxford 1993). It implies stereotypes of women's physical and mental capabilities, which justify male control over women with reference to their labour, sexuality and reproductive roles. Feminism introduced the distinction between sex and gender to deal with sexism or the general tendency to attribute women's subordination to their anatomy. For ages, it was believed that the different characteristics, roles and status accorded to women and men in society are determined by biology (that is sex), that they are natural and, therefore, not changeable (Ann Oakley 1985, cited in Bhasin 2000). However, people are born with sexual differences, which are biological differences, but are taught what the appropriate behaviour and attitudes, roles and activities are for them, and how they should relate to other people. Gender refers to these socio-cultural definitions of man and woman, the way societies distinguish between the two and assign to them social roles. Throughout their life, parents, teachers, peers, culture and society reinforce this. This learned behaviour is what makes up gender identity and determines gender roles (Williams et al. 1994).

10.3.2.2 Human Rights of Women

The United Nations Convention on the Elimination of All Forms of Discrimination against Women (CEDAW) defines discrimination against women as "any discrimination, exclusion or restriction made on the basis of sex which has the effect or purpose of impairing or nullifying the recognition, enjoyment or exercise by women, irrespective of their marital status, on a basis of equality of men and women, of human rights and fundamental freedoms in the political, economic, social, cultural, civil or any other field."

Boys and girls have the same rights but their problems may differ. A gender-sensitive approach implies understanding and consideration of the different realities, needs and interests of boys and girls, and men and women. Such an approach takes into consideration the power relations between male and female members of the family and the community in order to understand how these might influence the decision-making and the distribution of workload, income and resources in the family, community and society at large (UNICEF 2001).

10.3.3 Adultism and Rights of Child

(Refer to Chapters 1 and 2.)

10.3.4 Ageism and Rights of Elderly

10.3.4.1 Ageism

The older persons have traditionally carried a high status; the oldest man has generally been considered the head of the family. The technological advancement with industrialisation, urbanisation and liberalisation has been changing the socio-economic context of ageing. The fast moving world of technology in the liberalised economy values young and educated professionals. The experiential wisdom of the older person is not considered productive in this scenario. Moreover, the concept of retirement from work is leading to lowering of their status as non-productive dependents. It is the earning man, who is now considered the head of the family. Women, who were always subordinate to the men in the family, earlier had authority over younger women. The trends show inverting of hierarchies and ambiguity of roles rather than a movement towards an egalitarian family structure, due to growing consumerism (Tata Institute of Social Sciences 1999).

The marginalisation of the elderly is being justified by ageism, which is the holding of prejudicial views about individuals or groups based on their age (Marshall 1994). Ageism leads to dislike of old people based on the belief that old age causes the older persons to be unattractive, unintelligent, asexual, unemployable and senile (Comfort 1976, cited in Cockerham 1991). It assumes that the older persons have reduced physical and intellectual capabilities and are, therefore, dependent on the younger population. This is generally not true at the age of 60, just because it is generally the age of retirement from formal work. The young-old (61–75) are productive human resources, as seen in the informal sector, and the old-old (76–90) are capable of being useful to the society and are not dependent liabilities. The non-productive very old (91+), the disabled and the terminally ill; the landless and migrant; and the single older persons in cities, where community supports are weak, are more likely to be neglected, abused and rendered destitute (Tata Institute of Social Sciences 1999).

10.3.4.2 Human Rights of Older Persons

The United Nations 18 Principles for the rights of the older persons fall under the five clusters of:

Independence (access to basic services and care, opportunities to work or make income, access to education, safe living environments);
Participation (to form associations or movements of older persons);
Care (access to family, community and institutional care, health, social and legal services);
Self-fulfilment (have opportunities for development of potential and access to educational, cultural, spiritual and recreational resources of society) and
Dignity (to prevent exploitation, physical or mental abuse) (Atal 2001).

There is a need to accept old age as a developmental stage and not a problem or a disease, and older persons as human resources and not liabilities. Coordinated approaches are necessary to ensure that the following needs of older persons are met as human rights: self-fulfilment, health and nutrition; work and financial security; property and housing; adult education; recreation and mobility; family and community awareness and interaction, protection from neglect, violence and destitution; and death with dignity.

10.3.5 Democratic Family Decision-Making

Democratic decision-making is the affirmation of each family member's dignity, worth and welfare. All the members should be encouraged to participate in the family discussion, no matter how different their contributions might be. All the members, in turn, have a responsibility to contribute their best for the betterment of the group functioning. It is important to sit in a circle to assure that. When genuine respect is received from others, each person feels comfortable in revealing his or her ideas, confident that no one will ridicule or condemn them (Khavari and Khavari 1989).

In family decision-making, each member should avoid becoming attached to his or her own ideas or preferences. Once expressed, the idea no longer belongs to an individual, but becomes the property of the family, which means that the contributor can then look at the idea just as objectively as the other members. This leaves the family free to accept or reject the idea without fear of hurting the feelings of the one who suggested it. Even if a solution is not finally adopted as a solution or plan, the one who offered it retains dignity and a sense of worth if given a respectful and courteous hearing. All members should fully understand that rejection of an idea is not a rejection of its originator (Khavari and Khavari 1989).

Following are the steps for democratic decision-making:

1. The family members should be relaxed and seated in a circle for the decision-making.
2. Every member should share what the problem is from their point of view and listen to one another, with the intent to understand.
3. Explore the facts first, with reference to who, where, when, why and how.
4. Discuss feelings, opinions and perceptions attached to these facts and then carry out its analysis.
5. Carry out a brainstorming of suggestions for action without evaluating them. Sometimes one idea inspires a member to think of a way to make it work better, followed by even a better idea from someone else, creating group synergy.
6. Discuss the suggestions with reference to criteria such as the following:
   - the resources/capacity that the family has to implement each, and
   - the advantages and disadvantages that each may lead to with reference to the family and its members.
7. Create a solution that would satisfy all the members and meet the above criteria.
8. Allocate roles to implement the decision taken but make a joint commitment and take joint responsibility for its consequences.
9. Monitor the consequences of implementation of the decision and decide if there is a need to change it.
10. It is okay to make mistakes in decision-making and learn from them.

10.3.6 Activities

10.3.6.1 Activity 11: Self-Disclosure of Gender Experiences

Procedure:

1. Ask each participant, individually, to complete the following sentence: "Sometimes I'm glad I'm a girl/boy because ...". Ask them to list as many of the advantages of being a girl/boy as they can.
2. Then ask each participant to complete the following sentence: "Sometimes I wish I were a girl/boy because ...". Again they should list as many reasons as possible.

3. Allow all the participants to share their views and discuss the stereotypes that come up in the sharing session.
4. Ask questions and lead discussion for processing the activity (Source: "Stereotypes: Self disclosure" in Williams et al. 1994, pp. 127–128).

Estimated time: 30–45 minutes

Activity 12: Awareness of sexism in proverbs

Procedure:

1. Ask the participants to list the common sexist proverbs on girls and boys or men and women and put up on the board (for example girls/women can never keep a secret . . . so they should be kept out of confidential family matters).
2. The participants identify the assumptions of physical and mental capabilities of men and women.
3. The participants examine reasons for these assumptions.
4. Discuss counter evidence.

Estimated time: 30–45 minutes

Activity 13: Assessment of family roles and power

Procedure:

1. Ask each participant to fill up the following chart for assessment of family roles and power and share with their partner.

No.	Family activity	Role: Who carries it out?	Power: Who has the final say?
1	Cooking		
2	Looking after the sick and the old		
3	Shopping		
4	House cleaning		
5	Helping children with studies		
6	Working to earn		
7	Savings and investment		
8	Decision about career/marriages		

2. Ask questions and lead discussion for processing the activity.

Estimated time: 45 minutes

Activity 14: Gender quiz

Procedure:

1. Hand out the following gender quiz to each participant and ask them to write "Agree", "Disagree" or "Undecided" against each of the following statements:

No.	Gender statement	Agree – 1 Disagree – 2 Undecided – 3
1	Girls are born physically weaker than boys are	
2	By birth, girls are better at taking care of children and cooking than boys are	
3	Boys are better at mathematics than girls are and girls are better at languages than boys are	
4	Girls must get married after school, but boys may study further	
5	Girls must choose between a career and a family	
6	A marriage succeeds only if the girl is less educated than the boy is	
7	To be a good wife and mother, a girl must marry at an early age	
8	A woman becomes complete only when she becomes a mother	
9	Single women cannot raise their children well	
10	When a girl/woman is raped she is responsible for it	
11	Only men contribute to the country's economy	
12	A woman's work is less strenuous than a man's work	
13	Men are more sincere about work than women are as women tend to be preoccupied with household matters	
14	When women work outside their home, they tend to neglect and break their family	
15	Women make bad drivers	
16	Women keep on gossiping about each other	

2. A volunteer compiles the responses and prepares the aggregate scores.
3. Discuss agreements and disagreements along with reasons for gender roles and stereotypes and counter evidence.

Estimated time: 45 minutes

Activity 15: Understanding adultism

Procedure:

1. Ask the participants to reflect on whether they were/are told the following in their childhood/now and how they felt/feel about it:

   - You are only a child.
   - You will know when you grow up.
   - Stop acting like a child and grow up.
   - We know what is good for you.
   - You need not know this now.
   - You will not decide without asking us.

2. Ask questions and lead discussion for processing the activity.

Estimated time: 15 minutes

Activity 16: Understanding child rights

Procedure

1. Form four groups to discuss the following categories of child rights:

   - Child right to family care
   - Child right to development
   - Child right to participation
   - Child right to protection

2. The groups discuss the following questions on each of these categories and then share with the large group:

   - What does this right include?
   - When and why are these rights not achieved in our families?
   - How can these rights be achieved in our families?

3. Ask questions and lead discussion for processing the activity.

Estimated time: 30–45 minutes

Activity 17: Exercise on images of the older persons

Procedure:

1. Identify proverbs on older persons and put up this list on the board. Alternately distribute the following Elderly Quiz to elicit the participants' opinion regarding the stereotypes of the older persons. Participants write "Agree" or "Disagree" against each of the following statements
2. Participants identify the assumptions for the above stereotypes and images of the older persons, their reasons and discuss counter evidence.
3. Discussion may be conducted with the following arguments for the above statements:

   1. Most of the older persons in developing nations work in the unorganised sector where there is no retirement. Most of them work until they die.

No.	Statement	Agree – 1 Disagree – 2
1	Older persons cannot do any productive work	
2	Older persons are conservative, inflexible and resistant to change	
3	Older persons have completed enjoying life	
4	Older persons must give up worldly comforts and become religious	
5	Older persons must get involved in social work after retirement	
6	Older persons must spend their time taking care of their grandchildren	
7	Older persons spoil their grandchildren	
8	Older persons are a burden to the family	
9	Older persons do not contribute to society	
10	Older persons are incapable of creativity, of making progress, of starting afresh	
11	Older persons must dress in a drab/sober manner	
12	Older persons must stay only with people of their own age	

2. Older persons find a lot of sense in the way they have lived their own life, as it has been functional for them.
3. Right to enjoy life continues through the life span.
4. At all ages, human beings prefer worldly comforts. Religious orientation can come at any age.
5. It is healthy to keep oneself occupied with good work after retirement from a full time job.
6. Older persons are very fond of their grandchildren but they may have other interests too.
7. Older persons tend to pamper grandchildren and so do parents. Actually, grandparents are good buffers between parents and their children.
8. Older persons are sources of experiential wisdom and so an asset to the society.
9. Older persons have already contributed to the society for many years.
10. Creativity and making progress are not related to age, though starting afresh may be difficult in old age.
11. Age is not a determining factor for how one should dress up.
12. Society is made up of people in different age groups and that is the natural social mix. Segregation is not good by age or any other factor.

Estimated time: 45 minutes

Activity 18: Small group discussion on awareness about issues and rights of the older persons

Procedure:

1. Form small groups of participants and allot issues of elderly for discussion such as negative attitude of the young generation, sending them to old age homes, physical disabilities, financial dependence, family abuse, vulnerability to robbery and murder, and so on.
2. Ask the small groups to discuss these issues with reference to the rights of the older persons of independence, participation, care, self-fulfilment and dignity and present to the large group.
3. Ask questions and lead discussion for processing the activity.

Estimated time: 30 minutes

Activity 19: Role-play for democratic family decision-making

Procedure:

1. Form small groups of participants and allot each small group different situations that are pertinent to their daily family life experiences. Examples of such situations are:

   (1) Grandmother coming to stay in a nuclear family
   (2) Planning a family vacation
   (3) Budgeting of the bonus income for the family
   (4) Planning for a sister's wedding
   (5) Planning for a daughter's career
   (6) Selection of a new house
   (7) Impending transfer of one of the spouses

2. The small groups can prepare role-plays on democratic decision-making in these situations, and present to the large group.
3. Ask questions and lead discussion for processing the activity.

Estimated time: 30–45 minutes

References

Atal, Y. (2001). The United Nations and Ageing. In I. Modi (Ed.) *Ageing and Human Development Global Perspectives* (pp. 1–9). Jaipur: Rawat Publications.

Bhasin, K. (2000). *Understanding Gender*. New Delhi: Kali for Women.

Blood, R. O. and Wolfe, D. M. (1960). *Husbands and Wives: The Dynamics of Married Living*. New York, NY: Free Press.

Carter, B. and McGoldrick, M. (Eds.). (2005). *The Expanded Family Life Cycle: Individual, Family and Social Perspectives* (3rd ed.). New York, NY: Pearson.

Cockerham, W. C. (1991). *This Aging Society*. Englewood Cliffs, NJ: Prentice Hall, Inc.
Collins, D., Jordan, C. and Coleman, H. (2007). *An Introduction to Family Social Work* (2nd ed.). Belmont, CA: Thomson–Brooks/Cole.
Desai, M. (1994). Concepts and conceptual frameworks for understanding family. In *Enhancing the Role of the Family As an Agency for Social and Economic Development*. Bombay: Tata Institute of Social Sciences.
Duncan, S. F. and Goddard, H. W. (2005). *Family Life Education: Principles and Practices for Effective Outreach*. Thousand Oaks, CA: Sage.
Duvall, E. M. (1977). *Marriage and Family Development*. Philadelphia, PA: J.B. Lippincott.
Energize. (1991). *Energize*. Granville: Quest International.
Hepworth, D. H., Rooney, R. H., Rooney, G. D., Strom-Gottfried, K. and Larson, J. A. (2006). *Direct Social Work Practice: Theory and Skills* (7th ed.). Belmont, NY: Thomson Higher Education.
Johnson, D. W. and Johnson, F. P. (2009). *Joining Together: Group Theory and Group Skills* (10th ed.). Columbus, OH: Pearson.
Khavari, K. A. and Khavari, S. W. (1989). *Creating a Successful Family*. London: Sterling Publishers.
Kolenda, P. (1987). *Regional Differences in Family Structure in India*. Jaipur: Rawat Publication.
Leslie, G. R. and Korman, S. K. (1984). *The Family in Social Context*. New York, NY: Oxford.
Levy, M. J. (1949). *The Family Revolution in Modern China*. Cambridge, MA: Harvard University Press.
Marshall, G. (Ed.). (1994). *The Concise Oxford Dictionary of Sociology*. New York, NY: Oxford University Press.
McIntyre, J. (1966). The structure-functional approach to family study. In F. I. Nye and F. M. Berardo (Eds.) *Emerging Conceptual Frameworks in Family Analysis* (pp. 52–77). New York, NY: The Macmillan Co.
Mignon, S. I., Larson, C. J. and Holmes, W. M. (2002). *Family Abuse: Consequences, Consequences, Theories, and Responses*. Boston: Allyn and Bacon.
Nye, F. I. and Berardo, F. M. (1973). *The Family: Its Structure and Interaction*. New York, NY: The Macmillan Co.
Olson, D. H. (1988). *Family Perspectives in Child and Youth Services*. New York, NY: The Haworth Press.
Patterson, J. M. (1988). Families experiencing stress. *Family Systems Medicine*, 6, 202–237.
Reader's Digest Oxford. (1993). *Word Finder*. Oxford: Clarendon Press.
Rogers, E. M. and Sebald, H. (1962). A distinction between familism, family integration and kinship orientation. *Marriage and Family Living*, 24, 25–30.
Shah, A. M. (1973). *The Household Dimension of the Family in India*. New Delhi: Orient Longman.
Staley, J. (1982). *People in Development: A Trainer's Manual for Groups*. Bangalore: SEARCH.
Tata Institute of Social Sciences. (1999). *An Attempt to Develop Gerontological Social Work in India: A Seminar Report, The Indian Journal of Social Work*. Mumbai: Tata Institute of Social Sciences
Thompson, C. L. and Henderson, D. A. (2007). *Counseling Children*. Belmont, CA: Thomson-Brooks/Cole.
Tiny Tot Best of Moral Stories. (2002). Delhi: Tiny Tot Publications.
Tseng, W. and Hsu, J. (1991). *Culture and Family: Problems and Therapy*. New York, NY: The Haworth Press.
United Nations Children's Fund. (2001). *Pocket Guide for a Rights-Based Approach to Programming for Children: Application in South Asia*. Kathmandu: United Nations Children's Fund.
Wikipedia. (2008). *Patriarchy*. http://en.wikipedia.org/wiki/Patriarchy. Accessed 21 January 2008.
Williams, S., Seed, J. and Mwau, A. (1994). *The Oxfam Gender Training Manual*. United Kingdom: Oxfam.

Chapter 11
Parenting Education

11.1 Concepts of Parenting Education

11.1.1 Importance and Steps of Parenting Education

Parents are the primary socialising agents in a child's early life, and socialisation is the principal means for shaping the attitudes and behaviours acquired early in life that persist throughout adulthood (Zimmerman 2001). Parent education refers to a systematic and conceptually based programme, intended to impart information, awareness or skills to the participants on aspects of parenting (Fine 1980). After years of doing therapeutic work with parents, Ginott (cited by Duncan and Goddard 2005), who has carried out therapeutic work with parents for many years, noted that most parents need parenting education rather than therapy as they are only ill-informed. They should be treated as students instead of patients. Parent education should ideally be conducted for mothers and fathers and so is best conducted as evening or weekend sessions.

Ginnot (cited by Duncan and Goddard 2005) suggested four steps in the process of supporting parents: recitation, sensitisation, learning of concepts and teaching and practice of better skills.

1. *Recitation*: In this stage, parents are encouraged to talk about their challenging experiences as parents. This allows parents to discover that all parents have problems. It also allows the parenting educator to model attention, understanding and acceptance. Many parents have never had someone sensitively listen to them before. It is important for parents to feel heard and understood.
2. *Sensitisation*: After parents begin to feel accepted, valued and safe, the educator turns the attention of the parents to understanding their children's feelings.
3. *Learning of Concepts*: Parents can learn principles that will help them be more effective and apply them to situations in their homes.
4. *Teaching and Practice of Better Skills*: Participants learn how to use their new skills and get practice in applying the principles.

M. Desai, *A Rights-Based Preventative Approach for Psychosocial Well-Being in Childhood*, Children's Well-Being: Indicators and Research 3,
DOI 10.1007/978-90-481-9066-9_11,

11.1.2 Content of Parenting Education

According to Popple and Vecchiolla (2007), parenting education generally focuses on

1. Child development (what behaviours are normal at various ages),
2. Ways for parents to set goals and establish clear communication,
3. Methods of managing behaviours and
4. Discipline techniques.

A module on parenting education needs to start with life-skill enrichment of parents as individuals as discussed in the following chapters:

- Enrichment of Self-Awareness
- Enrichment of Thinking Skills
- Enrichment of Emotional Intelligence
- Enrichment of Interpersonal Relationship Skills
- Enrichment of Interpersonal Communication Skills.

It can then cover the following topics:

1. Enrichment of life skills;
2. Enrichment of marital relationship skills;
3. Awareness of child rights (covered in Chapter 2);
4. Assertive parenting skills; and
5. Age-appropriate development needs.

11.2 Marital Relationship Skills

The quality of the marital relationship of parents is an important determinant of parenting skills, especially for the parenting partnership.

11.2.1 What Is Marriage

A marriage is a legally recognised union between two people, generally a man and a woman, in which they are united sexually, cooperate economically and may give birth to, or adopt and rear children (Strong et al. 2008, p. 8). Strong et al. (2008, p. 9) observe that the following factors are common in marriages across cultures:

- It establishes rights and obligations connected to gender, sexuality, relationship with kin and in-laws and legitimacy of children.
- It allows the orderly transfer of wealth and property from one generation to the next.

11.2.2 Attachment with Parents in Infancy

Hazan and Shaver (1987, cited by Nelson-Jones 1999) suggest three styles of adult loving that depend upon styles of attachment with parents in infancy:

- Secure attachment based on a sense of confidence and security in intimacy;
- Anxious/ambivalent attachment characterised by dependency, lack of confidence in attachment and feeling unappreciated by others; and
- Avoidant attachment is characterised by lack of acceptance of others, avoidance of closeness and anxiety in intimate situations.

11.2.3 Marital Relationship Skills

A married couple needs to develop

- An identity as a married couple which defines boundaries with reference to regulating distances with others outside the marriage
- A separate and connected cohesion, retaining individual-level identity, and structure and flexibility as a couple
- Egalitarian and strengths-based perception of each other
- Acceptance and respect for and celebrating differences with one another
- Empathy and unconditional love for each other
- Assertive, open, direct and clear communication with each other
- Sensitive listening to each other
- Giving positive feedback to each other
- Requesting behaviour change to each other
- Satisfactory sexual relationship
- Joint activities
- Win–win as the goal in the relationships
- Collaborative conflict management with each other
- Partnership in parenting.

Intimacy is most important in a love relationship. According to Alberti and Emmons (1998), intimacy is a quality of relationship between two people who care deeply about each other, which is characterised by mutual attraction, open and honest communication, commitment to continuation of the partnership, enjoyment of their life together, a sense of purpose for this relationship and mutual trust which honours and respects each other. This model of intimacy embodies the idea of acceptance of self, of the partner, and of the relationship.

Darnell (2001) recommends being non-judgemental, putting others first, and expresses appreciation as necessary for learning to love the partner:

Being Non-Judgemental: Being judgemental includes our notions of good and bad, right and wrong, should and should not, which can generate considerable negative feeling and assumptions about our significant others. It can interfere with true acceptance of the other person and even of our own feelings. This does not mean that we stop discriminating whether we like or dislike what they are doing. It also does not mean becoming passive and accommodating to whatever goes on. In fact, by being non-judgemental, we feel less victimised by any aversive behaviour on their part and feel free to be more loving and more proactive when we disagree with what they are doing.

Putting Others First: We need to enjoy giving in a relationship, putting the other's needs first. However, we should not overaccommodate or overfunction simply out of habit or fear of disapproval or rejection.

Express Appreciation: Sometimes we assume that our loved ones know how we appreciate them. Sometimes we allow our frustrations to interfere with expressing our appreciation. We must let the significant other know how we appreciate them. Even if the desired outcomes do not occur, we need to acknowledge their good intentions and efforts.

Gottman (cited by Ford 2006) recommends the following seven principles for making a marriage work:

1. Enhance your love maps by continually updating your knowledge about your partner.
2. Nurture your fondness and admiration for each other.
3. Turn towards each other instead of away by staying connected.
4. Let your partner influence you.
5. Solve your solvable problems.
6. Overcome gridlock by moving to discussion.
7. Create shared meaning.

Fisher (cited by Ford 2006) offers the following suggestions for making marriages last:

- Keep infatuation alive by scheduling time together and apart.
- Approach your marriage as you would a friendship.
- Allow for the differences between men and women.
- Do not try to force your partner to change.
- Communicate by sharing thoughts and feelings.
- Be faithful.

A couple should not decide to have babies because of social pressure, a status symbol, to save the marriage or because of the love they will receive from the baby. The couple should determine their readiness for parenting in terms of biological, social and emotional and financial readiness (Mawhinney and Petersen 1990).

11.3 Assertive Parenting Skills

11.3.1 Self-Identity as Parents

Anderson and Sabatelli (2007, p. 199) note that the beginning of parenthood, rather than marriage, is the most accurate marker event for achievement of adult status in our society. Marriages can end but parenthood is life-long. When a couple moves from just a couple to a couple rearing children, the family moves from an adult-focused to a child-focused system. This change has implications for changing self-identity for parents from a spouse to a parent of young dependent children to parents of children growing towards independence. Generally, parents make these shifts depending on their observation and experience of their own parents.

With the birth of the first child, parents have to make the following changes:

1) make readjustments in the conjugal sub-system to,
2) make space for a new parenting sub-system with their children,
3) make adjustments between work and family life and
4) make readjustments in their filial system to make space for their parents' grandparental sub-system.

Collins et al. (2007) note that parents need to understand the changes needed in parental lifestyle with change in the child's developmental stage. When the children move to the stage of adolescence, parents have to make the following changes:

(1) make readjustments in their parenting sub-system to allow the adolescent children for more independence,
(2) refocus on their conjugal sub-system and career and
(3) make readjustments in their filial system accommodating for care-giving of and losing ageing parents.

11.3.2 Assertive Parenting Style

Parenting styles can be classified into passive, aggressive and assertive where assertive parents are the effective parents.

- Aggressive parents keep their children in control and end up with children who are either frightened and intimidated or rebellious and defiant.
- Passive parents allow their children to control them, devalue themselves and then lose patience with them.
- Assertive parents are clear, firm, determined and fairly confident, and relaxed (Biddulph and Biddulph 2007).

For assertive parenting style, parents need to develop

- Self-identity and self-esteem as parents
- Assertiveness as parents
- Proactive, rational, realistic, flexible, creative, self-responsible and positive thinking skills as parents
- Emotional intelligence as parents.

For assertive parenting style, parents need to develop

- Egalitarian and strengths-based perception of their child
- Sensitivity and empathy for their child
- Unconditional love for their child
- Appreciation for child's play
- Assertive communication with their child
- Skills to promote their child's life skills
- Positive disciplining their child's behaviour
- Collaborative conflict management with their child.

11.3.3 Appreciation for Child's Play

Children play because it is fun, play is child's work and it contributes to their development immensely. Parents should plan for the following range of play media that encourage the child to use and explore all developmental domains appropriate for the child's age group:

1. Real-life toys: Doll house with dolls, furniture and household items, cars, buildings, animals, medical kit, school kit, money and so on.
2. Creative expression and emotional release media: Chalks and blackboards, crayons, paints, brushes, white and coloured paper, scissors, puppets, clay, sand tray and so on.
3. Acting-out and aggressive-release media: Inflatable punching toy, pounding bench and so on (Barlow et al. 1985, cited by Thompson and Henderson 2007).
4. Story books and games (Geldard and Geldard 2002).

While selecting the media:

- Focus on the features of the play and not on the features of the toy.
- Select toys that let the child tell his/her story (Daswani 2007).

Parents need to

- Encourage children to play, laugh and use their imaginations.
- Respect playtime and its rituals as much as the other routines.

- Let the child select the game to play.
- Let them get dirty in the sand, water, water colours and so on.
- Let them teach you how to use their toys.
- Show them what and how they played as a child.
- Many everyday objects, if safe, can become the toy of the moment.
- Children need time for self-initiated play (Daswani 2007).

11.3.4 Assertive Communication with the Child

11.3.4.1 Problems in Communication

According to Gordon (2000), parents tend to use the following verbal messages to children when they come to them with feelings or problems:

- Judging, criticising, disagreeing, blaming
- Ordering, directing, commanding
- Warning, admonishing, threatening
- Exhorting, moralising, preaching
- Advising, giving solutions
- Lecturing, teaching, giving logical arguments
- Name-calling, ridiculing, shaming
- Interpreting, analysing, diagnosing
- Withdrawing, distracting, humouring, diverting
- Questioning, interrogating.

These responses make the child "hear" the following about his/her thought processes:

- You do not take me seriously.
- You do not think my judgement is legitimate.
- You do not trust me to work out this problem myself.
- You think I am doing something bad or wrong (adapted from Gordon 2000).

These responses make the child "hear" the following about his/her feelings:

- You do not care about how I feel.
- You do not think my feelings are important.
- You do not accept my feeling the way I do (adapted from Gordon 2000).

Children's reactions to these messages therefore are

- They stop talking.
- They become defensive.
- They argue/counterattack.
- They feel inferior/guilty (adapted from Gordon 2000).

11.3.4.2 Positive Communication

Parents need to use the following skills:

- Assertive, open, direct and clear communication with their children
- Sensitive listening to their children
- Giving positive feedback to their children
- Giving negative feedback to their children.

When children talk, parents need to listen to them actively and ask questions in order to understand their thoughts and feelings and give feedback that conveys acceptance and respect. This approach conveys the following to the child:

- Your ideas are worthy of being listened to.
- I want to hear your point of view.
- I want to know you better.
- You have a right to express the way you feel (adapted from Gordon 2000).

According to Miller (2007), children need to feel affirmation, affection and acceptance through unconditional positive regard in the following ways:

- Affirmation for being: I am glad you are who you are.
- Affirmation for becoming independent: It is okay to try new things on your own.
- Affirmation for learning to Think: It is okay to make mistakes as long as you accept responsibility for making amends.
- Affirmation for developing an individual identity: You can express your own thoughts and feelings without fear of rejection, it is okay to disagree.

Active listening:

- Fosters catharsis.
- Helps child be less afraid of negative feelings.
- Promotes a relationship of warmth between parents and child.
- Facilitates problem solving by the child.
- Influences the child to be more willing to listen to the parents' thoughts and ideas (adapted from Gordon 2000).

Miller (2007) recommends the following for assertive communication:

- Use of simple language and short statements is effective.
- Honesty is essential even about sad events.
- Directness or getting right to the point is essential.
- Tact keeps channels of communication open.
- Concreteness makes communication clear.
- Respect is an integrated part of assertive communication.
- Optimism boosts cooperation by sharing hope.

- Flexibility is necessary to distinguish assertiveness from stubbornness.
- Confidence strengthens assertive communication by projecting assurance that what is being said is really meant.
- Persistence conveys that we really mean what we say.
- Assertiveness with empathy is strength and love rolled into one.

11.3.5 Developing Child's Life Skills

11.3.5.1 Build Self-Esteem in the Child

Parents need to encourage the child to develop self-esteem by

- Praising the child when he does something well.
- Rewarding efforts and small steps and not just success.
- Avoiding praising only perfection (Marion 2007).

11.3.5.2 Develop Child's Emotional Intelligence

For development of child's emotional intelligence parents need to

- Teach children to use words to describe their emotions.
- Create a safe emotional climate to talk about negative and positive emotions (Marion 2007).

11.3.5.3 Promote Children's Independence in Problem Solving

Parents need to help their child move from dependence to independence to interdependence with the parents and other people. Gordon (2000) notes that all children have mostly untapped potential for finding good solutions for the problems they face so parents should let children own their problems and find their own solutions. If parents hand them pre-packaged solutions children remain dependant and fail to develop their own problem-solving skills. Instead of taking over their children's problems and come up with solutions, they should be facilitators or catalysts or helping agents, helping the child work through the problem-solving process on his/her own (Gordon 2000).

11.3.6 Positive Disciplining of the Child

11.3.6.1 History of Disciplining Methods

Biddulph and Biddulph (2007) trace the following history of disciplining methods used by parents:

- *Hitting and Hurting* made children fearful or broken spirited or they became angrier and hit back. Children learn that it is okay to hit if you are bigger.
- *Shaming and Blaming* took the place of hitting and hurting which resulted in a damaged self and children became what they were called.
- *Rewards and Consequences* with reference to star charts, pocket money and bearing the natural consequences work but not enough.
- *Time Out* or sending the children to their room to cool off works as it gives time for parents to cool off too. However, it does not involve thinking about change.
- *Stand and Think* is a thinking and teaching method of disciplining where the indiscipline is dealt with.

According to Miller (2007), punishment is intended to retaliate or pay a child back for something he/she has done. It is used to bully or coerce children into behaving the way we want them to behave. Biddulph and Biddulph (2007) give the following explanation for why parents put children down:

- You repeat what was said to you
- You just thought it was the right thing to do
- You are stressed out.

11.3.6.2 Positively Dealing with the Child's Problem Behaviour

Biddulph and Biddulph (2007) recommend the following "Not to Dos" with children:

- Do not use put-downs
- Do not compare
- Never talk to other people about children's faults in their presence or hearing
- Do not use guilt to control children.

Marion (2007) recommends the following positive discipline strategies:

- Help children save face and preserve their dignity.
- Set the expectations for desired behaviour clarifying boundaries or limits.
- Encourage positive behaviours and deemphasise negative behaviours.
- Give meaningful feedback to children.
- Redirect very young children from a forbidden or dangerous activity.

According to Marion (2007, p. 280), children manifest behaviour problems when their following needs are not met:

- Feeling of being loved and appreciated
- Feeling of being safe and secure

- Exercise and physical activity
- Sound sleep and rest and play
- Adequate nutrition, including enough water
- Basic medical care

Miller (2007) identifies the following reasons for children's problem behaviour which can be prevented:

- Inappropriate expectations
- Misunderstanding expectations
- Immature self-control
- Boredom, fatigue and discomfort
- Desire for recognition and discouragement
- Frustration and rebellion

According to Miller (2007), mildly annoying behaviour that is neither harmful nor unfair can be ignored in the following ways:

- Focus attention elsewhere.
- Discreetly redirect to more positive substitute behaviour.
- Assist the child in recognising the general effects of positive behaviours.

Miller (2007) recommends that child's harmful or unfair behaviour needs to be immediately interrupted in the following ways:

- Redirect inappropriate behaviour firmly and respectfully.
- Explain the potential consequences of unacceptable behaviour.
- Emphasise unconditional caring and affection.
- Maintain and express confidence that a problem will be resolved.
- Protect children's dignity and privacy.

Grunwald and McAbee (1985, cited by Collins et al. 2007) recommend the following principles of natural and logical consequences:

- The consequences should be directly related to the behaviour.
- The consequence should be meaningful to the child.
- The consequence of the behaviour should be known ahead of time.
- The child should be aware that there is a choice between appropriate behaviour and behaviour that will lead to negative consequences.

11.4 Age-Appropriate Development Interventions

Developmental psychologists have defined developmental needs by age groups.

11.4.1 Development Needs in Infancy

Age Group: Birth to one and half years.

Developmental Tasks: The main developmental tasks in infancy are:

1. Satisfaction of the sensory-motor needs.
2. Satisfaction of the oral needs.
3. Development of trust in their parents and environment and learn that the world is safe, consistent and predictable (adapted from Thompson and Henderson 2007).

Intervention Needed: To achieve these tasks in infancy parenting education is needed on:

1. Giving importance to breast-feeding and supplementary diet and nutrition.
2. Providing safe, responsive, affectionate and consistent care-giving in infancy (adapted from Thompson and Henderson 2007). O'Connell et al. (2005) recommend that in infancy, parents may communicate love and tenderness via all the child's senses:
   (a) Communicating through the sense of touch by hugging, cuddling and rocking
   (b) Communicating through the visual (care-giver's face) and taste senses (milk)
   (c) Communicating through the sense of hearing by talking, singing and story-telling

11.4.2 Development Needs in Toddlerhood

Age Group: One and half to 3 years

Developmental Tasks: The main developmental tasks in toddlerhood are

1. Satisfaction of the sensory-motor needs through handling of objects.
2. Satisfactory toilet training.
3. Gaining a sense of self-control as well as control over their environment (adapted from Thompson and Henderson 2007).

Intervention Needed: To achieve these tasks in toddlerhood parenting education is needed on

1. Allowing children to experience success in doing things for themselves.
2. Providing satisfactory toilet training without giving the child a sense of shame.
3. Disciplining children without giving them a sense of shame and doubt (adapted from Thompson and Henderson 2007).

11.4.3 Development Needs in Preschoolage

Age Group: 3–6 years

Developmental Tasks: The main developmental tasks in the preschoolage are

1. Development of skills in the areas of language, numbers, classification and interrelationships,
2. Social development,
3. Development of a sexual identity and
4. Development of a sense of initiative as opposed to feelings of guilt about never doing anything right (adapted from Thompson and Henderson 2007).

Intervention Needed: To achieve these tasks in preschoolage parenting education is needed on

1. Providing opportunities to develop language, numbers, classification and interrelationships, social development and development of a sexual identity through preschool education.
2. Allowing children's initiatives, give them choices and encourage them to participate in family activities.
3. Having realistic expectations in order to prevent guilt (adapted from Thompson and Henderson 2007).
4. Free play in this age group is important for learning the tasks of autonomy and initiative (O'Connell et al. 2005).

11.4.4 Development Needs in Middle Childhood

Age Group: 6–12 years

Developmental Tasks: The main developmental tasks in the middle childhood are

1. Development of ego and superego and
2. Learning a range of academic, social, physical and practical skills needed in an adult world (adapted from Thompson and Henderson 2007).

Intervention Needed: To achieve these tasks in middle childhood:

- Parenting education is needed on meeting the needs of children in middle childhood and
- Children should be provided with PEG programmes on psychosocial skills and skills of interaction with the environment.

11.4.5 Developmental Needs in Adolescence

Age Group: 12–18 years

Developmental Tasks: The main developmental tasks in the adolescence are

1. Understanding of sexuality and
2. Development of a self-identity and the direction of how it fits into their future (adapted from Thompson and Henderson 2007).

Intervention Needed: To achieve these tasks in early adolescence:

- Children should be provided with development programmes on sexual rights and responsibilities, enrichment of vocational selection and awareness of citizens' rights and responsibilities and
- Parenting education is needed on meeting the needs of children in adolescence.

References

Alberti, R. and Emmons, M. (1998). *Complete Guide to Assertive Living*. Mumbai: Jaico Publishing House.

Anderson, S. A. and Sabatelli, R. M. (2007). *Family Interaction: A Multigenerational Developmental Perspective* (4th ed.). Boston, MA: Pearson.

Biddulph, S. and Biddulph, S. (2007). *The Complete Secrets of Happy Children*. Sydney: Harper Collins Publishers.

Collins, D., Jordan, C. and Coleman, H. (2007). *An Introduction to Family Social Work* (2nd ed.) Southbank, VIC: Brooks/Cole.

Darnell, D. (2001). *Learning to Love*. University of New York at Chapel Hill, Counselling and Psychological Service.

Daswani, S. (2007). Parental Involvement in Children's Play. In K. P. Nonis and S. Daswani (Eds.) *The Power of Movement: How to Enhance Children's Cognitive, Social, Emotional and Physical Development* (pp. 1–14). Singapore: Prentice Hall.

Duncan, S. F. and Goddard, H. W. (2005). *Family Life Education: Principles and Practices for Effective Outreach*. Thousand Oaks, CA: Sage.

Fine, M. J. (1980). The Parent Education Movement: An Introduction. In M. J. Fine (Ed.) *Handbook on Parent Education* (pp. 3–27). New York: Academic Press.

Ford, L. (2006). *Human Relations: A Game Plan for Improving Personal Adjustment*. (4th ed.). Upper Saddle River, NJ: Prentice Hall.

Geldard, K. and Geldard, D. (2002). *Counselling Children: A Practical Introduction*. London: Sage.

Gordon, T. (2000). *Parent Effectiveness Training: The Proven Program for Raising Responsible Children*. New York: Three Rivers Press.

Marion, M. (2007). *Guidance of Young Children* (7th ed.). Upper Saddle River, NJ: Pearson/Merrill/Prentice Hall.

Mawhinney, V. T. and Petersen, C. J. (1990). *Child Development: Parenting and Teaching* (2nd ed.). Cincinnati, OH: South-Western Publishing Co.

Miller, D. F. (2007). *Positive Child Guidance* (5th ed.). Southbank, VIC: Thomson.

Nelson-Jones, R. (1999). *Creating Happy Relationships*. London: Continuum.

O'Connell, A., O'Connel, V. and Kuntz, L. A. (2005). *Choice and Change: The Psychology of Personal Growth and Interpersonal Relationships* (7th ed.). Upper Saddle River, NJ: Prentice Hall.

Popple, P. R. and Vecchiolla, F. (2007). *Child Welfare Social Work: An Introduction*. Boston: Pearson Allyn and Bacon.

Strong, B., DeVault, C. and Cohen, T. F. (2008). *The Marriage and Family Experience: Intimate Relationships in a Changing Society* (10th ed.). Belmont, CA: Wadsworth.

Thompson, C. L. and Henderson, D. A. (2007). *Counseling Children*. Southbank, VIC and Belmont, CA: Thomson/Brooks/Cole.

Zimmerman, S. L. (2001). *Family Policy: Constructed Solutions to Family Problems*. London: Sage.

Part III
Secondary and Tertiary Prevention for Psychosocial Well-Being in Childhood

Introduction to Part III

Introduction to Secondary Prevention

Secondary prevention is prevention of neglect of children in at-risk situations due to individual, parental or situational characteristics.

Goals of Secondary Prevention of Neglect in Childhood

Secondary prevention may aim at the following goals:

- Prevention of vulnerability of children in at-risk situations to neglect, abuse and commercial exploitation,
- Promotion of their psychosocial well-being,
- Promotion of their age-appropriate developmental opportunities and
- Promotion of their rights to family care, development, participation and protection.

Interventions for Secondary Prevention

Secondary prevention of neglect of children in at-risk situations may be achieved through the following interventions with them and their families:

- Case management:
  - Direct intervention for giving information and advice, teaching and training in psychosocial skills and counselling
  - Linking with natural support systems, self-help groups, flexitime supplementary childcare and other formal systems of state and voluntary organisations

- Psycho-educational group work: In psycho-educational group work at this level also, children and their families are treated as students who are learning rather than patients who need to be treated.

These children should be prevented from entering the juvenile justice system.

Introduction to Tertiary Prevention

Tertiary prevention is prevention of abuse, commercial exploitation and conflict with law in childhood through the juvenile justice system and through the substitute childcare systems if necessary.

Goals of Tertiary Prevention of Abuse and Commercial Exploitation in Childhood

Tertiary prevention of abuse and commercial exploitation in childhood may aim at the following goals:

1. Prevention of
    - Further abuse and commercial exploitation of the same children,
    - Effects of abuse and commercial exploitation on mental and physical health of children,
    - Abused and commercially exploited children facing conflict with law and
    - The cycle of abuse by preventing the survivors of abuse and commercial exploitation growing up to be offenders of children as adults;
2. Promotion of their psychosocial well-being;
3. Promotion of their age-appropriate developmental opportunities; and
4. Promotion of their rights to family care, development, participation and protection.

Goals of Tertiary Prevention of Conflict with Law in Childhood

Tertiary prevention of conflict with law in childhood may aim at the following goals:

1. Prevention of
    - First-time offence leading to more offences
    - Status offence leading to property crime, and
    - Property crimes leading to violent crimes;
2. Prevention of their vulnerability, neglect, abuse and commercial exploitation;

3. Promotion of their psychosocial well-being;
4. Promotion of their age-appropriate developmental opportunities; and
5. Promotion of their rights to family care, development, participation and protection.

Systems and Interventions for Tertiary Prevention

The existing systems for tertiary prevention of abuse, commercial exploitation and conflict with law in childhood are the juvenile justice system and substitute childcare such as foster family care, child adoption and institutional childcare, often working independently. The rights-based preventative approach for children's psychosocial well-being requires that

1. The juvenile justice system should be used only for restorative justice to children facing abuse and commercial exploitation and for children who have harmed others.
2. Children should be removed from their homes for placement in the appropriate substitute childcare only if the family preservation services fail and only though the juvenile justice system.

Tertiary prevention may be achieved by carrying out the following interventions with them and their families:

- Case management:
  - Advocacy intervention for restorative justice through the juvenile justice system
  - Linking with natural support systems, self-help groups, integrated supplementary and substitute childcare and other formal systems of state and voluntary organisations
  - Direct intervention for giving information and advice, teaching and training in psychosocial skills and counselling
- Psycho-educational group work

In psycho-educational group work at this level also, children and their families are treated as students who are learning rather than patients who need to be treated.

Teaching–Learning Objectives

Part III focuses on the rights-based secondary prevention of neglect of children at risk situations and tertiary prevention of abuse, commercial exploitation and conflict with law in childhood. The teaching–learning objectives for this Part are to

1. Learn to carry out the stages of casework process and conduct case management with children and their families with reference to direct work and system linkage;
2. Examine the types, causes and consequences of situations where children are at risk of neglect, including the emergency situations, and learn to carry out rights-based intervention with them for secondary prevention;
3. Learn to carry out child advocacy interventions for restorative justice in the juvenile justice system for tertiary prevention;
4. Learn to carry out rights-based placement of children in foster family care, child adoption and institutional childcare, aiming at tertiary prevention;
5. Examine the types, causes and consequences of abuse and commercial exploitation in childhood, and learn to carry out rights-based intervention for tertiary prevention; and
6. Examine the types, causes and consequences of conflict with law in childhood and learn to carry out rights-based intervention for tertiary prevention.

Chapter Plan

The Chapter Plan of Part III is therefore as follows:

12. Process of Casework with Children and their Families
13. Case Management with Children and Their Families
14. Children at Risk of Neglect and Secondary Prevention
15. Children in Emergency Situations and Secondary Prevention
16. Systems for Tertiary Prevention for Children
17. Abuse in Childhood and Tertiary Prevention
18. Commercial Exploitation in Childhood and Tertiary Prevention
19. Conflict with Law in Childhood and Tertiary Prevention

Tutorial Plans

Case Discussions

1. Eight small groups may be formed to take responsibility to plan and coordinate a tutorial session for each of the following topics.

    (1) Process of Casework with Children and Their Families
    (2) Case Management with Children and Their Families
    (3) Children at Risk of Neglect and Secondary Prevention
    (4) Children in Emergency Situations and Secondary Prevention
    (5) Systems for Tertiary Prevention for Children
    (6) Abuse in Childhood and Tertiary Prevention
    (7) Commercial Exploitation in Childhood and Tertiary Prevention
    (8) Conflict with Law in Childhood and Tertiary Prevention

2. Each small group may prepare a plan to demonstrate and plan the other students' implementation of the application of theories to case situations by

   a. reading the relevant Lecture Notes, Textbooks, and supplementary books and
   b. viewing the relevant Audio-Visuals from the Library if available,
   c. in consultation with the Professor.

3. The tutorial plan may be prepared in the following format.

   - Name of the Tutorial Session
   - Names of Student Members
   - Tutorial Objectives
   - Tutorial Schedule (to include activities, names of students who will carry them out, feedback on the activities and time estimate)
   - Plan for Demonstration of a Case by the Planning Group
   - Case Studies for the Other Groups

4. After the tutorial the report of the tutorial may be submitted in the same format, with an additional paint of 'Self-Learning of the Planning Group'.

Visits

1. Make visits in small groups to the following child welfare/protection organisations in their city:

   - Juvenile/Children's Court
   - Foster Family Care Project
   - Child Adoption Agency
   - Children's Institution
   - Government Department of Child Welfare/Protection

2. Take permission from the social worker and the client to make observations on psychosocial intervention and/or case management meetings carried out by the social worker.
3. Write individual reports on the organisation and the observations made.
4. Make a group presentation to the larger class through role-plays.

Recommended Reading

Copen, L. M. (2000). *Preparing Children for Court: A Practitioner's Guide*. Thousand Oaks, CA: Sage.

Downs, S. W., Moore, E. and McFadden, E. J. (2009). *Child Welfare and Family Services: Policies and Practice* (8th ed.). Boston, MA: Pearson Allyn and Bacon.

Doyle, C. (2006). *Working with Abused Children: From Theory to Practice* (3rd ed.). Basingstoke and New York: Palgrave Macmillan.

Hepworth, D. H., Rooney, R. H., Rooney, G. D., Strom-Gottfried, K. and Larson, J. A. (2006). *Direct Social Work Practice: Theory and Skills* (7th ed.). Belmont, NY: Thomson Higher Education.

Hess, K. M. and Drowns, R. W. (2004). *Juvenile Justice*. Southbank, VIC: Thomson Wadsworth.

Kadushin, A. and Martin, J. A. (1988). *Child Welfare Services* (4th ed.). New York, NY: Macmillan.

Popple, P. R. and Vecchiolla, F. (2007). *Child Welfare Social Work: An Introduction*. Boston, MA: Pearson Allyn and Bacon.

Rose, S. R. and Fatout, M. F. (2003). *Social Work Practice with Children and Adolescents*. Boston, MA: Pearson Education, Inc.

Save the Children. (2005). *The Right not to Lose Hope: Children in Conflict with the Law*. London: Save the Children.

Thompson, C. L. and Henderson, D. A. (2007). *Counseling Children*. South Melbourne, VIC and Belmont, CA: Thomson/Brooks/Cole.

United Nations Children's Fund and International Social Service. (2004). *Care for Children in Emergency Situations: Implications for International Standards*. New York, NY and Geneva: United Nations Children's Fund and International Social Service.

Wilson, C. and Powell, M. (2001). *A Guide to Interviewing Children: Essential Skills for Counsellors, Police, Lawyers and Social Workers*. London: Routledge.

Chapter 12
Process of Casework with Children and Their Families

12.1 Concepts of Process of Casework

The process of casework is a problem-solving process. This process may be blocked by a number of factors, including lack of knowledge, inadequate resources or experiencing emotional responses that impair the ability to solve the problem (Turner and Jaco 1996, cited by Rose and Fatout 2003). The problem-solving method requires realistic, proactive, rational, creative and positive thinking skills. Following are the steps recommended for problem solving:

1. Identify the real problem and not just its symptoms;
2. Understand one's perception, opinions, feelings and action about the problem;
3. Explore alternatives for the solution to the problem;
4. Select the best solution with reference to the following criteria:
    - the resources/capacity that one has to implement each alternative and
    - the advantages and disadvantages that each alternative may lead to with reference to self and others.
5. Make a commitment to implement the solution selected and take responsibility for its consequences;
6. Monitor the consequences of implementation of the solution; and
7. If the first solution fails, learn lessons from it and rethink the solution as a circular process.

The casework process is a continuous and integrated series of purposeful activities with the client. This process comprises of stages of intake and engagement, assessment, planning, implementation, evaluation and termination, used by the worker in a spiral-like manner (Compton et al. 2005).

M. Desai, *A Rights-Based Preventative Approach for Psychosocial Well-Being in Childhood*, Children's Well-Being: Indicators and Research 3,
DOI 10.1007/978-90-481-9066-9_12,

12.2 Interview with Children and Their Families

12.2.1 Social Work Interview

According to Kadushin and Kadushin (1997), an interview is a dyadic or group conversation with a deliberate purpose that the participants accept. So

1. The interviewer selects the content to facilitate it's achievements. The content of the interview is likely to have unity, a progression and thematic continuity.
2. One person has to take responsibility for directing the interaction so that it moves towards the goal. One person is designated as an interviewer and the other interviewee. The role relationships are structured.
3. The relationship between the interviewer and the interviewee is not reciprocal.
4. The actions of the interviewer must be planned deliberate and consciously selected to further the purpose of the interview.
5. The interviewer has an obligation to maintain contact until the purpose is achieved.
6. An interview requires exclusive attention to the interaction.
7. The interview is generally a formally arranged meeting.
8. Interviewee participants usually differ in terms of background, experience and lifestyle.
9. Interviewing in social work is the skill of facilitating disclosure of personal information for professional purposes.
10. Interviewing speech seeks to be more formal, precise, structured, explicit and organised.
11. The interviewer has to record what went on during the interview in order to make subsequent use of it in helping the interviewee.

As dialogues, social work interviews have the following four requirements according to Egan (2002):

- Turn Taking: Dialogue is interactive.
- Connecting: What each person says should be connected in some way to what the other person is saying.
- Mutual Influencing: Each party should be open to being influenced by what the other person says.
- Co-creating Outcomes: Good dialogue leads to outcomes that benefit both parties.

As the social work interview is concerned with problems relating to how clients deal with their social environment, it differs from other kinds of interviews in that it is apt to be diffuse, not standardised, interviewee controlled, with no set agenda, focused on affective material and concerned with the interpersonal interaction of the participants. As a result, social workers generally cannot determine in advance much of what they have to do in the interview; they must respond to the situation as it develops. The general purposes of most social work interviews are informational, assessment and therapeutic. The same interview often serves more than one purpose (Kadushin and Kadushin 1997).

12.2.2 Interview Setting

The case worker's office should be planned for privacy and as a friendly, comfortable, relaxed and a safe place for the interview with the child (Thompson and Henderson 2007).

12.2.2.1 Desk

Direct intervention with the child seems to work better if he/she can control the distance between him/her and the counsellor. Having a desk between the two creates formal distance and having no desk between the two creates an intimidating feeling. A better arrangement is using the corner of a desk as an optional barrier that allows the child to retreat behind the desk corner or to move around the corner when he or she feels comfortable doing so (Thompson and Henderson 2007).

12.2.2.2 Play Media

The social worker should be prepared with activities, toys and settings that will be interesting, engaging and developmentally appropriate for the child (Dishion and Stormshak 2007). The following range of play media appropriate for different age groups could be selected and displayed in the office:

1. Real-life toys: Doll house with dolls, furniture and household items, cars, buildings, animals, medical kit, money and so on.
2. Creative expression and emotional release media: Chalks and blackboards, crayons, paints, brushes, white and coloured paper, scissors, puppets, clay, sand tray and so on.
3. Acting-out and aggressive-release media: Punching toy, pounding bench and so on.
4. Story books and games (Geldard and Geldard 2002).

While selecting the media:

- Focus on the features of the play and not on the features of the toy.
- Select toys that let the child tell his/her story (Daswani 2007).

12.2.3 Planning an Interview

Adequate ventilation and light, comfortable room temperature, sufficient space, chairs that adequately support the back, privacy, freedom from distraction and open space between participants are necessary for productive interviews (Hepworth et al. 2006).

According to Sheafor and Horejsi (2006), just as there should be an overall intervention plan, there should be a plan for each interview with the client, with reference to the overall plan. This plan must be tentative and flexible in order to respond to client concerns that could not be anticipated. It should include

- The goals of the interview,
- Who needs to be present,
- Face-to-face or telephone mode,
- One-on-one, family or group session,
- Time needed,
- Where and when and arrangements to be made,
- Techniques to be used,
- Factors related to the client's emotional and physical state, values and religious beliefs and social and family network to be considered,
- Need for documentation.

12.2.4 Interview Transitions

Shebib (2003) identifies the following types of interview transitions:

- Natural transitions take place as the discussion flows seamlessly from one topic to another.
- Strategic transitions take place when worker makes choices among topic alternatives.
- Control transitions are used to manage the direction of the interview.
- Phase transitions bridge the work of one phase to another.
- Connect (Linking) transitions are used to join or blend ideas.

Kadushin and Kadushin (1997) provide the following guidelines for transitions:

- Planning a transition involves a decision about why this transition would further the interview's objective.
- Having decided that a transition is necessary, be sensitive to a point in the interaction that would be appropriate for introducing the transition.
- Prepare the interviewee for your intention to make a transition.
- If the reasons for the transition are not obvious, explain the rationale.

- Make the transition in a manner that is the least disruptive for the flow of the interview.
- Do not impose the transition if the interviewee signals a lack of readiness to make the change.

12.2.5 Summarising

According to Shebib (2003), summarising is an active interviewing skill that can serve a number of purposes:

- It is a way of confirming understanding and checking assumptions.
- It is a way or organising complex data and content by tying disjointed but related ideas together.
- It can be helpful in working with clients who are overly verbose, are prone to introduce irrelevant material, or wander from topic to topic.

According to Egan (2002), summarising proves particularly useful at the beginning of a new session when a session seems to be going nowhere and when a client gets stuck.

12.3 Initial Stages of Casework with Children and Their Families

In order to implement appropriate casework with children and their families, it is important to first go through the initial stages of intake and engagement, assessment and planning.

12.3.1 Engagement

12.3.1.1 General

The first stage of casework process is intake and engagement. According to Hull and Kirst-Ashman (2004), engagement focuses on establishing a professional relationship between the worker and the client, which is characterised by a clear purpose, a commitment to meeting client needs, ethical standards of practice and worker emphasis on communicating warmth, genuineness and empathy. The latter is important for building and rapport and trust and can be conveyed by

- Greeting clients in such a way as to encourage them to talk. While greeting the clients, it is important to extend the courtesy of asking the clients how they prefer to be addressed (Hepworth et al. 2006).
- Demonstrating effective attending skills that communicate your interest in the client's situation.

12.3.1.2 Engagement with Parents

Before beginning to work individually with the child, it is generally useful to consult with the parents without the child being present. They also need to be told that the social worker will develop an exclusive relationship with the child which is not influenced by the parents (Geldard and Geldard 2002). Dishion and Stormshak (2007, pp. 80–82) offer the following basic initial interviewing strategies that specifically address the emotional issues of seeking help for parenting:

- Support parents' strengths and efforts.
- Paraphrase parents' concerns and show empathy and understanding of the history and ecology of the problem.
- Reflect discrepancies of conflicting and competing emotions.
- Link concerns to assessment.
- Frame the situation optimistically.
- Normalise problems by sharing that there are others who share the same issues and struggles.

12.3.1.3 Engagement with Children

Children may start with the fear of the unknown and may resist by

- Refusing to talk/share, deny that there is a problem.
- Avoid eye contact.
- Come late or miss appointments.
- Exhibit negative body language (Thompson and Henderson 2007).

As the primary goal during the engagement stage is building rapport and trust, the social worker may do the following:

- Articulate the nature of the social worker's relationship with the child with reference to helping the child.
- Follow the child's lead in beginning the "getting to know you" process and not start by asking about his or her problem or other personal questions.
- Invite the child to select and get engaged with the toy, media, story book or game that he/she finds interesting (adapted from Dishion and Stormshak 2007, p. 83).

According to Geldard and Geldard (2002, pp. 12–16), the child–counsellor relationship should be purposeful, exclusive, safe, authentic, confidential and non-intrusive, as discussed below.

Purposeful Relationship: Children need to know the exact purpose of meeting the counsellor. The counsellor should therefore know what information the child has been given before the first session and clarify, affirm or correct perceptions about what will happen.

Exclusive Relationship: The social worker should develop an exclusive relationship with the child which is not influenced by others, mainly the parents.

Safe Relationship: In order to give the child a sense of security and predictability, a structure is important which includes

- Giving the information about the expected length of each session and
- Setting behavioural limits to protect the child, the counsellor and property from damage.

Authentic Relationship: The child–counsellor relationship should be a genuine and honest relationship which allows the child to be natural and spontaneous.

Confidential Relationship: The exclusive relationship has to respect confidentiality. The child should be ensured that the fears, anxieties and negative thoughts towards parents or others will not be disclosed to them without the child's permission. The child should have control over factors such as who will tell whom and when. This will make the child feel safe in making disclosures.

Non-intrusive Relationship: Too many questions should not be asked to disclose information which is private and scary to share, as it may be intrusive and may silence the child.

12.3.1.4 Engagement with Families

When it is necessary to engage the whole family, Hepworth, et al. (2006) recommend that the social worker should meet the following objectives:

- Establish a personal relationship with individual members and an alliance with the family as a group.
- Clarify expectations and explore reservations about the helping process.
- Clarify roles and the nature of the helping process.
- Clarify choices about participation in the helping process.
- Elicit the family's perception of the problem.
- Identify needs and wants of family members.
- Define the problem as a family problem.
- Emphasise individual and family strengths.
- Ask questions to elicit information about the patterned behaviours of the family.
- Draw the family's attention to repetitive communications and discuss whether they wish to change these patterns.
- Begin assisting members to relate to one another in more positive ways.
- Establish individual and family goals.
- Gauge motivation of family members to return for future sessions and negotiate a contract.
- Negotiate tasks to be accomplished during the week.

- Families can develop their own sets of indicators for desirable behaviour change.
- End the session by summarising problems discussed, goals formulated and progress achieved.

The social worker will often encounter a persistent tendency of some members to blame others. The worker's tasks in this situation are twofold:

1. Ensure that you do not collude with family members in labelling others as problems.
2. Model the circular orientation to causality of behaviour and emphasise that family members reciprocally influence one another in ways that perpetuate patterns of behaviour (Hepworth et al. 2006).

According to Kilpatrick and Holland (2006), the process of preparing the family for success can be initiated by

1. Defining all members in the family as being hurt by their circumstance and that blaming will not solve the problem.
2. Normalising the family problem, by conveying that all families have problems and families in similar situations have been successful in overcoming their conflicts.
3. Emphasising the family's strengths and positive motivation, the fact that they have attended a session shows that they still have some concern for their family and hold some hope for change.

12.3.2 Assessment

12.3.2.1 General

In casework, assessment involves acquiring an understanding of the problem, what causes it and what can be changed to minimise or resolve it (Barker 1999, cited by Kirst-Ashman and Hull 2006). Kirst-Ashman and Hull (2006) emphasise the following in assessment:

- Involvement of the client is essential.
- Highlighting strengths makes assessment different from diagnosis.
- It is a continuous activity.
- It involves judgement through critical thinking skills.

12.3.2.2 Assessing the Problem

Initial Issues: According to Hepworth et al. (2006), initially three issues should be assessed in all situations:

- What does the client see as his or her primary problems or concerns? Start where the client is.
- What (if any) potentially serious health or safety concerns might require the social worker's and client's attention? Assessment of the severity of the problems is necessary to determine whether clients have the capacity to continue functioning in the community or whether strong supportive or protective measures are needed.
- What (if any) current or impending legal mandates must the client and the worker consider?

Self-Assessment: Children/Parents' self-assessment of the problem provides an opportunity to the social worker to

- Appreciate their approach to behaviour change.
- Assess their level of insight.
- Learn more about the dynamics of the family (adapted from Dishion and Stormshak 2007, pp. 116–117).

The child will have a personal perception of themselves and their problem which will not be the same as the parents' perception. The child may be invited to tell his/her story for which verbal communication alone will not be adequate. Inviting them to tell their story through the use of play or other suitable media may be preferable especially when children have poor communication skills or high levels of emotional distress (Geldard and Geldard 2002).

According to Boyden and Levison (2000), social meanings have a very important bearing, in that the effects of adversity on children are determined not simply by the objective nature of the situation or event so much as by children's subjective experience of that situation. They also emphasised the significance of children's own ideas about their circumstances since these fundamentally influence children's responses. In other words, potentially hazardous or stressful situations normally present far less risk to children when they are culturally endorsed, for example, child marriage and child labour in the family occupation.

Description of the Problem: Other aspects considered important in understanding the problem by Hepworth et al. (2006) are listed below:

- Site, temporal context, severity and frequency of problematic behaviours
- Duration of the problem
- Exception or when the current concern did not exist
- Client's emotional reactions to the problem
- Coping effort and the resources and strengths that clients have used previously when dealing with issues.
- Needs based on life stage and stresses based on life transitions

Problems as Violation of Child Rights: Children's problems can be assessed as violation of their following child rights:

- Child right to family care
- Child right to development
- Child right to participation
- Child right to protection

12.3.2.3 Assessing the Strengths

Saleeby (2006) recommends exploring strengths in the following:

- Personal qualities, traits and virtues that people possess: A sense of humour, caring, creativity, loyalty, insight, independence, spirituality, moral imagination, patience and so on (Wolin and Wolin 1983, cited by Saleeby 2006).
- The talents that people have are as follows: Playing a musical instrument, telling stories, cooking, home repair, writing, carpentry and so on.

According to Saleeby (2006), to discover strengths in the clients, the following kinds of questions can be asked

- *Survival questions*: How have you managed to survive thus far, given all the challenges you have had to contend with? What have you learnt about yourself and about your world during your struggles? What strengths, insights or skills have you gained? People do not just learn from successes, they also learn from their difficulties and disappointments.
- *Support questions*: What people have given you special understanding, support and guidance? Cultural stories, narratives and myths, accounts of origins and migrations or trauma and survival may also provide sources of meaning and inspiration in times of difficulty or confusion.
- *Exception questions*: When things were going well, what was different? What parts of your world and your being would you like to recapture, reinvent or relive?
- *Possibility questions*: What are your hopes, visions and aspirations? What personal qualities and people are helping you move in this direction?
- *Esteem questions*: When people say good things about you what are they likely to say?
- *Perspective questions*: What are your ideas or theories about your current situation?
- *Change questions*: What are your ideas about how things might change? What has worked in the past to being about a better life for yourself?

12.3.2.4 Comprehensive Assessment

1. Preliminary Demographic Information:

   - Age-based developmental needs
   - Sex
   - Ethnic background
   - Education
   - Household composition and socio-economic status through a household grid

2. Assessment of the Problem from the Child's and the Parents' Points of View:

   - Perception of his/her problems and factors causing the problem
   - Emotional reaction to the problem
   - Coping behaviour and problem-solving patterns
   - Nature of social support from parents, siblings, relatives, classmates, teachers, friends, boy/girl friend and neighbours through an individual social support map
   - Need and utilisation of the public services for welfare and/or protection (police, courts) if any

3. Areas of Child's Individual Assessment:

   - Medical Assessment
     - Neuro-behavioural disorders if any
     - Physical health
     - Physical abilities/disabilities
     - Signs of abuse if any
   - Timeline to map critical events and conditions in the child's lifecycle
   - Self-development
     - Group self-identity and connectedness
     - Values
     - Individual self-identity
     - Self-esteem
   - Thinking patterns
     - Irrational versus rational
     - Rigid versus creative
     - Protective versus self-responsibility
     - Negative versus positive
   - Emotional functioning
     - Awareness of emotions in self and others
     - Experience and expression of negative emotions
     - Experience and expression of positive emotions

- Interpersonal relationship patterns
  - Boundary in relationships
  - Perception of others
  - Feelings for others
  - Conflict management patterns
- Interpersonal communication patterns
  - Verbal language
  - Body language
  - Listening
  - Feedback
- Interaction with the systems in the environment through the child's ecomap
  - Interaction with the family
  - Interaction with the school
  - Interaction with the health systems
  - Interaction with the recreation systems
- Summary matrix of strengths and needs for change in the child and his/her environment

4. Areas of Assessment of the Child's Family:

- Family structure
  - Family history (through a family genogram)
  - Household composition (through a household grid)
  - Family ideologies
  - Family functional orientation
  - Family rules
  - Family role allocation
  - Family power analysis
- Family development
  - Timelines
  - Family development stages
  - Family developmental tasks
  - Family developmental transitions
  - Family adaptability
- Family interactions and relationships
  - Family interactions and relationships
  - Boundary, cohesion and adaptability
  - Relational dialectics
  - Family activities

  - Family conflict patterns
  - Family communication patterns
- Family's interaction with the environment through a family ecomap
  - Harmony with community
  - Sources and Types of Social Support (through a Social Support Map)
  - Satisfaction with socio-economic services
  - Need and utilisation of public services for welfare and protection
- Effects of the family on the child and vice versa

5. Overall Assessment:

   A summary matrix of strengths and needs for change in the child, child's family and its environment is useful to plan intervention. This would then help make decisions on the goals for change at the child's family or environment levels and the strengths to be used to meet the child's unmet needs and solve the problems.

12.3.2.5 Sources of Assessment

According to Hepworth et al. (2006), following are the most common sources of information to carry out an assessment of the clients:

- Interview with clients
- Direct observation of non-verbal behaviour
- Direct observation of interaction between the client and family members
- Home visits
- Collateral information from relatives, friends, physicians, teachers, employers and other professionals
- Tools for assessment
- Personal experiences of the practitioner based on direct interaction with the client

12.3.2.6 Observation of Children

Because young children have limited verbal ability, much of the information you gather about him or her will need to be based on observation of his or her non-verbal behaviour in play and interactions with others. However, conclusions should not be drawn based on a single observation or in the same setting (Sheafor and Horejsi 2006). Areas for observation of children are the body language including general appearance, dress and adornment, facial expressions, gestures and posture, behaviour, use of space and use of time, motor skills, play, and communication and interactions with others. The child may be observed in various settings such as the school, playground, home and neighbourhood (Rose and Fatout 2003).

12.3.2.7 Observation of Family

Observations of the family include

- Observing individuals
- Observing transactions between individuals
- Observing the family character (Wise 2005).

Carter and McGoldrick (2005) note the following main characteristics of the family as a social system:

1. The family as a whole is more than the sum of its parts. The focus is therefore on the overall patterns in the family relationships and not on the individual's intra-psychic processes.
2. Family members' behaviours are best explained by circular causality. So cause and effect thinking, which asks why and looks for someone to blame for a problem is not useful.
3. A change in one family member affects all of the family members. Family intervention can, therefore, focus on one person, who is the most motivated and functional family member, who can take action to change his or her part in the family process.

12.3.2.8 Home Visits

Home visits are significant in assessing the child's family and other environmental factors, which is not possible in an agency situation. Wasik and Bryant (2001) opines that home-visiting provides a unique opportunity for observation, as homes provide knowledge about living conditions, families and communities. The organisation of the home and the resources available for daily living enable one to understand more about an individual's or family's strengths and coping strategies available for supports and limitations imposed by the home environment. He recommends that a home visitor should be sensitive to the standards of dress of the community that he/she is visiting and flexible and responsive to the immediate needs of families as well as to their long-term goals.

12.3.2.9 Tools for Assessment

Tools for assessment of children can be background sheets or other forms that clients complete, timelines, genograms, ecomaps, social support maps or tests or assessment instruments. Most of these can provide the baseline data in the stage of assessment and can be used to monitor and evaluate changes over time (Kirst-Ashman and Hull 2006).

Timelines: Timelines can be used to map critical events and conditions in the lifecycle of the individual or the family (Thomlison 2007). It is a self-assessment tool that demonstrates how the client has responded to positive and negative events in their life and clarifies their areas of strengths and needs (Kaplan and Girard 1994).

Genogram: A genogram is a graphic representation of a family tree that displays detailed data on relationships among individuals. It goes beyond a traditional family tree by allowing the user to analyse hereditary patterns and psychological factors that punctuate relationships. Genograms allow a therapist and his/her patient to quickly identify and understand various patterns in the patient's family history which may have had an influence on the patient's current state of mind (Genopro 2008).

Ecomap: An ecomap is a tool of assessment that graphically displays the person-in-environment perspective by focusing on the relationships between the client and the major systems in the client's environment. The client can be an individual or a family. The systems include the neighbourhood and ethnic community, support systems, socio-economic services and public services. In collaboration with the client, the social worker develops an ecomap by placing the client in the centre and showing the following:

- Whether the relationship of the client with each of these systems exists or not,
- Whether the relationship is positive (+) or negative (–),
- Whether the relationship is weak (dashed line) or strong (solid line) or stressful (zigzag line) and
- The direction of the relationship (through an arrow) (Hartman 1995, cited by Poulin 2005).

The worker and the client review the completed ecomap to see its effect on the problem faced by the client as well as the client's strengths (Poulin 2005).

Social Support Map: Social network mapping is a tool for assessing a client's social support networks and the nature of support from the client's point of view (Tracy and Whittaker 1990, cited by Miley et al. 2007).

The sources of support for children may be identified from the parents, siblings, friends, classmates, teachers, neighbours or relatives. For each support system, the following may be examined:

- Type of support received
- Frequency of support received
- Opportunities for reciprocal exchanges
- Constraints faced if any

Following are different types of support that can be assessed:

- Concrete instrumental support
- Information, knowledge and skills
- Emotional support
- Affiliational support (Rothery and Enns 2001, cited by Thomlison 2007).

12.3.3 Planning

Planning in casework required the use of the problem-solving method for goal setting and action planning. Contracting is also an important task in the planning stage.

12.3.3.1 Goal Setting

Goal setting serves many important purposes in casework: Giving direction, defining roles, motivating and measuring progress (Shebib 2003) and defining action programmes for reaching these goals. Egan (2002) recommended that the goals may be identified as outcomes that are clear, specific, realistic, sustainable and flexible. They may be formulated within a time frame with reference to immediate outcomes, intermediate outcomes and final outcomes. The solution-focused treatment model recommends the use of a miracle question to establish goals. Sklare (2005, cited by Thompson and Henderson 2007) recommends that with children this question may be stated in magic terms.

12.3.3.2 Action Planning

Shebib (2003) recommends a series of steps for action planning and implementation leading to the client's goals: Identify alternatives for action, evaluate alternatives and choose an action strategy, and develop and implement plans and evaluate outcomes.

1. Identifying alternatives for action serves two purposes: First, it holds clients back from impulsive action based on the first alternative available, which may simply be a repeat of previous unsuccessful attempts at change. Second, it helps to ensure that clients have choices based on a full range of possibilities. When there is choice, clients can make more rational decisions.
2. The next step is to assist clients in evaluating alternatives and making choices based on some criteria such as relevance, effectiveness, capacity of the client to implement, consistence with the values and beliefs of the clients and potential cost.
3. Developing and implementing plans involves four steps: Sequencing plans, developing contingency plans, putting plans into action and evaluating.

According to Hepworth et al. (2006), many clients feel overwhelmed and intimidated when facing the prospect of tackling goal implementation. For this reason, the task-centred model considers it important to

- Break the goals into constituent parts, partialise goals into general tasks and sequence them, so that the clients gain a sense of efficiency.
- Decide and focus on general tasks that are most significant in moving towards the client's goal. It is important to settle on tasks that have an excellent chance

for successful accomplishment by the client. Success with one task engenders confidence and encourages clients to tackle another task.
- The process of partialising continues with the development of specific tasks, which may be behavioural or cognitive.
- Assist clients in planning and preparing to implement each task, by enhancing the client's commitment to carry out the task, plan the details of carrying out the task, analysing and resolving obstacles, rehearsing or practicing behaviours involved in tasks and summarising the task plan.

12.3.3.3 Contracting

Contracting with clients is intended as a facilitative tool that enables both client and practitioner to reach agreement about the goals and tasks of their work together. Contracting is a natural culmination of the assessment phase and the introduction of the change-oriented (goal attainment). Although contracts may not be legally binding, the social worker must commit to outline the work to be done, thereby obtaining informed consent from clients (Hepworth et al. 2006).

According to Sheafor and Horejsi (2006) the contract should include the following elements:

- Problems or concerns to be addressed
- Goals and objectives of the intervention
- Activities the client will undertake
- Tasks to be performed by the worker
- Identification of other persons, agencies or organisations expected to be participate and clarification about what they will be expected to contribute to the change process

Hepworth et al. (2006) recommend that means of monitoring progress, housekeeping items, such as the time frame, provisions for cancelling or changing scheduled sessions and financial arrangements and stipulations for renegotiating the contract should also be part of the contract.

12.4 Concluding Stages of Casework with Children and Their Families

12.4.1 Evaluation

12.4.1.1 Purpose and Levels

Evaluation in casework is useful to

- Assess the effectiveness of the intervention.
- Assess the efficiency of the intervention.

- Building case theory.
- Review the theories behind the intervention.
- Make improvements in the intervention approach.

Evaluation can be carried out at the formative level (monitoring) as well at the concluding level of casework intervention (summative evaluation). Evaluation can focus on effectiveness or efficiency of social work intervention.

Rosen and Proctor (1979) have classified outcome at three levels:

1. Intermediate outcomes, which are presumed to contribute to or create a facilitative climate for continuation of the programme. Assessment of the intermediate outcome may be done through monitoring.
2. Instrumental outcomes, which, when achieved, are assumed to lead necessarily to the achievement of the programme goals without the help of the programme;
3. Ultimate outcomes are indicators of achievement of the programme goals. The instrumental outcome may be assessed at the conclusion stage, whereas a follow up study is needed to assess the ultimate outcome of practice.

12.4.1.2 Formative Evaluation/Monitoring

According to Morris and Fitz-Gibbon (1978), formative evaluation of practice implementation is known as monitoring. They further specify that monitoring often means assuming a role in the planning, development and refinement. Monitoring can meet the following goals:

- Evaluate the implementation of intervention with reference to the goals and action plans.
- Ascertain the process of change and the intermediate outcome of the intervention
- Document the intervention efforts that help to study what led to the final outcome of the intervention.
- Identify obstacles and make changes/improvements in the intervention approach.

12.4.1.3 Evaluation of Effectiveness

Evaluation of effectiveness in casework is generally done of the outcome with reference to (1) the pre-intervention assessment, (2) the goals set if these goals are clear, specific and realistic (Hepworth et al. 2006) and (3) client's satisfaction.

According to Kirst-Ashman and Hull (2006), the common evaluation designs for generalist social work practice are single-system designs, goal-attainment scaling, target-problem scaling, task-achievement scaling and client satisfaction questionnaires. An aggregate periodic review of the case records of the agency is another useful design for evaluation.

Single-System Designs: Single-system design facilitates a formative type of evaluation of practice with a system, be it an individual, family, group, organisation, community or other collectivity. The heart of single-system design is collecting repeated information on the target problem alike time series research (Bloom and Fischer 1982). The steps in single-system research are

1. A measurable goal is identified.
2. Baseline data is collected on the goal prior to the intervention called Phase A.
3. A record of the frequency of the behaviour is kept during and following the intervention called Phase B.
4. A graphical representation of the change is prepared (Kirst-Ashman and Hull 2006).

Goal-Attainment Scaling: When the client has multiple goals or the goals are not easily measurable, goal-attainment scaling can be used to evaluate the effectiveness of intervention. For each goal, a scale of outcome is developed ranging from

1. The least favourable outcome,
2. The less than expected outcome,
3. The expected level of success,
4. The more-than-expected level of success, to
5. The most favourable outcome (Kirst-Ashman and Hull 2006).

Target-Problem Scaling: In target-problem scaling, the problem is identified, a plan is implemented and changes in the target problem are measured to determine if the problem has changed in severity (Kirst-Ashman and Hull 2006).

Task-Achievement Scaling: Task-achievement scaling is a method of evaluating the degree to which an identified set of tasks has been accomplished that cannot be measured by single-system designs or goal-attainment scaling. The focus is on results and not efforts. A five-point scale is used ranging from

- Completely achieved (4),
- Substantially achieved (3),
- Partially achieved (2),
- Minimally achieved (1) to
- No opportunity to work on the task (0) (Kirst-Ashman and Hull 2006).

Client Satisfaction Questionnaires: Examples of client satisfaction questions:

- How would you rate the overall quality of service provided?
- Did you get the kind of service you wanted?
- To what extent did the social worker meet your needs?
- If a friend had a similar need, would you recommend this centre to him/her? (Kirst-Ashman and Hull 2006).

Aggregate Review of the Case Records of the Agency: An aggregate periodic review of the case records of the agency is useful for several purposes:

1. It is another way to examine whether the programme reaches the designated target population;
2. It is useful to analyse the problems people come with;
3. It can show the trend in people's problem manifestations over a period of time;
4. The process of the practitioner's intervention can be examined through such a review; and
5. The process of change and the outcome of the intervention can be analysed through such a review.

A valuable outcome of such a review is that it also helps in arriving at an improved case recording system.

12.4.1.4 Evaluation of Efficiency

Efficiency of intervention may be evaluated by a cost benefit analysis of the outcome with reference to the resources or efforts put in.

12.4.1.5 Evaluation Through Follow-Up

Follow-up is important for evaluating the ultimate outcome of an intervention. Blythe and Tripodi (1989, cited by Kirst-Ashman and Hull 2006) provided the following list of possible intervention outcomes that may be discovered during follow up:

1. The client may be functioning at the same level as at the time of termination.
2. The client may have improved since termination. This may be due to delayed impact of the intervention or to other non-intervention factors.
3. The client may have deteriorated may be due to premature withdrawal of the intervention of other unknown factors.
4. The client may have relapsed.

12.4.2 Termination

Termination is the process of formally ending the individual social worker–client relationship which may be planned or unplanned.

12.4.2.1 Planned Termination

According to Hull and Kirst-Ashman (2004), termination should be based on clear evidence that the goals of practice have been achieved. Following are the tasks recommended by them at the stage of termination:

- Deciding when to terminate.
- Summarising progress.
- Evaluating achievement of goals/objectives.
- Maintaining and continuing progress.
- Resolving emotional reactions of the worker and client.
- Making appropriate referrals.

Toseland and Revas (1998, cited by Hull and Kirst-Ashman 2004) suggested the following tasks to help clients maintain and generalise changes:

- Helping clients select relevant and appropriate situations to work on.
- Helping clients build confidence in their own abilities.
- Using multiple situations and settings when helping members learn new behaviours.
- Extending treatment through use of follow up sessions.
- Reducing setbacks in other environments.
- Helping clients confront future problems by teaching them a problem-solving process.

12.4.2.2 Unplanned Termination

Sheafor and Horejsi (2006) identified the following situations when the termination may be unplanned and unexpected:

- The client withdraws, for personal or financial reasons.
- The worker accepts employment elsewhere.
- The helping process is blocked by a problem in the worker–client relationship necessitating transfer to another worker.
- The client requires specialised services that are best provided by another social worker, professional or agency.

In the case of termination by the worker, the worker has an obligation to make the termination or transfer as positive an experience as possible.

Chart 12.1 Summary of the Process of Casework

Process of Engagement

Engagement with Parents

- Support parents' strengths and efforts.
- Paraphrase parents' concerns and show empathy and understanding.
- Frame the situation optimistically.
- Normalise problems by sharing that there are others who share the same issues and struggles.

Engagement with Children

- Articulate that the nature of the social worker's relationship with the child is purposeful, exclusive, safe, authentic, confidential and non-intrusive.
- Follow the child's lead in beginning the "getting to know you" process.
- Invite the child to select and get engaged with the toy, media, story book or game that he/she finds interesting.

Engagement with Family

- Define all members in the family as being hurt by their circumstance and that blaming will not solve the problem.
- Normalise the family problem.
- Emphasise the family's strengths and positive motivation.

↓

Process of Assessment

Assessing the Problem

- Initial health, safety and legal matters
- Self-assessment
- Site, temporal context, severity and frequency of problematic behaviours
- Duration of the problem
- Exception or when the current concern did not exist
- Client's emotional reactions to the problem
- Coping effort and the resources and strengths that clients have used previously when dealing with issues.
- Needs based on life stage and stresses based on life transitions
- Problems as violation of child rights

Assessing the Strengths

Ask:
- Survival questions
- Support questions
- Exception questions
- Possibility questions
- Esteem questions
- Perspective questions
- Change questions

Comprehensive Assessment

1. Preliminary Demographic Information
2. Areas of Child's Individual Assessment:
   - Medical Assessment
   - Timeline to map critical events and conditions in the child's lifecycle
   - Self-development
   - Thinking patterns
   - Emotional functioning
   - Interpersonal relationship patterns
   - Interpersonal communication patterns
   - Interaction with the systems in the environment through the child's ecomap
3. Areas of Assessment of the Child's Interaction with the Family:
   - Family structure
   - Family development
   - Family interactions and relationships

- Family's interaction with the environment through a family ecomap
- Effects of the family on the child and vice versa

↓

Process of Planning

Goal Setting →

- Effective goals are clear, concrete, specific, realistic, sustainable and flexible.
- Goals may be formulated within a time frame with reference to immediate outcomes, intermediate outcomes and final outcomes.

Action Planning →

For each goal:

- Identify alternatives for action
- Evaluate alternatives and select the best
- Develop sequenced detailed action plans
- Analyse and resolve obstacles
- Rehearse or practice behaviours involved
- Develop contingency plans
- Enhance the client's commitment to carry out the plan

Contracting

The contract should include:

- Problems or concerns to be addressed
- Goals set
- Tasks the client will undertake
- Tasks to be performed by the worker
- Identification of other persons, agencies or organisations expected to be participate and their roles
- Means of monitoring progress
- Time frame
- Stipulations for renegotiating the contract

↓

Process of Implementation

(Discussed in the next chapter)

↓

Process of Evaluation

Formative Evaluation/Monitoring →

- Evaluate the implementation of intervention with reference to the goals and action plans.
- Ascertain the process of change and the intermediate outcome of the intervention

Evaluation of Effectiveness →

Evaluate the effectiveness of the outcome with reference to:

- Pre-intervention assessment

Evaluation of Efficiency

Evaluate the efficiency of intervention by a cost benefit analysis of:

- The outcome with reference to

• Document the intervention efforts that help to study what led to the final outcome of the intervention. • Identify obstacles and make changes/improvements in the intervention approach.	• Goals set • Client's satisfaction	• The resources or efforts put in

↓

Process of Termination When Goals Have Been Achieved

- Summarise progress.
- Evaluate achievement of goals/objectives.
- Make suggestions to maintain and continue progress.
- Resolve emotional reactions of the worker and client.
- Make appropriate referrals.

References

Bloom, M. and Fischer, J. (1982). *Evaluation Practice: Guidelines for the Accountable Professional*. Englewood Cliffs, NJ: Prentice Hall.

Boyden, J. and Levison, D. (2000). *Children As Economic and Social Actors in the Development Process*. Stockholm: Ministry of Foreign Affairs.

Carter, B. and McGoldrick, M. (Eds.) (2005). *The Expanded Family Life Cycle: Individual, Family and Social Perspectives* (3rd ed.). New York, NY: Pearson.

Compton, B. R., Galaway, B. and Cournoyer, B. R. (2005). *Social Work Processes* (7th ed.). Belmont, CA: Thomson/Brooks Cole.

Daswani, S. (2007). Parental involvement in children's play. In K. P. Nonis and S. Daswani (Eds.) *The Power of Movement: How to Enhance Children's Cognitive, Social, Emotional and Physical Development* (pp. 1–14). Singapore: Prentice Hall.

Dishion, T. J. and Stormshak, E. A. (2007). *Intervening in Children's Lives: An Ecological, Family-Centered Approach to Mental Health Care*. Washington, DC: American Psychological Association.

Egan, G. (2002). *The Skilled Helper: A Problem-Management and Opportunity-Development Approach to Helping* (7th ed.). Pacific Grove, CA: Brooks/Cole.

Geldard, K. and Geldard, D. (2002). *Counselling Children: A Practical Introduction*. London: Sage.

Genopro. (2008). *Introduction to the Genogram*. http://www.genopro.com/genogram/. Accessed 19 May 2008.

Hepworth, D. H., Rooney, R. H., Rooney, G. D., Strom-Gottfried, K. and Larson, J. A. (2006). *Direct Social Work Practice: Theory and Skills* (7th ed.). Belmont, NY: Thomson Higher Education.

Hull, G. H. and Kirst-Ashman, K. K. (2004). *The Generalist Model of Human Service Practice*. Singapore: Thomson.

Kadushin, A. and Kadushin, G. (1997). *The Social Work Interview: A Guide for Human Service Professionals* (4th ed.). New York, NY: Columbia University Press.

Kaplan, L. and Girard, J. L. (1994). *Strengthening High-Risk Families: A Handbook for Practitioners*. New York: Lexington Books.

Kilpatrick, A. C. and Holland, T. P. (2006). *Working with Families: An Integrative Model by Level of Need* (4th ed.). Boston, MA: Pearson/Allyn and Bacon.

Kirst-Ashman, K. K. and Hull, G. H., Jr. (2006). *Understanding Generalist Practice* (4th ed.). Belmont, CA: Brooks/Cole.

Miley, K. K., O'Melia, M. and DuBois, B. (2007). *Generalist Social Work Practice: An Empowering Approach*. Boston, MA: Allyn and Bacon.

Morris, L. L. and Fitz-Gibbon, C. T. (1978). *How to Measure Programme Implementation*. London: Sage.

Poulin, J. (2005). *Strengths-Based Generalist Practice: A Collaborative Approach*. Belmont, CA: Brooks/Cole.

Rose, S. R. and Fatout, M. F. (2003). *Social Work Practice with Children and Adolescents*. Upper Saddle River, NJ: Pearson Education, Inc.

Rosen, A. and Proctor, E. K. (1979). Specifying the treatment process: The basis for effectiveness research. *Journal of Social Service Research*, 2(1), 25–43.

Saleeby, D. (2006). Introduction: Power in the people. In D. Saleeby (Ed.) *The Strengths Perspective in Social Work Practice* (4th ed., pp. 1–24). Boston, MA: Pearson.

Sheafor, B. W. and Horejsi, C. R. (2006). *Techniques and Guidelines for Social Work Practice* (7th ed.). Boston, MA: Allyn and Bacon.

Shebib, B. (2003). *Choices: Counseling Skills for Social Workers and Other Professionals*. New York: Allyn and Bacon.

Thomlison, B. (2007). *Family Assessment Handbook: An Introduction and Practical Guide to Family Assessment* (2nd ed.). Belmont, CA: Thomson Brooks/Cole.

Thompson, C. L. and Henderson, D. A. (2007). *Counseling Children*. Belmont, CA: Thomson/Brooks/Cole.

Wasik, B. H. and Bryant, D. M. (2001). *Home Visiting: Procedures for Helping Families* (2nd ed.). Thousand Oaks: Sage Publications Inc.

Wise, J. B. (2005). *Empowerment Practice with Families in Distress*. New York: Columbia University Press.

Chapter 13
Case Management with Children and Their Families

13.1 Concepts of Case Management

13.1.1 Importance of Case Management

According to Kirst-Ashman and Hull (2006), the following factors are operating to increase the importance of case management for social workers:

- Increased emphasis on maintaining clients in the least restrictive environment;
- The goal of keeping people out of institutions;
- Efforts to reduce or contain costs of providing services;
- Increased attention to rights of clients who often lack awareness of available resources;
- Awareness that some clients cannot follow through on the ordinary referral because of their limited capacities;
- Increased focus on how the environment contributes to client problems; and
- Expansion of human service programmes and increased complexity and fragmentation of services.

13.1.2 Definition of Case Management

According to the Standards of Social Work Case Management developed by the National Association of Social Workers in the United States in 1992:

> Social work case management is a method of providing services whereby a professional social worker assesses the needs of the client and the client's family, when appropriate, and arranges, coordinates, monitors, evaluates, and advocates for a package of multiple services to meet the specific client's complex needs. A professional social worker is the primary provider of social work case management. Distinct from other forms of case management, social work case management addresses both the individual client's bio-psychosocial status as well as the state of the social system in which case management operates. Social work case management is both micro and macro in nature: intervention occurs at both the client and system levels. It requires the social worker to develop and maintain a therapeutic relationship with the client, which may include linking the client with systems that provide

M. Desai, *A Rights-Based Preventative Approach for Psychosocial Well-Being in Childhood*, Children's Well-Being: Indicators and Research 3,
DOI 10.1007/978-90-481-9066-9_13,

him or her with needed services, resources, and opportunities. Services provided under the rubric of social work case management practice may be located in a single agency or may be spread across numerous agencies or organizations.

13.1.3 Principles of Case Management

Gerhart (1990, cited by Kirst-Ashman and Hull 2006) articulates the following principles of case management:

1. Individualisation of services
2. Comprehensiveness of services
3. Parsimonious services
4. Fostering autonomy
5. Continuity of care

13.1.4 Tasks of Case Managers

Kirst-Ashman and Hull (2006) list the following tasks of case managers:

1. Assessment of the client's needs, social network capabilities and the abilities of social service providers.
2. Development of a comprehensive service plan that includes multidisciplinary professional involvement and maximum client involvement.
3. Intervention directly with the client to strengthen skills and capacities for self-care and/or indirectly with systems impinging on the client.
4. Monitoring of service plan implementation and tracking of client status, service delivery and involvement of social network members.
5. Evaluation of service plan effectiveness and its impact on client functioning, on the social network's capacity to support the client and on the ability of the social service professional to work with the client.

13.1.5 Principles of Teamwork for Case Management

When diverse resources work together in common planning, decision making and consolidated action, they need to work as a team. Timberlake et al. (2008) list the following principles of effective teamwork for case management:

- The client system must sanction the team with the understanding that there will be open communication among members.
- All members of the team must clearly know their own professional identities and the distinctive contribution they and their agencies can make to the team.

- Collaboration necessitates revisions in policy, job descriptions and accountability requirements.
- Members of the team must respect each discipline, understand the service orientation, recognise the competencies, trust the communications and rely on the work of each team member.
- The team must meet on a regular basis for shared communication, planning and evaluation.
- The team must define each person's tasks, roles, goals and methods.
- The team as a whole must systematically review its own process, its accomplishments and failures.
- The team must assume collective responsibility for service outcome.

13.1.6 Techniques of Case Management

The techniques of case management intervention with children and their families may be broadly divided into techniques of direct intervention and techniques of system linkage.

13.2 Techniques of Direct Intervention with Children and Their Families

The main techniques used in direct intervention with children and their families are:

- Giving Information and Advice
- Teaching and Training in Psychosocial Skills
- Counselling.

13.2.1 Giving Information and Advice

The social worker needs to provide information to the client that he or she needs to carry out the tasks identified. The information should be provided in a logical, organised, step-by-step fashion and the client should be invited to ask questions to clarify any uncertainty. Complicated multiple step instructions may need to be written down (Sheafor and Horejsi 2006).

Advice-giving refers to worker statements that recommend what a client should do. It is inappropriate in a counselling-therapy setting but appropriate in a referral, brokering, or advocacy setting. The worker should not offer advice until he/she has determined that the client genuinely wants it and unless he/she has the expertise in that area. The client's receptivity to advice may be tested by asking questions such as "Have you asked others for suggestions?" and "May I tell you what other people do in that situation?". When advice is given, present it in a way that says 'This is what I would do' or "This is what others have done", explaining the reasons. The responsibility for deciding what to do should be left to the client (Sheafor and Horejsi 2006).

13.2.2 *Teaching and Training Psychosocial Skills*

Much of case management practice involves teaching clients problem solving and conflict management skills to deal with troublesome life situations, change dysfunctional behaviour and learn effective patterns of social interaction (Sheafor and Horejsi 2006).

13.2.2.1 Psychosocial Skills

Specifically, the clients need to develop the following psychosocial skills:

- Self-awareness
- Thinking skills
- Emotional intelligence
- Interpersonal relationship skills
- Interpersonal communication skills
- Family life education.

The teaching-training methods may be comprised of decision analysis, role play and use of the client–worker relationship as follows.

13.2.2.2 Decision Analysis

Decision analysis is a means by which the worker helps the client consider a range of alternative behaviours in certain situations.

13.2.2.3 Role-Play

Role-playing is often used to assess the nature of the client's interpersonal processes and to practice new social skills (Walsh 2006). Behavioural rehearsal is a technique of role-playing that is drawn from behavioural therapy. It teaches a client how to handle a specific interpersonal exchange for which he or she feels unprepared. It can make use of modelling and coaching. Role reversal is a technique where one person is asked to take on the perspective of another person in an effort to better understand him or her, especially in a conflict situation. It allows the individuals to experience how his or her own behaviour, as dramatised by another, affects others. It can provide insight and maybe even a little humour (Sheafor and Horejsi 2006).

13.2.2.4 Use of the Client–Worker Relationship

Focus on the relationship between the worker and the client works as a model of the client's typical ways of thinking and feeling in other relationships (Walsh 2006).

13.2.3 Counselling Children

Counselling is treating the client's psychosocial problems. The brief practice models of counselling that are discussed in this section are cognitive restructuring, solution-focused treatment and crisis intervention. Across treatment modalities, the focus of these models on immediate or focused concerns, an active stance by the practitioner, and conscious use of time limits were found to be productive (Hepworth et al. 2006).

13.2.3.1 Cognitive Restructuring with Children

Cognitive restructuring is a technique used in cognitive behavioural therapy, solution-focused treatment and emotional management by reframing cognitive distortions.

Cognitive Distortions: Thompson and Henderson (2007) identify the following common cognitive distortions in children:

- It is awful if others do not like me.
- I am bad if I make a mistake.
- Everything should go my way; I should always get what I want.
- Things should come easily to me.
- Adults should be perfect.
- There is only one right answer.
- I cannot help being the way I am; I will always have to be this way.

Reframing Cognitive Distortions: According to Sheafor and Horejsi (2006), the social worker can help a client modify distortions in self-talk, by asking the client to notice that, when you hold to the facts and avoid using inaccurate words, you begin to feel differently and things do not seem as bad as before. Through reframing comments and actions, the social worker gives the client credit for the positive aspects of his or her behaviour relative to the presenting problem. This strategy introduces clients to new ways of looking at some aspect of themselves or the problem (Walsh 2006).

According to Littlejohn and Domenic (2001, cited by West and Turner 2006), reframing can be done from:

- Negative to positive statements
- Past to the future
- Hostile to neutral
- Individual to community interests
- Complaint to request.

Hepworth et al. (2006) recommend the following steps in cognitive restructuring:

1. Accept that self-statements determine emotional reactions to events.
2. Identify dysfunctional beliefs and thought patterns.
3. Identify situations involving dysfunctional cognitions.
4. Replace dysfunctional cognitions with functional self-statements.
5. Identify rewards and incentives for successful coping efforts.

Sheafor and Horejsi (2006) recommend a five-step approach to help a client modify distortions in self-talk, by asking the client to

1. Identify what you are feeling and thinking right now.
2. Get in touch with your self-talk.
3. Examine the objective reality of your situation. Once the facts have been identified, relax, take a deep breath and repeat them out loud three times.
4. Notice that, when you hold to the facts and avoid using inaccurate words, you begin to feel differently and things do not seem as bad as before.

Once the client is able to describe his or her patterns of maladaptive self-talk, the cognitive restructuring techniques of self-instruction, visualisation and journaling may prove helpful:

- Self-instruction comprises of positive self-talk, covert speech and countering negative talk, in the form of a set of statements that are repeated by the client on a regular basis, perhaps three times a day and especially in times of distress.
- Visualisation is a technique in which a client is taught to prepare himself or herself to deal with a worry-causing event by repeatedly imagining this event and mentally rehearsing the steps necessary to handle it successfully.
- Journaling is a technique of keeping a daily log of significant thoughts and feelings (Sheafor and Horejsi 2006).

13.2.3.2 Solution-Focused Counselling with Children

Solution-focused treatment emphasises the construction of solutions and deemphasises the problems. The client begins with a problem statement but quickly moves to solutions. In this model, the cause of the problem and the solution are not necessarily connected. It assumes that change can occur when clients are motivated and empowered to construct solutions. Clients and families are considered experts because they have the knowledge, resources and strengths needed to formulate solutions. It is strongly influenced by the views of Milton Erikson that people are constrained by the social construction of their problems. According to this view, people have untapped unconscious resources which can be released by shifting their perspectives (Hepworth et al. 2006). It is similar to cognitive restructuring because the professional has an active role in first helping clients to question self-defeating constructions and then assisting them to construct new and more productive perspectives (Nichols and Schwartz 2004, cited by Hepworth et al. 2006). It assumes that people respond better to a present and future counselling orientation than they do to a past orientation focused on why they have a problem they cannot solve (Thompson and Henderson 2007).

According to Walsh (2006), the solution-focused practice is influenced by the following theories:

- The systems thinking as developed at the Mental Research Institute (MRI) in Palo Alto views clinical problems as developing because people establish patterns of interaction in relation to a life problem such as underreacting, overreacting, avoiding, denying and even taking actions that worsen the situation. In a sense, the problem becomes the sum of the failed solutions. MRI interventions represent efforts to identify and explore a client's vicious cycle and find new ways of interrupting the problem cycle.
- The communications theory about words having an impact on people's attitude towards self and the world influenced the shift from problem-talk to solution-talk.
- The crisis theory providing focused, effective and short-term intervention for people in need of immediate relief.

The following types of questions are employed to enable clients to arrive at specific goals and to think of exceptions to problems:

- Miracle Questions: For example, "If a miracle happened overnight and your problem was solved what would you be doing differently?"
- Scaling Questions: For example, "On a scale of 0–10, where 0 is the worst that things could be and 10 is the day after the miracle, where are you right now?
- Exception Questions: Ask about instances of exceptions to the problem situation (Thompson and Henderson 2007).

Kilpatrick and Holland (2006) list the following assumptions of solution-focused family interventions:

- The unsolvable problems presented by the client are reframed to be solvable.
- The problem is defined as a part of the change process.
- Only a small change is needed that will snowball into dramatic changes.

Campbell et al. (1999, adapted by Thompson and Henderson 2007) present the following five types of statements that assist clients in moving away from the problem impasse towards solutions:

1. Normalising statements let clients know that they are not alone in experiencing their problem.
2. Restructuring statements are used to rephrase the impasse as directions for the future.

3. Affirmation statements reinforce positive steps the client has already taken.
4. Bridging statements connect clients' attributes to with the next steps for achieving goals.
5. Between-session homework statements serve to connect the sessions and move clients towards their goals.

13.2.3.3 Crisis Intervention

A crisis is defined by James and Gilliland (cited by Hepworth et al. 2006) as a perception of an event or situation that creates an intolerable difficulty that exceeds the resources or coping mechanism of the person. A crisis can be developmental, which is predictable, or situational, which is unexpected (Walsh 2006). Examples of developmental crisis situations for children are starting or changing schools. Situational crisis situations that children and adolescents may experience are loss, bereavement, grief, family violence, parental separation/divorce, potential suicide, abuse (Rose and Fatout 2003), commercial exploitation and disasters.

People's reactions to crises typically go through several stages:

1. The initial rise in tension is accompanied by shock and perhaps even denial of the crisis-provoking event.
2. To reduce the tension, the individual resorts to his or her usual emergency problem-solving skills. When they fail to alleviate the tension, heightened tension ensues.
3. The individual experiences tension so severe that the person feels confused, overwhelmed, helpless, angry or perhaps acutely depressed. The length of this phase varies according to the nature of the hazardous event, the strengths and coping capacities of the person and the degree of responsiveness from social support systems. The person may suffer a mental breakdown, or in extreme situations, attempt suicide. Prolonged crisis-related stress without relief has the potential to severely affect cognitive, behavioural and physical functioning (Hepworth et al. 2006).

Crisis assessment emphasises emotional reactions, coping capacity, the conditions that prompted the occurrence of the crisis, and clients' perception of the situation, social supports and strengths. The temporal focus is on the here and now and the goals are limited to alleviating distress and enabling clients to regain equilibrium. It delineates tasks that the client can perform to achieve a new state of equilibrium. Although crisis professionals are active and directive in defining tasks, clients are encouraged to participate to the extent that they are capable of doing so. After completion of the essential tasks, the worker moves into the final major activity of anticipatory guidance that assists clients to anticipate future crisis situations and to plan coping strategies that will prepare them to face future stresses (Hepworth et al. 2006). The skills required for crisis intervention are poise, creativity, flexibility, quick mental reflexes, tenacity, courage, a clear sense of reality, strong resilience and energy (Rose and Fatout 2003, p. 129).

James and Gilliland (2001, cited by Hepworth et al. 2006) recommend six-step problem-solving model for crisis intervention:

1. Define the problem.
2. Ensure client safety.
3. Provide support.
4. Examine alternatives. The social worker should think of alternatives and the extent to which they promote:
   (1) situational supports, involving people who care about what happens to the client,
   (2) coping mechanisms, represented by actions, behaviours or environmental resources that clients may use to get past the crisis situation and
   (3) positive and constructive thinking patterns that effectively alter how the client views the problem, lessening his or her level of stress and anxiety.
5. Make plans.
6. Obtain commitment.

13.2.3.4 Play Therapy

Advantages of Play Therapy: Incorporating play into counselling with children has several advantages:

1. The child is given freedom to make choices.
2. Play evokes fantasies and unconscious feelings.
3. Play offers familiar tools for children to use.
4. The only limits required are to keep the child and others safe from harm.
5. Play therapy allows the child a safe place to act out feelings, to gain understanding, and to change (Bradley and Gould 1993, cited by Thompson and Henderson 2007).

Schaefer (1993, cited by Thompson and Henderson 2007) identified the following therapeutic powers of play:

1. Overcoming resistance
2. Communication of self-expression
3. Competence and self-esteem
4. Creative thinking for problem solving
5. Catharsis to release strong emotions
6. Abreaction or adjustment to difficulties by symbolically reliving them
7. Role-play of new behaviours
8. Fantasy to make sense of painful reality
9. Metaphoric teaching through stories, playing and artwork
10. Attachment formation
11. Relationship enhancement
12. Positive emotion

13. Mastering developmental fears through repeated play activities
14. Game play help develop ego strength and interaction skills.

Qualities of a Play Therapist: According to Kottman (2001, cited by Thompson and Henderson 2007), the effective play therapist will most likely be a person who has the following qualities:

- Playful and fun-loving attitude
- Willingness to use play and metaphors as communication tools
- Flexibility and ability to deal with ambiguity
- Comfort with children and experience interacting with them
- Ability to set limits and maintain personal boundaries.

Play Toys and Media: The following categories of play media appropriate for different age groups could be arranged in the room after making sure that they are safe:

1. Real-life toys: Doll house with dolls, furniture and household items, cars, buildings, animals, medical kit, school kit, money and so on.
2. Creative expression and emotional release toys: Chalks and blackboards, crayons, paints, brushes, white and coloured paper, scissors, puppets, clay, sand tray and so on.
3. Acting-out and aggressive-release media: punching toy, pounding bench and so on.
4. Story books and games (Geldard and Geldard 2002).

Play Stages: Orton (1997, cited by Thompson and Henderson 2007) suggests an integrated approach to the therapeutic play process that moves through five stages:

1. Relationship: If a strong relationship is built, the child feels accepted and understood.
2. Release: The child uses play to express feelings and to ease tension through cathartic release.
3. Re-creation: The child begins to explore significant events or relationships that trigger uncomfortable thoughts and feelings.
4. Re-experiencing: Children begin to understand the links between past events and to connect that knowledge with current thoughts, feelings and behaviours.
5. Resolving: Resolving is reached when children are able to act on their understanding and to experiment with various solutions.

Play Therapy Skills: Kottman (2001, 2004, cited by Thompson and Henderson 2007) identified the following basic skills for play therapy:

- Tracking: Describe what the child is doing
- Restating content: Paraphrasing

- Reflecting feelings
- Returning responsibility to the child to build self-reliance, self-confidence and self-responsibility
- Using the child's metaphor without imposing the counsellor's interpretation of the meaning
- Setting limits in the play area to keep the child safe, increase self-control and enhance self-responsibility by:
  - Protecting the child from hurting self or others
  - Keeping the child from damaging the play setting
  - Maintaining the toys and play media
  - Staying in the session for the scheduled amount of time.

Assessment of Progress: Barnes (cited by Thompson and Henderson 2007) has suggested the following criteria for assessing progress in play therapy:

1. The child comes to the sessions looking more hopeful and relaxed.
2. The child appears to have increased confidence.
3. The child can summarise what has happened and what has been learned.
4. The child's interactions with parents appear more relaxed.
5. Play patterns, interactions and/or body language have changed.
6. The child openly raises a problem or concern.

13.2.4 Working with Parents/Families

13.2.4.1 Positive Beliefs About Families

Collins, Jordan, and Coleman (2007, pp. 23–26) note that negative attitudes to families, make the social worker blame the parents, fail to respect or embrace diversity, impose singular or restrictive views and erect barriers that prevent an open understanding and acceptance of the struggles of family life and its members. By comparison, positive attitudes to families form a necessary base for constructive family social work. They recommend the following beliefs to guide family social work:

1. A child's emotional and behavioural difficulties should be viewed within the context of the family and the larger social environment.
2. Most family difficulties do not appear overnight but have developed gradually over the years.
3. All people need a family.
4. Families want to be healthy.
5. Families want to stay together and overcome their differences.
6. Parents need understanding and support for the challenges involved in keeping relationships satisfying and for raising children.

7. Parents can learn positive, effective ways of responding to their children if they have opportunities for support, knowledge and skills.
8. Parents' basic needs must be met before they can respond effectively and positively to the needs of their children.
9. Every family member needs nurturing.
10. Family members regardless of gender or age deserve respect from each other.
11. A difference exists between thoughts and actions in parenting.
12. A difference exists between being a "perfect" parent and a "good enough" parent.
13. Families require fair and equal treatment from environmental systems.

13.2.4.2 Intervention with Families

In the early stages of family intervention, the social worker may ask family members to talk directly to him or her about sensitive issues, rather than to one another, to minimise interpersonal tensions. If tensions are so high that productive interactions cannot proceed, the worker can use displacement stories as a means of taking the family's focus off itself and giving it some distance from its own concerns. The story selected has to be of a hypothetical family with similar problems and the worker asks the family to share observations and suggest interventions (Kilpatrick and Holland 2006).

According to Hepworth et al. (2006), on-the-spot interventions are a potent way of modifying patterns of interaction by intervening immediately based on communication that takes place in the sessions. They provide the following guidelines for making such interventions:

1. Focus on process rather than content.
2. Give feedback that is descriptive and neutral rather than general or evaluative.
3. Balance interventions among the family members to divide responsibility.

Hepworth et al. (2006) suggest that the social worker can facilitate positive interactions in following ways:

- Coach family members to own their feelings.
- Translate complaints into requests for change.
- Clarify positive intentions.

The social worker may carry out the role of a mediator in resolving family conflicts. The mediator facilitates separating people from the problem by asking each participant to describe the problem and to state his or her feelings about the problem. The mediator's skills are to help clarify perceptions, to reframe the problem presented in the interests of the participants present and to validate each participant by using reflective listening techniques. Each party needs to feel heard by the mediator. Each party is encouraged to use "I" statements than "you" statements (Parsons et al. 1994).

According to Compton and Galaway (1989, cited by Parsons et al. 1994, pp. 274–275), the techniques used in mediation include the following:

- Bring about convergence of the perceived values of both parties to the conflict.
- Assist the parties in identifying common interest in a successful outcome.
- Help the parties identify that they have more at stake in a continuing relationship than the issue of the specific conflict.
- Facilitate communication by encouraging them to talk to one another.
- Help each party recognise the legitimacy of the other's interests.
- Avoid a situation in which issues of winning and losing are paramount.
- Break the conflict down to separate issues.

Parsons et al. (1994, p. 275) recommend the following skills for mediation among others:

- Reframing partisan, persuasive and emotionally laden statements into less toxic, more interests-based language.
- Promoting each participant's listening by reflecting and asking each participant to reflect back what he or she heard.
- Moderating so that one person does not dominate the conversation or does not dominate the other party.

13.3 Techniques of System Linkage for Children and Their Families

13.3.1 Need for and Problems in System Linkages

13.3.1.1 Need for System Linkages

Intervention with children for secondary and tertiary prevention requires coordination of services by systems such as supplementary and substitute child welfare systems, juvenile justice system, legal advocacy, education, vocational guidance, psychiatric and physical health services, and so on.

13.3.1.2 Problems in System Linkages

Each of these systems operates within a value, practice and policy context. Accordingly, these systems differently perceive the child's/family's needs for resources and can support or have conflict with them (Thomlison 2007). Shulman (1984, cited by Yanca and Johnson 2008) has identified three blocks in the interactions of clients with environmental systems:

The Complexity of Systems: The very institutions set up to solve problems have become so large, complex and impersonal that it has become difficult for people to understand how to approach these systems and use the resources they provide.

Self-Interest: The self-interest of the systems often is in conflict with the interest of others.

Communication Problems: Often there is a lack of adequate communication or there is inaccurate communication among the systems. As a result, the systems cannot work together.

Social disadvantages often make accessibility to, utilisation and satisfaction with services difficult for marginalised groups. Distance, inconvenience of timings, cost, administrative formality, legal barriers, discrimination and emergency situations are found to be barriers to access to social services, as mentioned below:

Distance: Kabeer (2004) notes that services of various kinds tend to be concentrated in locations, which privilege the wealthy and in urban and easily accessible rural areas. The poor generally have to travel longer distance to access services.

Administrative Formality: The use of social services often requires a certain amount of administrative formality. For instance, users may need some form of identification, insurance numbers, identity cards or registration with a specific facility. This inevitably entails paperwork and can disadvantage some groups of people, especially illiterate persons, some very old people or those with mental or psychological problems who do not live with caring relatives (UNESCAP 2002).

Legal Barriers: Non-availability of legal documents often becomes a barrier to access to services. Governments can review the regulations on service provision to identify those elements – whether laws, regulations, standards or procedures – that tend to exclude the poor (UNESCAP, UNDP and ADB 2005).

Discrimination: Users are discriminated against due to their race, religion or caste (Kabeer 2004).

Affordability: People may simply not be able to afford the services, especially the poor in developing countries. Even when ostensibly free at the point of use (like many health and welfare services), there is a hidden cost, for example, of transport to the service, time lost from work, costs of childcare and costs of prescribed medicines (UNESCAP 2002). Besides reducing the direct costs, Governments can also try to reduce opportunity costs. The most direct way of doing this is by extending the network of services to bring them closer to communities. But it is also possible to consider mobile services, such as satellite clinics, that might reach distant villages once a month (UNESCAP, UNDP and ADB 2005).

Emergency Situations: During wars or civil conflicts and natural disasters, social service delivery systems are often disrupted or even abandoned in the case of some war zones, or the civil aid functions usurp the wider welfare aspects following natural disasters (UNESCAP 2002).

13.3.1.3 Implications of the Problems with System Linkages

When organisations provide only the primary service for which they are established and do not provide related services or coordinate with other organisations that provide related services, they only partly meet the needs of the people. As a result, people either do not get all their needs met, or face a fragmented social service delivery system, in which they have to deal with problems such as discontinuity and inaccessibility of services.

Sometimes with intervention of more than one system, things get worse rather than better because people's lives continue to be controlled by others, and they experience system-induced traumas. These may be repeated, insensitive and humiliating interviews; a frightening medical examination; a confrontation involving the perpetrator or the victim's family; an unpleasant placement experience; treatment that the child finds unhelpful or traumatic and court testimony. Often the most problematic aspects of intervention are, not knowing what is going to happen and having no say in decisions. It is important that the intervention not exacerbate the child's sense of powerlessness (Faller 1993).

13.3.1.4 Techniques of System Linkage

The main techniques of system linkage are:

- Information and Referral
- Inter-Organisational Collaborations
- Utilising and Enhancing Natural Support Systems
- Forming Self-Help Groups
- Conflict Mediation.

13.3.2 Information and Referral

To perform the role of information about and referral to the formal systems, social workers must have thorough knowledge of the available formal systems and their benefits, eligibility criteria and application procedures, so that they can make appropriate referrals. Working relationships with key contact persons are essential to making successful referrals (Hepworth et al. 2006). According to Sheafor and Horejsi (2006), the social worker should:

1. Understand the client situation,
2. Assess the various resources available to meet client needs and
3. Connect the client with the resource.

In some instances, it will help to accompany family members to the resource on their first visit.

13.3.3 Inter-organisational Collaboration

Inter-organisational collaboration involves creating a shared vision and developing new goals. Ownership and control of the project are balanced and risks and benefits are shared (Hepworth et al. 2006). Miley et al. (2007) list the following benefits of inter-agency collaboration:

- Broad base of ownership and a diverse pool of expertise
- Distribution of costs and responsibilities of new ventures among the coalition members.
- More power to influence decision-makers, legislators, the media and the general public.

13.3.4 Linkages with Natural Support Systems

Relatives, friends and neighbours are natural support systems that can be activated in times of adversity. Members of these systems can often be available immediately when a crisis occurs and can provide ongoing support (Hepworth et al. 2006). Natural helpers, colleagues and informal networks are also useful support systems. Support occurs when relationships are based on reciprocity, mutuality and shared power in an atmosphere where people can offer what they have to offer and receive the resources they seek. Social workers can encourage the clients' social support systems to develop purposefully, by enhancing their interactional skills and activating natural helpers (Miley et al. 2007).

Nonetheless, informal resources should not be strained, be exhausted or cause a hardship to the providers. They cannot provide long-term solutions to social problems. Instead, the preferred approach should focus on coordination between formal and informal resources (Hepworth et al. 2006).

13.3.5 Linkages with Self-Help Groups

Self-help groups (SHGs) are non-hierarchical groups of persons with similar concerns or problems joining together to be a helpful resource for one another. The caring that occurs in SHGs creates an empathic environment for exchanging ideas and providing relevant information, offers strategies for coping and problem resolution and empowers group members to confront troubling issues (Miley et al. 2007). Social workers need to form SHGs or link clients with SHGs.

13.3.6 Conflict Mediation

According to Parsons, Jorgensen and Hernandez (1994), the social worker takes up the role of a conflict mediator when the need is to reconcile opposite or disparate

Chart 13.1 Summary of Techniques of Case Management with Children and their Families

Giving Information and Advice
- Give information in a logical, organised, step-by-step fashion.
- Give advice only when the client genuinely wants it and if the worker has the expertise in that area.
- Let client take the final decision.

Teaching and Training in Psychosocial Skills

Use:
- Decision analysis
- Role-play, behavioural rehearsal, role reversal
- Client–worker relationship

DIRECT INTERVENTION WITH CHILDREN AND THEIR FAMILIES TO STRENGTHEN SKILLS AND CAPACITIES FOR SELF-CARE

Counselling Children
Use brief practice models of counselling:
- Cognitive restructuring
- Solution-focused treatment
- Crisis intervention
- Play therapy

Working with Parents/Families
Make on-the-spot interventions to facilitate positive interactions:
- Focus on process rather than content.
- Give descriptive and neutral feedback rather than general or evaluative.
- Balance interventions among the family members to divide responsibility.
- Coach family members to own their feelings.
- Translate complaints into requests for change.
- Clarify positive intentions.
- Mediate in resolving family conflicts.

Information and Referral
- Understand the client situation.
- Assess the various resources available to meet client needs.
- Connect the client with the resource.
- If necessary, accompany the client to the resource on their first visit.

Inter-Organisational Collaborations
Use inter-organisational collaboration for:
- Broad base of ownership and a diverse pool of expertise
- Distribution of costs and responsibilities among the collaborators
- More power to influence legislators, the media and the public.

SYSTEM LINKAGE FOR CHILDREN AND THEIR FAMILIES

Linkages with Natural Support Systems
Activate linkages with:
- Relatives
- Friends
- Neighbours
- Natural helpers
- Colleagues
- Informal networks

Linkages with Self-Help Groups
- Form SHGs or
- Link clients with SHGs

Conflict Mediation

Mediate in conflict between:
- The clients and the service providers
- Between systems on behalf of clients

points of view and engage the disputants in a unified action. Such mediation may be needed not only between the clients and the service providers but also between systems on behalf of clients. Occasionally, breakdowns occur between clients and service providers so that clients do not receive the needed services to which they are entitled. Clients may not have adequately represented their case, may have withdrawn application or the service provider may have withheld services (Hepworth et al. 2006). A set of antecedents exist for evolution of a conflict among systems, such as competition of scarce resources, lack of role clarity, or other situations that create a "we/they" mindset, for example, between two childcare agencies or between management and staff of one agency (Parsons et al. 1994).

References

Collins, D., Jordan, C. and Coleman, H. (2007). *An Introduction to Family Social Work* (2nd ed.). South Melbourne VIC: Thomson Brooks Cole.

Faller, K. C. (1993). *Child Sexual Abuse: Intervention and Treatment Issues*. Washington, DC: US Department of Health and Human Services.

Geldard, K. and Geldard, D. (2002). *Counselling Children: A Practical Introduction*. London: Sage.

Hepworth, D. H., Rooney, R. H., Rooney, G. D., Strom-Gottfried, K. and Larson, J. A. (2006). *Direct Social Work Practice: Theory and Skills* (7th ed.). Belmont, NY: Thomson Higher Education.

Kabeer, N. (2004). *Imagining "The Social": Social Policy Analysis for the Poor in Poor Countries*. Brighton: Institute of Development Studies.

Kilpatrick, A. C. and Holland, T. P. (2006). *Working with Families: An Integrative Model by Level of Need* (4th ed.). Boston, MA: Pearson Allyn and Bacon.

Kirst-Ashman, K. K. and Hull, G. H., Jr. (2006). *Understanding Generalist Practice* (4th ed.). Belmont, CA: Brooks/Cole.

Miley, K. K., O'Melia, M. and DuBois, B. (2007). *Generalist Social Work Practice: An Empowering Approach*. Boston, MA: Allyn and Bacon.

National Association of Social Workers. (1992). *Standards for Social Work Case Management*. http://www.naswdc.org/practice/standards/sw_case_mgmt.asp#def. Accessed 4 January 2007.

Parsons, R. J., Jorgensen, J. D. and Hernandez, S. H. (1994). *The Integration of Social Work Practice*. Belmont, CA: Brooks/Cole.

Rose, S. R. and Fatout, M. F. (2003). *Social Work Practice with Children and Adolescents*. Boston, MA: Allyn and Bacon.

Sheafor, B. W. and Horejsi, C. R. (2006). *Techniques and Guidelines for Social Work Practice* (7th ed.). Boston, MA: Allyn and Bacon.

Thomlison, B. (2007). *Family Assessment Handbook: An Introduction and Practical Guide to Family Assessment* (2nd ed.). Belmont, CA: Thomson/Brooks/Cole.

Thompson, C. L. and Henderson, D. A. (2007). *Counseling Children*. Belmont, CA: Thomson/Brooks/Cole.

Timberlake, E. M., Zajicek-Farber, M. L. and Sabatino, C. A. (2008). *Generalist Social Work Practice: A Strengths-Based Problem Solving Approach*. Boston, MA: Allyn and Bacon.

United Nations Economic and Social Commission for Asia and the Pacific. (2002). *Access to Social Services by the Poor and Disadvantaged in Asia and the Pacific: Major Trends and Issues*. New York: United Nations Economic and Social Commission for Asia and the Pacific.

United Nations Economic and Social Commission for Asia and the Pacific, United Nations Development Program and Asian Development Bank. (2005). *A Future Within Reach*. New York: United Nations Economic and Social Commission for Asia and the Pacific.

Walsh, J. (2006). *Theories for Direct Social Work Practice* (1st ed.). Belmont, CA: Thomson/Brooks/Cole.

West, R. and Turner, L. H. (2006). *Understanding Interpersonal Communication: Making Choices in Changing Times*. Southbank, VIC: Thomson.

Yanca, S. J. and Johnson, L. C. (2008). *Generalist Social Work Practice with Families*. Boston, MA: Pearson Allyn and Bacon.

Chapter 14
Children at Risk of Neglect and Secondary Prevention

14.1 Concepts of Children at Risk of Neglect and Secondary Prevention

14.1.1 Children at Risk of Neglect

Children may be at risk of neglect due to the following individual, parental and/or other situations:

1. Children with special needs
    - Children with neuro-behavioural disorders
    - Children with disability and/or chronic illness
2. Parental characteristics
    - Children of incapable parents
        - Children of substance users
        - Children of HIV/AIDS-infected/terminally ill parents
    - Children of parents facing conflict
        - Children of battered women
        - Children of divorce
    - Children of unavailable parents
        - Children of single-parent families
        - Children of prisoners
        - Child-headed households
        - Street children
    - Children of unwilling parents
        - Children born out of wedlock
        - Abandoned children

M. Desai, *A Rights-Based Preventative Approach for Psychosocial Well-Being in Childhood*, Children's Well-Being: Indicators and Research 3,
DOI 10.1007/978-90-481-9066-9_14,

3. Situational characteristics
   - o Children in poverty groups
   - o Children of migrants
   - o Children in emergency situations (discussed in Chapter 15)

14.1.2 Secondary Prevention

14.1.2.1 Goals

Secondary prevention is prevention of neglect of children in at risk situations. Secondary prevention may aim at the following goals:

1. Prevention of their vulnerability, neglect, abuse and commercial exploitation
2. Promotion of their psychosocial well-being
3. Promotion of their age-appropriate developmental opportunities and
4. Promotion of their rights to family care, development, participation and protection

14.1.2.2 Interventions

Secondary prevention of neglect of children in at-risk situations may be carried out through the following rights-based interventions:

- Case management
  - o Direct intervention for giving information and advice, teaching and training in psychosocial skills and counselling
  - o Linking with natural support systems, self-help groups, flexitime supplementary childcare and other formal systems of state and voluntary organisations
- Psycho-educational group work

14.2 Children with Special Needs

14.2.1 Situational Analysis

Children with special needs are different from their peers in terms of abilities or behaviour that affect their daily life, family life, education, public life and so on. They may be broadly divided into children with neuro-behavioural disorders and those with disabilities and/or chronic illness.

14.2.1.1 Children with Neuro-behavioural Disorders

According to Lesser and Pope (2007), neuro-behavioural disorders are a result of the linkage between brain dysfunction and behavioural manifestations. The neuro-behavioural disorders can be classified into learning disorders and brain-based disorders.

Learning disorders: The learning disorders mainly include learning disabilities and attention deficit disorder (ADD):

- Learning disabilities include language-based learning disabilities and non-verbal learning disabilities. The former mainly includes dyslexia which is a language and reading disability. Children with learning disabilities generally have a measured intelligence in the normal range but academically achieve well below the expected level (Thompson and Henderson 2007)
- ADD traits flow from lack of inhibitions – impulsiveness is inadequate inhibition of internal stimuli, distraction is inadequate inhibition of extraneous stimuli and hyperactivity is physically checking out those stimuli. These create a wide range of executive dysfunctions (Kutscher 2004)

Brain-based disorders: The brain-based disorders include autism, mental retardation and other genetic disorders:

- Autism is a developmental disability that significantly affects verbal and non-verbal communication and social interaction, as well as presence of restricted and/or repetitive behaviour, interests and activities
- Mental retardation or mental disability implies significantly sub-average general intellectual functioning and a reduced rate of learning, deficits in adaptive behaviour and adverse effects on educational performance (Thompson and Henderson 2007)

14.2.1.2 Children with Disabilities and/or Chronic Illness

The terms disability and chronic illness are often associated and/or used interchangeably. Illness can cause a disability; a disability can cause an illness; or the two may occur together (Lesser and Pope 2007). The World Health Organization (2006, cited by Lesser and Pope 2007) defines the terms impairment, disability and handicap as follows:

- Impairment is a disturbance in body structure or processes that is present at birth or results from later injury or disease – a loss or abnormality of psychological, physiological or anatomical structure of function
- Disability is a limitation in expected functional activity due to an underlying impairment – a restriction or lack of ability to perform an activity within the range considered normal
- Handicap is a social disadvantage experienced by people as a result of impairment or disability that occurs because they do not meet social expectations for performance

Rolland (1988, 1989, cited by Lesser and Pope 2007) has grouped chronic illness and disability into three categories:

1. Progressive permanent disabilities include conditions such as diabetes, cancer, HIV/AIDS
2. Constant permanent disabilities include blindness and visual impairment and deafness
3. Relapsing or episodic syndromes include disorders such as multiple sclerosis

Ableism is prejudice against the differently abled or disabled and discrimination in favour of the able-bodied. An ableist society treats able-bodied people as the standard of "normal living". This results in public and private places and services, education and social work being built to serve "normal" people. Some persons believe it is ableism that prevents disabled people from participating in the social fabric of their communities, rather than impairments in physical, mental or emotional ability (Association for the Advancement of Assistive Technology 2005).

Children who live with a disability are among the most stigmatised and marginalised of all the world's children. While all children are at risk of being victims of violence, disabled children find themselves at significantly increased risk because of stigma, negative traditional beliefs and ignorance. Lack of social support, limited opportunities for education, employment or participation in the community further isolates disabled children and their families, leading to increased levels of stress and hardship. Disabled children are also often targeted by abusers, who see them as easy victims (Groce 2005).

14.2.2 Interventions

Mackelsprang and Salsgover (1999, cited by Lesser and Pope 2007) highlight the following practice principles that are relevant for children with special needs:

- Assume that they are capable or potentially capable
- Reject pathological interpretations or that disability requires grief and mourning
- Consider that disability is a social construct and that practice with them must include attention to eliminating environmental, attitudinal and policy barriers to their full participation in the society
- Appreciate the history of oppression that persons with disabilities have faced.
- View disability as different and not dysfunctional and in so doing work towards helping persons adopt disability-affirming identities

Interventions needed with children with special needs are compiled by Thompson and Henderson (2007, p. 604) as follows:

- Recognise that the child is a person first
- Work towards an understanding of the child's specific exceptionality and the unique social, learning or behavioural problems that may accompany this exceptionality
- Enhance self-esteem and other psychosocial skills

- Facilitate adjustment to exceptionality
- Coordinate the services of other professionals working with the special needs of the child

Interventions needed with parents of children with special needs are compiled by Thompson and Henderson (2007, pp. 604–605) as follows:

- Help them understand the special needs of the child, prognosis, strengths and limitations
- Assist them in working through feelings and attitudes that may inhibit the child's progress
- Help them set realistic expectations of the child
- Encourage them to view their child as a unique individual with rights and potentials and the ability to make choices about his or her own life

14.3 Children of Substance Users

14.3.1 Situational Analysis

Parents who abuse substances, especially if they are addicted, are often unable to provide consistent, nurturing care that promotes their child's development. Use of psychoactive drugs also increases the risk of abuse. Some parents recruit their children into selling drugs, prostitution or other extremely damaging activities in order to obtain money to buy drugs or alcohol (Downs et al. 2009).

Children of substance abusers lack a positive role model as they are exposed to an environment of guilt, anger and justification of unpleasant realities. Lying begins with denial of unpleasant realities, broken promises and inconsistencies, to cover up the addiction and protect the dignity of the family. Other problems that these children face are loss of self-esteem, difficulty in having fun, fear and anxiety, lack of care and warmth, living in fantasies and difficulties with intimate relationships. Some become angry and aggressive at an early age and get branded as troublemakers. Some of these children take up adult responsibilities, whereas others are likely to take up substance abuse in childhood, adolescence or adulthood. Almost all of them develop personality traits, behaviours and coping styles that are unhealthy for a wholesome and well-balanced development (Tata Institute of Social Sciences 1998). The unspoken rules for children of the families of substance users as compiled by Thompson and Henderson (2007) are denial, lack of trust, lack of emotions and lack of fun.

14.3.2 Interventions

James and Gililand (2005, cited by Thompson and Henderson 2007) summarise treatment goals for children from substance abusing families as follows:

1. Give them emotional support
2. Provide accurate, non-judgemental information about substance abuse
3. Correct their perceptions of being the cause of the parental problems and the attached guilt and shame
4. Help them learn to cope with possible situations that may occur because of the abuse
5. Reduce their isolation

14.4 Children of HIV/AIDS-Infected/Terminally Ill Parents

14.4.1 Situational Analysis

The HIV/AIDS pandemic is threatening the physical health and survival of millions of children around the world. Stigma and discrimination, often associated with HIV infection, can lead to exclusion and isolation and ruin a child's chances to receive an education. Children whose families are affected by HIV/AIDS experience severe emotional and psychological distress. Economic hardship resulting from their parents' inability to work may cause children to drop out of school or become child labourers. They are often forced to assume the burden of caring for sick parents or for their younger siblings. HIV/AIDS is also destroying their families and depriving them of parental love, care and protection. Children orphaned by HIV/AIDS are more exposed to exploitation, abuse and violence. Conversely, many situations in which children have inadequate protection – including sexual exploitation, trafficking, violence, armed conflict, recruitment in armed forces or groups, displacement, detention and imprisonment, child marriage and female genital mutilation/cutting – also make them more vulnerable to HIV infection (UNICEF 2006).

14.4.2 Interventions

The following interventions are recommended by UNICEF (2006) for children of HIV/AIDS-infected parents.

Attitudes, customs and practices: It is important to oppose the prejudice, shaming and stigma often experienced by children infected, orphaned or made vulnerable by HIV/AIDS. Violence (including armed conflict), sexual discrimination, sexual abuse and unequal power relations (e.g., marriages of young girls to much older husbands) all increase children's vulnerability to HIV infection.

Open discussion: There is a need to raise awareness, counter myths and remove taboos about HIV/AIDS by making it an acceptable topic of discussion and providing accurate information about the disease and its prevention. Voices and participation of children can help break the silence and stop stigmatisation.

Children's life skills, knowledge and participation: These are particularly important when dealing with the threat and impact of HIV/AIDS. To avoid the risk of infection, all children need to be taught about sexual health and be empowered to refuse unsafe or unwanted sex and to negotiate safer options. Children already affected or infected by HIV/AIDS need support so they can develop skills that will help them cope, make informed decisions and protect themselves from exploitation and abuse.

Capacity of families and communities: Resources and skills must be invested to monitor vulnerable households, support families willing to foster or adopt orphaned children and strengthen community-level services. To help protect children in armed conflict or humanitarian crises, international peacekeeping and humanitarian personnel should be trained in HIV/AIDS awareness and prevention.

Essential services, including prevention, recovery and reintegration: Access to education – a fundamental human right – must be guaranteed to children who have been infected or affected by HIV/AIDS. Education also reduces their vulnerability to exploitation. Community-based childcare and psychosocial support are necessary to help families and communities cope.

Inheritance rights: The inheritance rights of women and children who have lost providers and care-givers to AIDS should be addressed (UNICEF 2006).

14.5 Children of Divorce

14.5.1 Situational Analysis

The lives and relationships of children in a divorcing family are profoundly affected – socially, psychologically and even legally (Thompson and Henderson 2007). MacFarland and Tollerud (2004, cited by Thompson and Henderson 2007) suggest that the stresses of divorce begin with the conflict before the divorce and continue with the aftermath that may involve relocations, loss of friends, changes in socioeconomic status, redefining relationships with both parents and sometimes adjusting to the remarriage of one or both parents. Often, mothers who were totally involved in the care of children and home may have to go to work, and children may be asked to assume the role of the absent parent. Children may feel rejected and have conflicting loyalties.

Wallerstein and Blakeslee (2003, cited by Thompson and Henderson 2007) describe the following psychological tasks that the children of divorce must successfully resolve:

- Acknowledging the reality of the marriage breakup
- Disengaging from parental conflict and distress and resuming customary pursuits
- Resolution of loss of a parent and familiar surroundings
- Resolving anger and self-blame
- Accepting the permanence of divorce
- Achieving realistic hope regarding relationships

14.5.2 Interventions

Social workers may train the parents going through divorce to implement the following with their children:

1. Talk with the child about the divorce at his or her cognitive level. Emphasise that the child is not at fault. Avoid blaming or criticising the other parent
2. Plan for ways to make the child's life as stable and consistent as possible
3. Avoid using children as go-betweens to carry messages
4. Arrange for regular visits from the absent parent to assure the children that they are loved by both parents
5. Avoid asking children to assume responsibilities beyond their capabilities (Thompson and Henderson 2007)

14.6 Children of Prisoners

14.6.1 Situational Analysis

According to Prayas (2002), children of prisoners, that is, undertrial/unconvicted or sentenced persons could denote all of the following sub-groups:

- Children born to mothers while in custody
- Minors (which include infants being breast-fed) permitted to be taken into police or prison custody with their mothers
- Minors, taken into penal custody with their mothers, who have been later sent outside (before or after attaining the prescribed age-limit), while the mother remains incarcerated
- Minors taken into custody with their mothers, who live with their mothers (bail/discharge/acquittal/completion of sentence)
- Minors left outside when either or both parents are taken into custody

Children of prisoners, whether they accompany their mothers or are left outside when the parents are arrested, need attention.

14.6.2 Interventions

Article 9.3 of the UNCRC states that "Where ... separation results from any action initiated by a State Party, such as the detention, imprisonment, exile, deportation or death (including death arising from any cause while the person is in the custody of the State) of one or both parents or of the child, that State Party shall, upon request, provide the parents, the child or, if appropriate, another member of the family with the essential information concerning the whereabouts of the absent member(s) of the family unless the provision of the information would be detrimental to the well-being of the child. States Parties shall further ensure that the submission of such a request shall of itself entail no adverse consequences for the person(s) concerned."

The Friends World Committee for Consultation (2004) urges the Committee on the Rights of the Child to consider the need for development of a Bill of Rights for Children of Imprisoned Mothers, which could take as a starting point the San Francisco Partnership for Incarcerated Parents "Bill of Rights" for children of incarcerated parents, which states the following:

1. I have the right to be kept safe and informed at the time of my parent's arrest
2. I have the right to be heard when decisions are made about me
3. I have the right to be considered when decisions are made about my parent
4. I have the right to be well cared for in my parent's absence
5. I have the right to speak with, see and touch my parent
6. I have the right to support as I struggle with my parent's incarceration
7. I have the right not to be judged, blamed or labeled because of my parent's incarceration
8. I have the right to a lifelong relationship with my parent

For promoting the rights of children of prisoners, the following government systems need to comprise the case management team: Police, prison administration, judiciary, juvenile justice system, the child protection department, probation officers and children's institutions (adapted from Prayas 2002).

14.7 Child-Headed Households

14.7.1 Situational Analysis

According to the International Committee of the Red Cross (2004), in a striking number of situations, groups of children are left without any adult to care for them and assume responsibility as heads of households. Massacres, genocide and HIV pandemics have created enormous demographic pressure in many developing countries, worsening prospects for millions of children and young people of having healthy and meaningful lives. Pressure on families and communities has diminished protection and worsened neglect and emotional suffering for separated children. This heightens the risk of discrimination, exploitation and abuse. Studies of the problems faced by child-headed households indicate that these are often linked to the difficulty of meeting basic needs as shelter, food, health, education and vocational skills training. A Joint Working Paper on Improving Protection for Children Without Parental Care by International Social Service and UNICEF (2004) note that child-headed households have the advantage of keeping siblings together and allow for the continuity of their relationship with the community. However, these children are especially vulnerable to marginalisation, insecurity and exploitation.

According to Save the Children (2005), with increasing numbers of child-headed households and children being responsible for the care of a number of other children, the criminalisation of children who are out of "traditional care situations", together with the fact that most of their livelihood options are illegal, will result inevitably in these children increasingly coming into conflict with the law. Without a re-conceptualisation not only of children's social role but also of their legal role and status, children in these situations will find themselves increasingly vulnerable and marginalised. They will be left unable to protect their rights against unscrupulous adults and their views, roles and responsibilities as children and as carers will be left unrecognised and unsupported by laws and bodies used to dealing with children only through the agency of adults.

14.7.2 Interventions

Following are the guiding principles for protection of these children formulated by the International Committee of the Red Cross (2004):

- Governments need to develop new policies and adapt existing ones in order to meet the challenges of rapidly increasing numbers of orphans; examine the expansion and educational, health care and other social services to ensure that they identify and address the special needs of children without care-givers; and ensure that services are adequate to include the burgeoning number of children for whom such services are critical
- Communities and poor families housing orphans need to be supported through expansion of basic services and the development of "safety nets". Community-based organisations – including religious organisations – providing alternative care for orphaned children need to be supported
- Effective protection of the rights of child-headed households such as access to education, and laws on adoption and fostering and on inheritance and protection of property and access to land is essential for protecting separated children from exploitation and discrimination
- All assistance programmes for child-headed households, separated children and orphans should be integrated in any given community with overall assistance to children in need of special protection. Stigmatisation should be avoided and social integration of children orphaned by war, HIV/AIDS or other misfortunes should be facilitated

14.8 Street Children

14.8.1 Situational Analysis

14.8.1.1 General

Children living on the street mainly include the homeless, abandoned, missing and run-away children, who have no or infrequent ties with their families. Street children are considered "out of place", meaning being outside of the physical places that are traditionally attributed to childhood, such as homes or schools or defined recreational areas. Instead, street children find themselves operating and even living in areas that are considered "public" but, in fact, are generally reserved for the adult public (Save the Children 2005).

Ennew (1995, cited by John 2003) noted that street children are outside childhood and perceived as being outside adult control. In their lives they have agency, autonomy and recognition amid their peers. In fact, they have something children rarely have, namely, power. The way in which they operate illustrates the enterprise and initiative children can show in especially difficult conditions – conditions faced by increasing numbers of the world's children – and makes us think about what children are capable of. Street children do not enjoy rights of protection and provision, which makes them seem "unnatural children". As people, however, they work for themselves, care for and respect each other and do not, in fact, ask society to rescue them. The way they operate challenges the hegemony of Northern and Western childhood.

14.8.1.2 Conflict with the Law

Save the Children (2005) observes that street children are often left with no other alternatives but petty theft to meet their basic needs, including food and clothes. By criminalising most livelihood choices available to street children and targeting their survival behaviours, the law in turn drives them towards more risky and exploitative options. For many of the children who are displaced temporarily or more permanently to the streets by their life circumstances, the streets are increasingly "no-go" zones. The increased reliance on curfews, dispersal orders and anti-social behaviour orders that criminalise children's use of public places, as well as their behaviour in them when deemed socially "inappropriate", represents yet another form of social exclusion for these children which brings them into direct conflict with the law (Save the Children 2005).

The Human Rights Watch (1996) noted that factors that contribute to this phenomenon are police perceptions of street children, widespread corruption and a culture of police violence, the inadequacy and non-implementation of legal safeguards and the level of impunity that law enforcement officials enjoy. The police generally view street children as vagrants and criminals. While it is true that they are sometimes involved in petty theft, drug-trafficking, prostitution and other criminal activities, the police tend to assume that whenever a crime is committed on the street, street children either involve themselves or know the culprit. Their proximity to a crime is considered reason enough to detain them. Street children are also easy targets. They are young, small, poor, ignorant of their rights and often have no family members who will come to their defence. It does not require much time or effort to detain and beat a child to extract a confession, and children are unlikely to register formal complaints. Police have financial incentives to resort to violence against children. Many children report that they were beaten on the street because the police wanted their money. The prospect of being sent to a remand home, the police station or jail, coupled with the threat of brutal treatment, creates a level of fear and intimidation that forces children or in some cases, their families, to pay the police or suffer the consequences (Human Rights Watch 1996).

14.8.1.3 Exploitation of Street Children

In the absence of adult protection and guidance, street children take to begging, prostitution, drug use and other such behaviour as survival strategies. The street girls are subjected to a greater risk of sexual exploitation (Mehra 1996).

14.8.1.4 Substance Abuse

Save the Children (2005) notes that with limited legitimate options for livelihood, children surviving on the street are easy and useful targets for those running the drug trades. Substance abuse and trading by the children themselves become both a means for survival and a way to survive. The use of drugs provides these children with a means of temporary escape from the world they live in as well as, in some cases, a hunger suppressant that enables them to get by. Being "high" can be understood as a coping strategy for children as well as a major bonding factor with peers.

14.8.1.5 HIV/AIDS Among Street Children

Sexual activities and sharing needles with peers make street boys and girls vulnerable to HIV/AIDS. According to Mehra (1996), younger children, boys and girls, are particularly vulnerable to STDs and HIV/AIDS when they are subjected to forced sodomy, due to lesions and sores in the torn anal region. Children infected with HIV can be further infected through unsafe sex and this increases their chances of developing AIDS. The problem is compounded by lack of correct and adequate information about HIV/AIDS, lack of guidelines on clinical management of HIV/AIDS for all health-care functionaries, lack of access to health-care facilities and so on (D'Mello 2001).

14.8.2 Interventions

14.8.2.1 Level of Work

According to Cox and Pawar (2006), social workers work with street children at three levels:

1. Direct work with street children who are separated from their families and communities
2. Work with street children and their families when they are in regular contact with each other
3. Work with street children, their families and the community when the street children are drawn from a number of families living within a common community

14.8.2.2 Structures of Work

Following are the common structures of work with street children:

- Mobile services by street educators, or street-based social workers, have proved to be one of the best ways of working with street children
- Drop-in day centres and temporary night shelters
- Children's participation in designing, implementing and evaluating the projects and children's involvement in outreach activities, as peer counsellors, advocates, health educators and facilitators (Asian Development Bank 2003)

14.8.2.3 Immediate Needs

Street children's immediate needs can be met through the following services:

- Meals
- Washing and laundry facilities
- Formal and non-formal education and vocational training
- Livelihood programmes
- Recreational and relaxation opportunities

14.8.2.4 Health Care

Programmes should pay special attention to physical and mental health, either through their own specialists or by referring children to community services.

- Health services and health education for first aid for injuries from accidents or abuse, improving hygiene and nutrition, and protection from accidents, illnesses, sexually transmitted diseases, HIV/AIDS and substance abuse
- Counselling and mental health services
- Life-skills training (Asian Development Bank 2003)

14.8.2.5 Reintegration

Street children need to be reintegrated with their families and communities in the following ways:

- In principle, reuniting a child with his or her family is the most desirable outcome of a programme, assuming the child wishes to return and the family is capable and willing to receive him or her
- When a return to the natural family is inadvisable, alternatives such as foster home, adoption, or community home should be identified
- Community-level programmes may focus on local governance, basic services, job creation, education, advocacy among relevant stakeholders, improving schools and other basic services, as well as strengthening social capital

- Awareness raising in communities can help sensitise community members to the special requirements of vulnerable children and avoid stigmatising former street children (Asian Development Bank 2003)

Chart 14.1 Summary of Children at Risk of Neglect and Secondary Prevention

Children at Risk of Neglect

1. Children with special needs:
   - o Children with neuro-behavioural disorders
   - o Children with disability and/or chronic illness
2. Parental characteristics:
   - o Children of incapable parents
     - ■ Children of substance users
     - ■ Children of HIV/AIDS-infected/terminally ill parents
   - o Children of parents facing conflict
     - ■ Children of battered women
     - ■ Children of divorce
   - o Children of unavailable parents
     - ■ Children of single-parent families
     - ■ Children of prisoners
     - ■ Child-headed households
     - ■ Street children
   - o Children of unwilling parents
     - ■ Children born out of wedlock
     - ■ Abandoned children
3. Situational characteristics:
   - o Children in poverty groups
   - o Children of migrants
   - o Children in emergency situations

Goal of secondary prevention

- Prevention of children's vulnerability, neglect, abuse and commercial exploitation
- Promotion of their psychosocial well-being
- Promotion of their age-appropriate developmental opportunities
- Promotion of their rights to family care, development, participation and protection

Intervention for secondary prevention

Supplementary interventions

- Flexitime child day care/
- Night care

Supportive interventions

- Case management:
  - o Direct intervention for giving information and advice, teaching and training in psychosocial skills and counselling
  - o Linking with natural support systems, self-help groups, flexitime supplementary childcare and other formal systems of state and voluntary organisations
- Psycho-educational group work for enrichment of psychosocial skills of children and parents

References

Asian Development Bank. (2003). *Working with Street Children: Exploring Ways for ADB Assistance*. http://www.adb.org/Documents/Books/Street_Children/Working_Streetchildren/working_with_streetkids.pdf. Accessed 22 July 2009.

Association for the Advancement of Assistive Technology. (2005). *Ableism*. www.sagepub.com/upm-data/5900_Entries_Beginning_with_A_Albrecht_Pdf.pdf. Accessed 23 September 2006.

Cox, D. and Pawar, M. (2006). *International Social Work: Issues, Strategies, and Programs*. Thousand Oaks, CA: Sage Publications.

D'Mello, S. (2001). Strategies for protection of children affected by HIV/AIDS. In *Report of the Consultation Workshop on Directions for UNICEF Strategies for Child Protection in India for 2003–2007*. Mumbai: Tata Institute of Social Sciences.

Downs, S. W., Moore, E. and McFadden, E. J. (2009). *Child Welfare and Family Services: Policies and Practice* (8th ed.). Boston, MA: Pearson Allyn and Bacon.

The Friends World Committee for Consultation. (2004). *Children of Imprisoned Mothers*. Geneva: The Friends World Committee for Consultation.

Groce, N. E. (2005). *Violence Against Disabled Children: UN Secretary Generals Report on Violence Against Children Thematic Group on Violence Against Disabled Children*, Convened by UNICEF at the United Nations, New York.

Human Rights Watch. (1996). *Police Abuse and Killings of Street Children in India*. New York: Human Rights Watch.

International Committee of the Red Cross. (2004). *Inter-agency Guiding Principles on Unaccompanied and Separated Children*. Switzerland: International Committee of the Red Cross.

International Social Service and United Nations Children's Fund. (2004). *Joint Working Paper on Improving Protection for Children Without Parental Care: A Call for International Standards*. Geneva: International Social Service and United Nations Children's Fund.

John, M. (2003). *Children's Rights and Power: Charging up for a New Century*. New York: Jessica Kingsley.

Kutscher, M. L. (2004). *The ADHD eBook*. www.pediatricneurology.com. Accessed 8 May 2004.

Lesser, J. G. and Pope, D. S. (2007). *Human Behavior and the Social Environment: Theory and Practice*. Boston, MA: Pearson Allyn and Bacon.

Mehra, J. (1996). *Reducing Risk Behaviour Related to HIV/AIDS, STD and Drug Abuse Among Street Children: National Report*. New Delhi: Ministry of Welfare, UNDCP, UNICEF, WHO and NACO.

Prayas. (2002). *Forced Separation: Children of Imprisoned Mothers*. Mumbai: Prayas.

Save the Children. (2005). *The Right Not to Lose Hope: Children in Conflict with the Law*. London: Save the Children.

Tata Institute of Social Sciences. (1998). *Reaching Out to the Children of Alcoholics*. Mumbai: TISS, Department of Extramural Studies.

Thompson, C. L. and Henderson, D. A. (2007). *Counseling Children*. South Melbourne, VIC and Belmont, CA: Thomson/Brooks/Cole.

United Nations Children's Fund. (2006). *Child Protection Information Sheet*. New York: UNICEF.

Chapter 15
Children in Emergency Situations and Secondary Prevention

15.1 Concepts of Children in Emergency Situations and Secondary Prevention

15.1.1 Children in Emergency Situations

In almost all emergency situations such as environmental disasters, ethnic/armed conflicts, refugee situations and other crises, children are the most vulnerable, often deprived of care and protection. These emergency situations tend to have the following effects on children:

- Disruption of the major support systems of children such as family, friends and school and disruption of food habits, education and recreation, and cultural life.
- Aggravation of patriarchy, poverty and incapability of parents for childcare.
- Making children who are otherwise cared for, vulnerable to neglect, abuse and commercial exploitation.
- Separation of children from their family and other support systems/ homelessness.
- Impact on children's emotional and mental well-being.

15.1.2 Secondary Prevention

15.1.2.1 Goals

Secondary prevention for children in emergency situations may aim at the following goals:

1. Prevention of their vulnerability, neglect, abuse and commercial exploitation,
2. Promotion of their psychosocial well-being,

M. Desai, *A Rights-Based Preventative Approach for Psychosocial Well-Being in Childhood*, Children's Well-Being: Indicators and Research 3,
DOI 10.1007/978-90-481-9066-9_15,

3. Promotion of their age-appropriate developmental opportunities and
4. Promotion of their rights to family care, development, participation and protection.

15.1.2.2 Interventions

Secondary prevention of neglect of children in emergency situations may be carried out through the following rights-based interventions:

- Case management:
    - Direct intervention for giving information and advice, teaching and training in psychosocial skills and counselling
    - Linking with natural support systems, self-help groups, flexitime supplementary childcare and other formal systems of state and voluntary organisations
- Psycho-educational group work

15.2 Children Affected by Emergency Situations in General

15.2.1 Situational Analysis of Children in Emergencies

Some of the factors affecting children's situation in emergencies are discussed by UNICEF and International Social Service (2004) as follows:

Lack of Preparedness: While increasing emphasis is being placed on the need for preparedness in the case of emergencies, it is clear that a significant proportion of the immediate response – with its longer-term ramifications – continues to be carried out on an ad hoc, spontaneous basis, often involving numerous and diverse actors.

Numbers of Affected Children: The number of children requiring care provision can obviously create tremendous pressure on the existing and potentially feasible out-of-home solutions.

Reduced Capacity of the Community: Communities affected by emergencies are materially and psychologically in a much-diminished position to look after children who have lost – permanently or temporarily – their parents.

Lack of Professionals: Local professionals working in child protection and related spheres will inevitably be among those killed or otherwise affected by an emergency, and many may have fled the area. The burden placed on those remaining, in the face of unprecedented need for their services, will therefore be all the greater.

Partial or Total Destruction of Infrastructure: Over and above the destruction of basic health, education, water/sanitation facilities and administrative systems, communication of all kinds – transport, phone lines, radio – is often severely jeopardised in emergencies, adding to the difficulties of those attempting to organise and provide alternative care for children.

Weak or Non-existent Government Presence: Under-resourced governments, and those that have lost effective control of given regions, have little or no impact in emergencies, and will not be able to ensure adherence to pre-determined policies and priorities in the child protection sphere.

Major Presence of Foreign Organisations: Assistance and relief in emergencies invariably requires the intervention of non-domestic agencies: inter-governmental, governmental and international and foreign voluntary organisations. However, the wider the response and the weaker the national authorities, the greater is the risk that programmes for children requiring out-of-home care will be uncoordinated, in violation of children's rights, and contrary to the prevailing policy.

Any crisis has adverse effects on children's psyches. Common feelings associated with crisis are anxiety, fear, insecurity, anger and grief. The traumatic experiences lead to nervous breakdown during and after a crisis, leading to a stunted personality. Many of these effects on children may last a long time (Narayan 1994).

In emergency situations, a number of children become separated from their families. These children form one of the most vulnerable groups in these situations. According to the International Committee of the Red Cross (2004), they could be in any of the following situations:

- Separated children are those separated from both parents, or from their previous legal or customary primary care-giver, but not necessarily from other relatives. These may, therefore, include children accompanied by other adult family members.
- Unaccompanied children (also called unaccompanied minors) are children who have been separated from both parents and other relatives and are not being cared for by an adult who, by law or custom, is responsible for doing so.
- Orphans are children, both of whose parents are known to be dead. In some countries, however, a child who has lost one parent is also called an orphan.

15.2.2 Rights of Children in Emergency Situations

The rights of children in emergency situations can be drawn from the following rights identified for separated, unaccompanied and orphan children in emergency situations by the International Committee of the Red Cross (2004):

- The right to a name, legal identity and birth registration;
- The right to physical and legal protection;
- The right not to be separated from their parents;
- The right to provisions for their basic subsistence;

- The right to care and assistance appropriate to their age and developmental needs; and
- The right to participate in decisions about their future (International Committee of the Red Cross 2004).

15.2.3 Intervention

15.2.3.1 Psychosocial Intervention

Save the Children (2004b) recommends the following goals of psychosocial programmes for children in emergency situations:

- Restoring the normal flow of development;
- Protecting children from the accumulation of distressful and harmful events;
- Enhancing the capacity of families to care for their children; and
- Enabling children to be active agents in rebuilding communities and in actualising positive futures.

The following is a guiding framework prepared by Save the Children (2004b) for operationalising emergency psychosocial programming for children. As a crisis situation stabilises, additional activities should be added and approaches expanded for a broader reach.

- *Ensure children's safety and security* to help reduce stress and prevent further threats.
- *Provide information and encourage participation.* In many instances, children and adults who have experienced a crisis feel that they have lost control of their life. It is important to help them feel connected and informed.
- *Recreate "normal" routines.* Schedules and regular activities allow children and families to feel more secure. There may be a need to adapt former activities to the new environment as well as to a situation of ongoing stress. It is important for international staff to know as much as possible about daily life and culture before the crisis.
- *Design activities that support children and their families.* If parents are distressed, they do not have the capacity to provide the kind of support their children require. In some cases, parents may not understand why their children are behaving in new ways and may not know how to comfort and care for their child in the new environment.
- *Reassure people.* Children and adults often need reassurance that their reactions to traumatic events are normal reactions to highly abnormal events. Avoid using words like "victim" or "traumatised" in programming operations as these terms are widely misused and carry stigma in almost all cultures. Using labels such as these promotes a model of illness (which needs to be cured) as opposed to a model of well-being (in which inherent strengths and resources are enhanced).

- *Ensure that programmes are designed to be inclusive.* Girls and boys who do not normally participate in organised social activities are among the most vulnerable. These may include girls (of all ages), youth, children who are not attending school, orphans (including those orphaned by AIDS and/or infected with HIV), disabled children and working children. It is necessary to talk with children and adults about the importance of inclusiveness in the early design phase.
- *Identify referral services.* Although the vast majority of the population will be able to adjust to their new situation, a small group of people may be severely affected and require treatment. There will also be individuals who had pre-existing psychological or psychiatric illnesses whose care has been disrupted. It is important to discuss referral mechanisms with health-care workers and mental health-care workers prior to programme implementation.
- *Respect confidentiality and rights.* Children and their families have a right to expect and request that their information, including the stories of their lives, are kept confidential. It is important to disclose this right to them as well as to staff.

15.2.3.2 Guiding Principles on Unaccompanied and Separated Children

The Inter-agency Working Group on Unaccompanied and Separated Children has prepared the Guiding Principles on Unaccompanied and Separated Children, under the leadership of the International Committee of the Red Cross, in 2004 as summarised below.

Preserving Family Unity

The International Committee of the Red Cross (2004) stresses that efforts must be made in an emergency to protect family unity and avoid child–family separation as follows.

Preventing Separation: Sometimes children may get separated from their families in emergencies accidentally, when fleeing from danger or during evacuation. The separation may also take place deliberately when children are abandoned or given over to the care of another individual or a residential centre, perhaps in the belief that they will have a better chance of survival or access to services.

It is possible to prevent children from being separated from their families, even in extreme emergencies. Parents and school teachers should teach children their name, address and details of where they come from, to facilitate tracing should they become separated. Name tags may be useful to identify children, particularly young children, if they are forced to flee.

Planning Evacuation: Whenever possible, children should be evacuated from their place of residence together with adult family members. Evacuating children without family members should be the last resort and temporary. International humanitarian law provides guidance to facilitate the return of evacuated children to their families and country (Additional Protocol to the 1949 Geneva Conventions, Article 78). Some of the suggestions are listed below:

- Reception and care arrangements at the destination must be confirmed prior to evacuation. Ways must be found to maintain contact between child and family, and measures taken to ensure early reunification. If the principles devised to protect the best interests of the child cannot be respected, the evacuation should be reconsidered.
- Children should be given the opportunity to express their opinion, and it should be taken into consideration.
- The personal and family particulars of each child must be recorded in a personal profile and history file. This file should also include complete information as to the identity of the entrusting agency and copies of the parents' written consent. A copy of the file should travel with the child. Further copies should be given to the parents, national authorities, the organisation responsible for the evacuation and a neutral monitoring agency. Documentation for children should include sufficient travel documents to enable easy return to the place of origin.
- Any evacuation, whether for safety or for medical reasons, should be limited to a place as close as possible to the child's home and family.

Legal Identity and Birth Registration: The child's identity, including nationality as well as the identity of his or her family must be recorded and preserved. Organisations caring for separated children must seek to obtain the documentation needed to record children's identity and filiation, if known. If a child's identity is not known, the relevant authorities should take appropriate measures to ascertain it. A new identity should be established only as a last resort.

Care Arrangements

Emergency Care and Assistance: According to the International Committee of the Red Cross (2004), in emergencies, interim care must be provided for children separated form their families until they are reunited. Following are the guiding principles in such situations:

- All children need security and physical and emotional care in a setting that encourages their general development.
- Where possible, this care should be provided in families within the child's own community, with close monitoring.
- Interventions should build on and strengthen the systems that currently function in the community, and involve community leaders and local authorities, unless their views are not in the best interests of the child.
- Children must be kept informed of the plans being made for them, and their opinions taken into consideration.

- Cooperation between all agencies providing interim care is essential, using agreed guidelines for family- and community-based programmes or institutional care.
- The provision of interim care should be based on the best interests of the child and should not be used to promote political, religious or other agenda.
- The focus must be on temporary care, with commitment to carrying out family tracing.

Institutional Care: Even during emergencies, institutions should be viewed as a last resort, to be used only when children genuinely have no one to take care of them. There are times, however, when family-based care is not possible and temporary institutional care and protection is required (International Committee of the Red Cross 2004).

Adoption: Following are the guiding principles formulated for adoption of unaccompanied and separated children by the International Committee of the Red Cross (2004):

- Unaccompanied or separated children must not be adopted in haste at the height of the emergency.
- Priority must be given to adoption by relatives wherever they live. If this is not an option, preference will be given to adoption within the community from which the child comes, or at least within his or her own culture.
- Adoption should not be considered:
  - If there is reasonable hope of successful tracing and reunification with the child's family in the child's best interest;
  - If it is against the expressed wishes of the child or the parents;
  - Unless a reasonable time has passed during which all feasible steps to trace the parents or other surviving family members have been carried out.
- Adoption in a country of asylum is not normally desirable. This is particularly true if there is the possibility of voluntary repatriation "under conditions of safety and dignity" in the near future.
- No payment, either in cash or in kind, should be involved, with the exception of legitimate legal costs and adoption agency expenses.

15.3 Children Affected by Environmental Disasters

15.3.1 Concepts of Environmental Disasters

According to the Wikipedia, an environmental/natural disaster is the consequence or effect of a hazardous event, occurring when human activities and natural phenomenon become enmeshed. Environmental disasters can be in the form of droughts, floods, cyclones, tsunami, hurricanes, landslides, earthquakes and so on.

15.3.2 Intervention

Following are good practices on disaster preparedness of children, suggested by Jabry (2003):

- Children in disaster-prone areas should be made aware of what might happen, how to react appropriately, how to seek help and what they can do to safeguard themselves, their families, their property and their environment.
- Communities in disaster-prone areas should develop disaster preparedness plans which include children's input. These plans should clearly identify local risks and hazards, be produced in media that all community members can understand and access and ensure that everyone is familiar with them.
- International, national and local government and non-government organisations that carry out disaster-related work should ensure that they have sufficient staff trained in child health, child development, child protection and child consultation and participation skills. The experts can run short training sessions for the local staff.

Following are good practices on recovery of children from disaster, suggested by Jabry (2003):

- Children and adolescents can and should help in a variety of recovery tasks in the aftermath of a disaster and not thought of as being in the way, or just hanging around or non-contributors. They can help in caring for and entertaining younger children, making and distributing food and so on.
- Children's education in the aftermath of a disaster needs to be established as an urgent priority. Routines for children with reference to regular meals, story telling, sports, music and festivals should be established as soon as possible. It sends a clear signal to children that they are important and cared for and allow them to recover a semblance of structure and normalcy in their lives.

15.4 Children Affected by Ethnic/Armed Conflicts

15.4.1 Concepts of Ethnic/Armed Conflicts

The liberal process of development has led to commodification of relationships and increased poverty, which have resulted in enlarged social prejudices and conflict with reference to religions, castes, tribes and regions throughout the world. The outcome is frequent incidents of collective violence, involving the masses, across class and age.

15.4.2 Situational Analysis of Children in Ethnic/Armed Conflicts

A summary of the impact of armed conflict on children, according to a review of trends and issues identified through secondary research on children affected by armed conflict in South Asia (Boyden et al. 2001), is given below:

- Disruptions to the familial and material environment (displacement from homeland, family dispersal, separation and discord, female-headed households, impoverishment, destitution, loss of service access, such as school and health centres, and social interaction and the intimidatory presence of military personnel);
- Threats to the physical integrity of the child (child casualties, physical violations, sexual violence, civil and political violations and HIV/AIDS);
- Transformation in the children's roles and responsibilities (increasing social and economic responsibilities, involvement in exploitative and hazardous work, recruitment in armed struggle); and
- Differentials in children's vulnerabilities.

Mental impact of violence also includes development of hostility, prejudices, stereotypes and biases, which when formed in childhood, last for lifetime (Narayan 1994). During armed conflict, societal values tend to be quickly eroded, leading to a significant increase in criminal and anti-social activity. Often it is impossible to impose the rule of law. Armed forces – governmental or other – may abuse their power by, for example, abducting children from their care-givers or from residential facilities and camps. Taking advantage of the chaos, individuals and groups may also seek to exploit children who cannot be protected by their parents. The protective facet of childcare provision therefore takes on very special importance in emergency situations (UNICEF and International Social Service 2004).

Families and children are not just getting caught in the crossfire, they are also likely to be specific targets. There has been increasing use of young children as soldiers as they are easier to intimidate and do as they are told, do not run away and do not demand salaries. In large drawn-out conflicts, children who are orphaned, frightened, bored and frustrated often choose to fight. In these violent circumstances, women and girls suffer the added trauma of sexual abuse and rape (Singh 2001).

Sexual bartering, rooted in poverty, powerlessness and displacement, is a widespread phenomenon in conflicts, post-conflict and refugee settings, and increases the risk of HIV/AIDS transmission. The law in conflict-affected countries often fails to protect children, particularly girls and young women, from having to use sex to obtain basic goods and services. Behind the widespread lack of awareness is an almost total absence of sexual and reproductive health services in most conflict situations and refugee camps (Save the Children 2004a).

15.4.3 Child Rights for Protection in Ethnic/Armed Conflict

Article 38 of the UNCRC states the following:

1. State parties undertake to respect and to ensure respect for rules of international humanitarian law applicable to them in armed conflicts, which are relevant to the child.

2. State parties shall take all feasible measures to ensure that persons who have not attained the age of 15 years do not take a direct part in hostilities.
3. State parties shall refrain from recruiting any person who has not attained the age of 15 years into their armed forces. In recruiting among those persons who have attained the age of 15 years but who have not attained the age of 18 years, state parties shall endeavour to give priority to those who are oldest.
4. In accordance with their obligations under international humanitarian law to protect the civilian population in armed conflicts, state parties shall take all feasible measures to ensure protection and care of children who are affected by an armed conflict.

The Optional Protocol to the Convention on the Rights of the Child on the involvement of children in armed conflict of 2002 requires that the state parties shall take all feasible measures to ensure that members of their armed forces who have not attained the age of 18 years do not take a direct part in hostilities.

According to the Plan of Action for Implementing the World Declaration on the Survival, Protection and Development of Children in the 1990s, children need special protection in situations of armed conflict. Recent examples in which countries and opposing factions have agreed to suspend hostilities and adopt special measures such as "corridors of peace" to allow relief supplies to reach women and children and "days of tranquillity" to vaccinate and to provide other health services for children and their families in areas of conflict need to be applied to all such situations. Resolution of a conflict need not be a prerequisite for measures explicitly to protect children and their families to ensure their continuing access to food, medical care and basic services, to deal with trauma resulting from violence and to exempt them from other direct consequences of violence and hostilities. To build the foundation for a peaceful world where violence and war cease to be acceptable means for settling disputes and conflicts, children's education should inculcate values of peace, tolerance, understanding and dialogue.

The ILO Convention No. 182 includes forced or compulsory recruitment of children for use in armed conflict in the list of the worst forms of child labour, which are to be eliminated as a priority.

15.4.4 Intervention

Children who have been continually exposed to violence often express a significant change in their beliefs and attitudes, including a fundamental loss of trust in others. Rebuilding the ability to trust is a task for everyone, but especially for those closest to children in their daily life. The most effective way to do this is by establishing good relationships with children, through play, listening, supporting, keeping promises, involving children in real tasks and giving them proper feedback. Exploring a child's experience of violence and displacement and the meaning it holds in his/her life can be important to the process of healing and recovery. Yet it should take place in a stable, supportive environment with participation of care-givers who have a solid and continuing relationship with the child. In-depth clinical interviews intended to awake the memories and feelings associated with a child's worst moments might be very harmful, especially if conducted with an unprepared child by a stranger. This kind of interview risks tearing down a vulnerable child's defences and leaving him/her in a worse state of pain and agitation than before (Save the Children 2004b).

Save the Children (2004b) has proposed the following principles and approaches to work with children affected by war and displacement.

- Apply a long-term perspective that incorporates the psychosocial well-being of children.
- Adopt a community-based approach that encourages self-help and builds on local culture, realities and perceptions of child development.
- Promote normal family and everyday life so as to reinforce a child's natural resilience.
- Focus on primary care and prevention of further harm in the healing of children's psychological wounds.
- Provide support as well as training for personnel who care for children.
- Ensure clarity on ethical issues in order to protect children.
- Advocate for children's rights.

15.5 Child Refugees

15.5.1 Concept of Refugees

The UN 1951 Convention Relating to the Status of Refugees and its 1967 Protocol define a refugee as a person, who owing to well-founded fear of being persecuted for reasons of race, religion, nationality, membership of a particular social group or political opinion, is outside the country of one's nationality and unable or unwilling to avail the protection of one's country. Refugees also leave their country for reasons of insecurity arising out of armed conflict or civil strife (UNHCR Brochure).

15.5.2 Situational Analysis of Child Refugees

With mounting unemployment and growing socio-economic problems, refugees are no longer received with open arms in most countries. At best, they are tolerated as a further burden on dwindling resources; at worst they are met with open hostility and closed borders (UNHCR Brochure).

15.5.3 Rights of Child Refugees

Article 22 of the UNCRC states the following:

1. State parties shall take appropriate measures to ensure that a child who is seeking refugee status or who is considered a refugee in accordance with applicable international or domestic law and procedures shall, whether unaccompanied or accompanied by his or her parents or by any other person, receive appropriate protection and humanitarian assistance in the enjoyment of applicable rights set forth in the present Convention and in other international human rights or humanitarian instruments to which the said States are Parties.
2. For this purpose, state parties shall provide, as they consider appropriate, cooperation in any efforts by the United Nations and other competent intergovernmental organisations or non-governmental organisations cooperating with the United Nations to protect and assist such a child and to trace the parents or other members of the family of any refugee child in order to obtain information necessary for reunification with his or her family. In cases where no parents or other members of the family can be found, the child shall be accorded the same protection as any other child permanently or temporarily deprived of his or her family environment for any reason, as set forth in the present Convention.

15.5.4 Role of the United Nations Refugee Agency

The UN High Commissioner of Refugees (UNHCR) provides the refugees asylum and protection, humanitarian assistance and solutions by way of voluntary repatriation, local integration or resettlement. It provides support for primary education of refugee children. For UNHCR's purpose, an unaccompanied minor is one who is separated from both parents and for whose care no person can be found who by law or custom has primary responsibility. In order to improve and enhance the protection and care of refugee children, UNHCR has adopted a Policy on Refugee Children in 1993. Typically, UNHCR works closely with other agencies to ensure that unaccompanied children are identified and registered, and their families traced.

15.5.5 Intervention

15.5.5.1 Emergency Care

Following are the guiding principles of the International Committee of the Red Cross (2004) for protection of refugee children:

- Separated children seeking refugee status should be admitted to the territory of an asylum country.

- Refugee or asylum-seeking children should not be detained. However, in situations where they are detained, this detention must be used as a measure of last resort and should be for the shortest period of time (UNCRC, Article 37).

According to the guiding principles of the International Committee of the Red Cross (2004), unaccompanied refugee children staying with host families in the country of asylum face a heightened risk of exploitation and denial of basic rights. Monitoring is particularly difficult in such circumstances. In addition, it hinders the opportunity of returning home once repatriation becomes possible. Therefore,

- Special efforts should be made at the earliest possible stage to identify unaccompanied refugee children staying with host families in the country of asylum.
- Steps need to be taken in collaboration with UNHCR and responsible authorities to legitimise their civil status.
- The situation of unaccompanied refugee children in the care of host families must be closely monitored.
- Placement of children in their own refugee community should be promoted. Fostering by families in the host country should be discouraged.

15.5.5.2 Durable Long-Term Solutions

The guiding principles of the International Committee of the Red Cross (2004) state that, as is the case for all children, family reunification should be the priority for the separated refugee child, be it in the country of asylum, in the country of origin through voluntary repatriation or in a third country, as follows:

- The decision on the return of a child to the country of origin for family reunification should be based on the best interests of the child. Each case should be reviewed individually by balancing the desirability of family reunification with the following non-exhaustive list of factors:
  - Conditions in the proposed place of return in the county of origin in terms of threat to the child's physical security and/or the risk of persecution;
  - Conditions in the country of asylum;
  - The wishes of the child;
  - The wishes of the parents and their capacity to care for the child;
  - The quality of care arrangements in the country of asylum.
- Where relatives other than parents/primary care-givers have been traced in the country of origin but parents/primary care-givers have not yet been found, caution should be exercised before proceeding with this family reunification as it could result in permanent separation for the child's parents/primary care-givers.
- If reunification is not possible despite all efforts, finding an alternative placement for the child in the country of origin is the preferred solution provided that fundamental changes have taken place there that make voluntary repatriation possible.

- Placing the child in an adoption family in another country either through local integration in the asylum country or resettlement in a third country, that is, inter-country adoption, should be considered only if the child cannot be suitably cared for in the country of origin.

References

Boyden, J., de Berry, J., Feeny, T. and Hart, J. (2001). *Children Affected by Armed Conflict in South Asia: A Review of Trends and Issues Identified Through Secondary Research.* Oxford: Refugee Studies Research Centre, Oxford University.

International Committee of the Red Cross. (2004). *Inter-agency Guiding Principles on Unaccompanied and Separated Children.* Switzerland: International Committee of the Red Cross.

Jabry, A. (Ed.) (2003). *Children in Disasters: After the Cameras have Gone. A Report for Plan UK.* Nottingham: Design2Print Solutions Ltd.

Narayan, L. (1994). Dynamics of families facing societal violence and interventions. In M. Desai (Ed.) *Family and Interventions: A Course Compendium* (pp. 211–241). Bombay: Tata Institute of Social Sciences.

Save the Children. (2004a). *Promoting Psychosocial Well Being Among Children Affected by Armed Conflict and Displacement: Principles and Approaches.* www.scslat.org/eng/hacemos/2.php. Accessed 22 July 2009.

Save the Children. (2004b). *Psychosocial Care and Protection of Children in Emergencies a Field Guide.* http://www.savethechildren.org/publications/technical-resources/emergencies-protection/PSYCHOSOCIAL_CONTENTS.pdf. Accessed 22 July 2009.

Singh, D. (2001). *Child Rights and Social Wrongs: An Analysis of Contemporary Realties*, vols. 1–3. New Delhi: Kanishka Publishers.

United Nations Children's Fund and International Social Service. (2004). *Care for Children in Emergency Situations: Implications for International Standards.* New York and Geneva: United Nations Children's Fund and International Social.

Chapter 16
Systems for Tertiary Prevention for Children

16.1 Concepts of Systems for Tertiary Prevention for Children

16.1.1 Goals of Tertiary Prevention

Tertiary prevention is prevention of abuse, commercial exploitation and conflict with law in childhood through the juvenile justice system and through the substitute childcare systems if necessary.

16.1.1.1 Goals of Tertiary Prevention of Abuse and Commercial Exploitation in Childhood

Tertiary prevention of abuse and commercial exploitation in childhood may aim at the following goals:

1. Prevention of

   - Further abuse and commercial exploitation of the same children,
   - Effects of abuse and commercial exploitation on mental and physical health of children,
   - Abused and commercially exploited children facing conflict with law and
   - The cycle of abuse by preventing the survivors of abuse and commercial exploitation growing up to be offenders of children as adults

2. Promotion of their psychosocial well-being;
3. Promotion of their age-appropriate developmental opportunities; and
4. Promotion of their rights to family care, development, participation and protection.

M. Desai, *A Rights-Based Preventative Approach for Psychosocial Well-Being in Childhood*, Children's Well-Being: Indicators and Research 3,
DOI 10.1007/978-90-481-9066-9_16,

16.1.1.2 Goals of Tertiary Prevention of Conflict with Law in Childhood

Tertiary prevention of conflict with law in childhood may aim at the following goals:

1. Prevention of
   - First-time offence leading to more offences,
   - Status offence leading to property crime, and
   - Property crimes leading to violent crimes
2. Prevention of their vulnerability, neglect, abuse and commercial exploitation;
3. Promotion of their psychosocial skills;
4. Promotion of their age-appropriate developmental opportunities; and
5. Promotion of their rights to family care, development, participation and protection.

16.1.2 Systems and Interventions for Tertiary Prevention for Children

The existing systems for tertiary prevention of abuse, commercial exploitation and conflict with law in childhood are the juvenile justice system and substitute childcare such as foster family care, child adoption and institutional childcare, often working independently. The rights-based preventative approach for children's psychosocial well-being requires that

- The juvenile justice system should be used only for restorative justice to children facing abuse and commercial exploitation and for children who have harmed others. It should not be used for children at risk of neglect who need the secondary prevention services.
- Children should be removed from their homes for placement in the appropriate substitute childcare only if the family preservation services fail and only though the juvenile justice system.

Tertiary prevention may be achieved by carrying out the following interventions through these systems:

1. Child advocacy interventions for restorative justice:
   - Facilitate child rights in the judicial proceedings
   - Conduct victim–offender mediation
   - Rehabilitate the child
   - Treat and rehabilitate offenders of children
2. Integrated supplementary and substitute childcare
   - Flexitime child day care/night care
   - Foster family care

- Child adoption
- Institutional childcare

3. Case management for children and their families:

- Direct intervention for giving information and advice, teaching and training, and counselling
- System linkage with natural support systems, self-help groups and formal systems of state and civil society

4. Psycho-educational group work with children and offenders.

16.2 Juvenile Justice System

16.2.1 Concepts of Juvenile Justice System

The juvenile justice system has its origin in the late nineteenth and twentieth century when reformers enjoined the child welfare purpose to that of youth correction, by creating the juvenile courts. Their concern was directed towards the youthful lawbreaker and children whose circumstances were likely to lead them into 'delinquency', rather than those who were grossly neglected or in need of other protections (Downs et al. 2009). The prevalence of the juvenile justice system indicates the ambivalence of the state's legal role in relation to children. While the model of the vulnerable ignorant child positioned them as requiring protection, children were also portrayed as a source of disruption requiring control and discipline (Burman 2008). The juvenile justice system is an outcome of a view that society needs to protect children, through welfare, but it also needs to be protected from them, through justice, which Goldson (2002) calls an expression of the victim–threat dualism. One system was developed to deal with both, deprivation and depravation among children, as very often the two were not very different. As Bose (1992) pointed out there is a blurred borderline between the two. More often than not, situational factors result in one child being and another child not being apprehended as a 'delinquent'. However, as far as child abuse is concerned, research shows that it cuts across socio-economic class. It is therefore important to understand each of these two issues separately as well as the linkage between the two to plan a preventative intervention (Hess and Drowns 2004).

According to Harding (1991), in the juvenile justice system, extensive state intervention to protect and care for children is legitimatized by the paternalistic perspective, undervaluing the biological family bonds. Substitute care is favoured when the care of the natural family is found to be inadequate.

16.2.2 Retributive Versus Restorative Justice

The philosophy of the juvenile justice system has been retributive where the court proceedings often provoke stressful thoughts, fears and even nightmares for a child

(Ferrara 2002). Lack of confidentiality and insensitive treatment by law enforcement agencies, medical and social investigators and the courts are the main court-related problems due to which child victims do not come forward (UNICEF 2004). Such systems re-victimise the victims.

An overview of the differences between retributive and restorative justice is given in the following table given by Save the Children (2004).

Chart 16.1 Difference Between Retributive and Restorative Justice

Retributive Justice	Restorative Justice
Crime defined as violation of the law of the state	Crime defined as violation of the rights of one person by another
Focus on establishing blame or guilt on the past (did they do it?)	Focus on problem solving, on liabilities and obligations in future (what should be done?)
Adversarial relationships and process	Dialogue and negotiation
Imposition of pain to punish and deter/prevent	Restitution as a means of restoring both parties: reconciliation/restoration as goal
One social injury replaced by another	Focus on repair of social injury
Responsibility for action directed from state to offender: – victim ignored-offender passive	Victim's and offender's roles recognised in both problem and solution: – victim's rights/needs recognised – offender encouraged to take responsibility
Offender accountability defined as taking punishment	Offender accountability defined as understanding impact of action and helping decide how to make things right
Response focused on offender's past behaviour	Response focused on harmful consequences of offender's behaviour

While retributive justice is primarily concerned with punishing crime, restorative justice focuses on repairing the injury that crime inflicts. The four guiding principles of restorative justice are

- Repairing the harm done and restoring the balance within community and society
- Restitution for the victim
- Ensuring that the offender understands and is willing to take responsibility for his or her actions
- Helping to change and improve future behaviour of the offender concerned (Save the Children 2004).

Hess and Drowns (2004) note that restorative justice gives balanced attention to three primary interests:

- Sanctioning offender's accountability to victims
- Rehabilitation of the offenders through competency development
- Enhancement of community safety

16.2.3 Child Rights for Restorative Justice

The child rights perspective requires a restorative justice approach to children's legal matters as it puts the best interests of the child first and focuses on prevention as a primary objective.

16.2.3.1 Importance of Children's Views in Judicial Proceedings

Article 12 of the UNCRC states the following:

1. State parties shall assure to the child who is capable of forming his or her own views the right to express those views freely in all matters affecting the child, the views of the child being given due weight in accordance with the age and maturity of the child.
2. For this purpose, the child shall in particular be provided the opportunity to be heard in any judicial and administrative proceedings affecting the child, either directly or through a representative or an appropriate body, in a manner consistent with the procedural rules of national law.

16.2.3.2 Rights of Child Victims and Witnesses of Crime

In 2005, the United Nations (UN) adopted the Guidelines on Justice in Matters involving Child Victims and Witnesses of Crime, regardless of their role in the offence. These guidelines are applicable in the justice process that encompasses detection of the crime, making of the complaint, investigation, prosecution and trial and post-trial procedures, regardless of whether the case is handled in a criminal justice system for adults or juveniles, or in a customary or informal system of justice. These Guidelines discuss the following principles:

- The right to be treated with dignity and compassion
- The right to be protected from discrimination based on the child's age, gender, disability and birth; and parents' ethnicity, political or other opinion
- The right to be informed about the child's rights, the case and support services
- The right to be heard and to express views and concerns
- The right to effective and coordinated assistance by trained professionals
- The right to privacy and confidentiality
- The right to be protected from hardship during the justice process through child-sensitive procedures
- The right to safety before, during and after the justice process
- The right to reparation, including restitution from the offender and aid from the state, addressing the costs of the services used
- The right to special measures to prevent recurring victimisation or offending

16.2.3.3 Child-Sensitive Judicial Procedures

The child-sensitive procedures recommended by the UN Guidelines on Justice in Matters involving Child Victims and Witnesses of Crime (2005) include the following:

- Interview rooms designed for children,
- Interdisciplinary services for child victims integrated in the same location,
- Modified court environments that take the child witnesses into consideration,
- Recesses during a child's testimony,
- Hearings scheduled at times of day appropriate to the age and maturity of the child,
- An appropriate notification system to ensure that the child goes to court only when necessary and so on.

16.2.3.4 Multi-system Approach

The UN Guidelines on Justice in Matters involving Child Victims and Witnesses of Crime (2005) recommend a multidisciplinary approach in developing protocols for cooperation among the wide array of services such as victim support, advocacy, economic assistance, counselling, education, health, legal and social services, together with the police and the prosecutor.

16.2.3.5 Safeguards During Criminal Proceedings

Measures and protocols are needed to ensure appointing appropriate legal representation for the child and minimising direct contact between the child and the offender. One way to do this is to allow alternatives to court testimony as sources of evidence, such as giving witness statements via special audio or video facilities, or in camera (UNICEF 2005).

16.2.3.6 Civil Remedies

Laws should provide adequate remedies so that child victims receive compensation for their emotional and physical injuries. This should not be contingent on cooperation with law enforcement, nor should it depend on the victim's immigration status. Moreover, laws should ensure that civil claims can be brought against anyone who has exploited the person, including public officials. A comprehensive damages scheme would allow courts to take into account the special circumstances of the victim, and would provide for general, punitive and special damages (that is, expenses incurred due to the exploitation, such as the cost of repatriation) (UNICEF 2005).

16.2.4 Child Advocacy Interventions for Restorative Justice

Legislation for restorative justice for children may be facilitated by child advocacy centres that can be attached to children's/juvenile/other courts. These centres can carry out the psychosocial interventions at case and group levels through child rights principles and social work approaches. A multi-system approach may be facilitated through techniques of case management. Focus may be on the following areas of work:

- Facilitate child rights in the judicial proceedings.
- Conduct victim–offender mediation.
- Rehabilitate the child.
- Treat and rehabilitate offenders of children.

16.2.4.1 Facilitate Child Rights in the Judicial Proceedings

The child advocacy centres may facilitate child rights in the judicial proceedings by carrying out the following tasks:

- Provide legal aid to children and their families.
- Advocate for rescue of the child victims and arrest and prosecution of offenders of children.
- Ensure a safety plan for the child victims.
- Inform the children of their rights and role in regard to court proceedings and preparing them for the judicial process.
- Enable children to familiarise themselves with the court surroundings.
- Inform children of the different roles of the key persons at court, such as the judge, the defence lawyer and the prosecutor.
- Inform the court of the special needs of children in general and of individual children in specific cases.
- Allow the views, needs and concerns of child victims to be presented and considered in proceedings where their personal interests are affected.
- Facilitate cross-examination of the child by the police and the court and child's testimony.
- Advocate for child witness statements via special audio or video facilities, or in camera.
- Advocate for civil remedies/reparation/restitution by the offenders to the victims.

16.2.4.2 Victim–Offender Mediation

Victim–offender mediation is a common model of restorative justice in which a mediator facilitates a dialogue between the victim and the offender, parents may also be involved. The primary outcome sought is to allow the victim to relay the impact of the crime to the offender, expressing feelings and needs. The offender is expected to develop increased awareness of the harm of the offence, gains empathy with the victim, admits guilt and agrees on a reparative plan (Hess and Drowns 2004).

Victim–offender mediation can take place at any point during the process, from the arrest of an offender to before their release from prison. Some people are initially hesitant to use it for serious offences; however, it is important to understand its purpose, which is to be not simply an alternative to sentencing but a way of assisting victims to deal with the great anger or hurt they experience as a result of the crime and to avoid becoming bitter and resentful. This type of mediation can help not just victims, but also offenders and the wider community to cope with the psychological impact of crime, in a way that the formal criminal justice system does not (Save the Children 2004).

16.2.4.3 Rehabilitation of the Child

The child advocacy centres may carry out the following tasks to rehabilitate the child:

- Implement the protection order by juvenile/children's court.
- Link the children and their families with supplementary and/or substitute child welfare services.
- Link children and their parents with other formal systems as needed: Health and housing, education, vocational guidance and training, livelihood/employment for the adults, rest, recreation and cultural life.

16.2.4.4 Treatment of Offenders

Society places a high level of importance on treatment of the child victims and on the punishment of the offenders, but almost none on the treatment of the offenders. However, unless they are treated, they will continue their former patterns of abuse and exploitation (Winton and Mara 2001). A common characteristic exhibited by those who commit crimes against children is their distorted beliefs and attitudes, typically portraying children as being responsible for their own abuse/exploitation. Treatment programmes that challenge these cognitive distortions and encourage the development of empathy with children may help to prevent sex exploiters from re-offending (ECPAT International 2008).

16.3 Substitute Child Welfare

16.3.1 Concepts and History of Substitute Child Welfare

Substitute childcare is care of children away from their natural family, when the care of the natural parents is found to be inadequate. It is also known as out-of-home childcare. In the substitute childcare perspective, much greater faith is placed in the value of beneficent state action to protect children's welfare. It is based on a belief that the state not only has the duty to intervene but also the capacity to provide something better for the child. Harding (1991) observes that state intervention undervalues natural family bonds and provides alternatives which may be equally if not more problematic. The class element is at play here where middle-class decision-makers pass judgement on working-class parents and children from deprived homes are placed in somewhat better-off ones. As Mason (1991) notes, substitute care literature, state funding and practice have historically focused on methods of choosing substitute placements and processes for terminating rights of the natural parents, in case of adoption, and given only limited or no attention to the methods of rehabilitating the natural parents.

16.3.2 Concerns in Substitute Child Welfare

A Joint Working Paper on Improving Protection for Children without Parental Care by International Social Service and UNICEF (2004) identified the following areas of concerns with reference to provision of out-of-home care of children:

- *Unwarranted recourse to out-of-home care*: Many placements of children in out-of-home care could easily be avoided if the major emphasis were to be placed on providing support and services to enable parents to care for their children themselves.
- *Inappropriate decisions regarding type of care*: Foster-care and residential placements may be ordered without full consideration of the range of options available (and their specific advantages and disadvantages) and/or without due regard to the needs and circumstances of the individual child.
- *Recourse to residential care*: Unnecessary over-use of residential placements is a common feature of out-of-home care throughout the world because other options have not been developed.
- *Inadequate permanency planning*: Permanency planning should be an integral part of the individualised care plan that needs to be drawn up for each child before or shortly after out-of-home care commences, and reviewed regularly as the placement evolves.
- *Children and parents with no voice*: Very often, no mechanisms or processes are foreseen to enable the child and the family to participate systematically and effectively in decision-making about appropriate care options and the longer-term goal of a placement.

16.3.3 Child Right to Biological Parental Care

Article 9 of the UNCRC emphasises the child right not to be separated from his or her parents, as follows:

1. State parties shall ensure that a child shall not be separated from his or her parents against their will, except when competent authorities subject to judicial review determine, in accordance with applicable law and procedures, that such

separation is necessary for the best interests of the child. Such determination may be necessary in a particular case such as one involving abuse or neglect of the child by the parents, or one where the parents are living separately and a decision must be made as to the child's place of residence.

2. In any proceedings pursuant to paragraph 1 of the present article, all interested parties shall be given an opportunity to participate in the proceedings and make their views known.
3. State parties shall respect the right of the child who is separated from one or both parents to maintain personal relations and direct contact with both parents on a regular basis, except if it is contrary to the child's best interests.
4. Where such separation results from any action initiated by a state party, such as the detention, imprisonment, exile, deportation or death (including death arising from any cause while the person is in the custody of the State) of one or both parents or of the child, that state party shall, upon request, provide the parents, the child or, if appropriate, another member of the family with the essential information concerning the whereabouts of the absent member(s) of the family unless the provision of the information would be detrimental to the well-being of the child. State parties shall further ensure that the submission of such a request shall of itself entail no adverse consequences for the person(s) concerned.

Article 10 of the UNCRC emphasises the child right to reunification with his/her parents, as follows:

1. In accordance with the obligation of state parties under Article 9, paragraph 1, applications by a child or his or her parents to enter or leave a state party for the purpose of family reunification shall be dealt with by state parties in a positive, humane and expeditious manner. State parties shall further ensure that the submission of such a request shall entail no adverse consequences for the applicants and for the members of their family.
2. A child whose parents reside in different States shall have the right to maintain on a regular basis, save in exceptional circumstances personal relations and direct contacts with both parents. Towards that end and in accordance with the obligation of state parties under Article 9, paragraph 1, state parties shall respect the right of the child and his or her parents to leave any country, including their own, and to enter their own country. The right to leave any country shall be subject only to such restrictions as are prescribed by law and which are necessary to protect the national security, public order (order public), public health or morals or the rights and freedoms of others and are consistent with the other rights recognised in the present Convention.

According to Harding (1991), there is a need to advocate for the defence of the birth family and parents' rights perspective that encapsulates the idea that birth or natural families are important for both children and parents and should be maintained wherever possible. The role of the state should be supportive of families, providing various services that they need to remain together. There should be an emphasis on the rights of parents as people in their own right, with an explanation of poor quality childcare which is sympathetic to parental difficulties. Placing children in substitute care should be seen as generally undesirable. Where children do have to come into state care, considerable intervention should be devoted to helping their families and maintaining links with them so that the children can return home again.

16.3.4 Intervention

16.3.4.1 Principles for Child Placement in Substitute Care

The UN Declaration on Social and Legal Principles relating to the Protection and Welfare of Children, with special reference to Foster Placement and Adoption Nationally and Internationally of 1986, states the following:

Article 3: The first priority for a child is to be cared for by his or her own parents.

Article 4: When care by the child's own parents is unavailable or inappropriate, care by relatives of the child's parents, by another substitute – foster or adoptive – family or, if necessary, by an appropriate institution should be considered.

Article 5: In all matters relating to the placement of a child outside the care of the child's own parents, the best interests of the child, particularly his or her need for affection and right to security and continuing care, should be the paramount consideration.

Article 6: Persons responsible for foster placement or adoption procedures should have professional or other appropriate training.

Article 7: Governments should determine the adequacy of their national child welfare services and consider appropriate actions.

Article 8: The child should at all times have a name, a nationality and a legal representative. The child should not, as a result of foster placement, adoption or any alternative regime, be deprived or his or her name, nationality or legal representative unless the child thereby acquires a new name, nationality or legal representative.

Article 9: The need of a foster or an adopted child to know about his or her background should be recognised by persons responsible for the child's care unless this is contrary to the child's best interests.

UNICEF (2004) recommends the following three principles to guide decisions regarding long-term substitute care for children, once the need for such care has been demonstrated:

- Family-based solutions are generally preferable to institutional placements
- Permanent solutions are generally preferable to temporary ones
- National (domestic) solutions are generally preferable to those involving another country.

16.3.4.2 Family Preservation Services

Family preservation services aim at prevention of placement of the child in substitute care. Downs et al. (2009, pp. 243–244) have compiled the following common elements of intensive, family preservation services:

- Commitment to maintaining children in their own homes.
- Focusing on the entire family system rather than on individuals.
- Beginning service as soon as the referral has been made.
- Seeing and working with families in their own homes.
- Maintaining flexible hours 7 days a week, with round-the-clock response to family needs.
- Providing intensive service over a limited period (from 1 to 5 months).
- Keeping caseload size small – often two–three cases at a time.
- Providing comprehensive services meeting a variety of therapeutic, concrete and supportive needs. (These could include day care or night shelter, financial assistance.)
- Teaching family members skills.
- Offering counselling or therapy within the home.
- Basing services on client need rather than agency categories.

16.3.4.3 Permanency Planning

The uncertain and impermanent living arrangements of children in temporary substitute care have led to the concept of permanency planning which is defined as the systematic process of carrying out, within a brief time-limited period, a set of goal-directed activities designed to help children live in families that offer continuity of relationships with nurturing parents or caretakers and the opportunity to establish life-time relationships (Maluccio et al. 1986). If family preservation services do not work, childcare may be provided in a substitute or foster family, for a temporary period so that the child can be sent back when the natural family is rehabilitated. If the natural family cannot be rehabilitated, adoption may be facilitated as a permanent substitute family. If the child is not adoptable, the child may be institutionalised until he/she reaches adulthood.

16.3.4.4 Standards of Substitute Child Welfare

Social workers should ensure the following standards for out-of-home childcare laid down by SOS-Kinderdorf International (2005):

A Reliable, Nurturing and Lasting Relationship:

- In all forms of out-of-home care, the child is guaranteed a reliable, nurturing and lasting relationship, either through maintaining a sound and positive contact with the biological parents or, when this is not possible, through a stable substitute care-giver.

- The child–care-giver relationship provides affection, stability, safety and emotional support.
- The child–care-giver relationship is based on the child's individual needs and fulfilment of his/her rights.
- Babies and younger children in particular are offered a lasting relationship and bonding possibilities sensitive to their individual needs and vulnerability.
- Children who have been abused or undergone serial placements, who are often deeply injured and their ability to bond severely damaged, are specifically supported in restoring their confidence in relationships as an important part of their healing process.
- Special consideration is given to children in short-term or interim care for them to maintain their biological family ties and that an appropriate care-giver-to-child ratio is provided.
- Issues such as birth registration, inheritance rights and access to information are given appropriate attention.

Child Protection:

- Children are aware, competent and have access to information, complaint mechanisms and protection units.
- Children have access to appropriate therapeutic interventions.
- Care-givers demonstrate a clear rejection of corporal punishment.

Child Participation:

- Children in out-of-home care are able to voice their opinions, views and concerns and be consulted on all matters affecting them.
- Children are able to communicate freely and openly and are listened to.
- Children's views assist care-givers in identifying their needs.
- Children receive sufficient information to enable them to make their own choices.
- All information provided to children and received from them is treated with respect and confidentiality. Children have access to their files according to their maturity.

Working in Partnership with Biological Families:

- Regular contact is maintained between the child and his/her biological family where it is in his/her best interests
- The biological family is recognised as an equal partner in the child's care, and involved as much as possible in decision-making and joint activities.
- Biological parents should be able to maintain parental responsibility and receive specialised assistance when required.
- The child is encouraged to learn about his/her roots and background and to fully understand the care situation. Knowledge of his/her parents, family and history

of placement is supportive to his/her search for identity as a natural part of a child's development.

Life After Care: Accompaniment and Support:

- Out-of-home care programmes guarantee that the child receives appropriate support either until the child can be reintegrated into his/her biological family, or until he/she can live independently as a young adult.
- Careful and periodic assessment of the child's care situation and individual needs is given.
- Clear provisions for a well-developed aftercare process are foreseen.
- Children are properly prepared and equipped for life in the wider society.
- Carefully accompanying children through the transition period supports successful integration into different social structures, for example, employment, further education, independent living. Attention is given to children and young people with special needs.

16.4 Foster Family Care of Children

16.4.1 Concepts of Foster Family Care

16.4.1.1 Definition

Foster-care is a broad term that includes all care outside the child's home, including day care, foster family care, pre-adoption care and institutional care, but often used synonymously with foster family care (FFC). FFC is what the Child Welfare League of America, Inc. (1959) defined as a child welfare service, which provides substitute family care for a planned period for a child when his or her own family is going through a crisis and cannot care for him or her for a temporary period or when adoption of an adoptable child is delayed. FFC terminates when the natural family is rehabilitated and is ready to take the child back or when the adoptable child is adopted. While in FFC, child legally still belongs to the natural parents who retain their guardianship.

16.4.1.2 History

In the mid-nineteenth century, foster family care developed in the United States, under the auspices of voluntary organisations, which focused on removing children from single mothers who were living in urban poverty (Jiminez 2010).

16.4.1.3 Types

To advocate FFC as a substitute for institutional care, voluntary organisations are redefining foster-care to include day foster-care, night foster-care, weekend foster-care, short-term foster-care and long-term foster-care (Nayak 1999). Foster day care may be planned when the family situation is such that parents can receive the child back at night. For example, a family where father is ill and mother is working, the child may return home after spending the day in a foster family. Group foster homes involve the parenting of a small group of children under the care of a couple or single adult who are respected members of their own community. A group of five–seven children live in a family environment and for all practical purposes like a normal family. Based on individual needs, children are placed either on a short-term or on a long-term basis.

16.4.1.4 Limitations

In a 1959 study, Maas and Engler found that many children in foster-care lingered or drifted through the system for many years although their placement was initially thought to be temporary (Jiminez 2010). FFC does not remain a temporary service when efforts are not made to rehabilitate the natural family or when it is not possible for the natural family to take the child back, for example, orphans and abandoned children. In the latter situations, efforts should be made to refer the child for permanent substitute care, such as adoption. FFC is inappropriate for adolescents, as they are in the process of achieving independence from the family, and for physically handicapped or mentally ill children who may be difficult to handle in a foster family.

16.4.2 Child Rights in Foster Family Care

According to the Article 20 of the UNCRC:

1. A child temporarily or permanently deprived of his or her family environment, or in whose own best interests cannot be allowed to remain in that environment, shall be entitled to special protection and assistance provided by the State.
2. State parties shall in accordance with their national laws ensure alternative care for such a child.
3. Such care could include, inter alia, foster placement, kafalah of Islamic law, adoption or if necessary placement in suitable institutions for the care of children. When considering solutions, due regard shall be paid to the desirability of continuity in a child's upbringing and to the child's ethnic, religious, cultural and linguistic background.

The UN Declaration on Social and Legal Principles relating to the Protection and Welfare of Children, with special reference to Foster Placement and Adoption Nationally and Internationally of 1986, states the following:

Article 10: Foster placement of children should be regulated by law.

Article 11: Foster family care, though temporary in nature, may continue, if necessary, until adulthood but should not preclude either prior return to the child's own parents or adoption.

Article 12: In all matters of foster family care, the prospective foster parents and, as appropriate, the child and his or her own parents should be properly involved. A competent authority or agency should be responsible for supervision to ensure the welfare of the child.

16.4.3 Intervention

The FFC worker has the following tasks:

- Intake and assessment of the child and his/her natural family
- Selection of a foster family
- Placement of the child
- Facilitation of child's separation from the natural family
- Involvement of the natural parents
- Supervision of the foster family
- Psycho-educational group work
- Child's reunification with the natural family

16.4.3.1 Intake and Assessment of the Child and His/Her Natural Family

A foster family care project may get referral of cases from hospitals, orphanages, schools and other welfare agencies. The foster family care worker should, therefore, keep liaison with such agencies in the town/city. The crisis situation of the family should be assessed. The first effort should be made to see if the child's care can be facilitated without removing him/her from his or her natural family through family preservation services. The child may be considered for foster family care if the placement is required for a temporary period and if the natural parents show good potentials for rehabilitation that enables the return of the child. If the child is not adoptable for whatever reason, he/she may be placed in foster family care for an extended period.

16.4.3.2 Selection of a Foster Family

The foster family should have the same socio-economic and ethnic, religious, cultural and linguistic background as that of the child's natural family. Preference should be given to relatives for kinship care or other families known to the child from neighbours and friends. Foster families may be recruited by motivating extended family members or child-loving couples to open their homes to children in need. Foster families may be selected from those willing to take up children in foster-care. The family's physical health, mental health and motivation to take the child in foster-care should be assessed before making the placement.

16.4.3.3 Placement of the Child

The period of child's placement may be planned according to the rehabilitation possibilities of the natural family. When there is more than one child in the family, priority should be given to the placement of the younger children, because they need and would benefit the most from the placement. As far as possible, all the siblings should be placed with the same foster family. The natural parents should be asked to sign an agreement for placing their child in foster-care and the foster parents should be asked to sign an agreement for receiving the child in foster-care. The FFC agency may pay the foster parents to cover the cost of the maintenance of the child.

16.4.3.4 Facilitation of Child's Separation from the Natural Family

Fahlberg (1991, cited by Downs et al. 2009) summarised the factors that influence the child's reaction to separation as follows:

- The child's age and stage of development
- The child's attachment to the parent
- The parents' bonding to the child
- The child's perception of the reasons for separation
- The child's preparation for the move
- The 'parting message' the child receives
- The 'welcoming message' the child receives
- The environment from which the child is being moved
- The post-separation environment
- The child's temperament

Preparing the child for placement and helping him or her in adjustment with the foster family is thus very important. Keeping the child in the same school is extremely important unless placement in another school would be in the child's best interest or are the wishes of an older child. The school personnel should be educated about the impact of foster-care on children (Downs et al. 2009).

16.4.3.5 Involvement of the Natural Parents

The social worker must involve the child's natural parents as partners in the planning of the placement and a valuable resource for the child. Parents should also be prepared for the painful feelings surrounding placement. They need support to overcome the guilt feeling and loneliness resulting from placing the child. The social worker should make sure that the parents retain some of their parental obligations. This may be assured by having them contribute something to the foster family for looking after the child's needs and by encouraging them to make regular visits to the child. They should be encouraged to participate in the child's medical appointments, school conferences, sports and other after-school activities and other important events in the child's life during the child's foster placement (Downs et al. 2009).

16.4.3.6 Supervision of the Foster Family

The social worker helps the foster family through its new role. The social worker supervises the placement to make sure that the child's needs for physical care, education, recreation and so on are met. Close supervision and support to foster families is considered an intrinsic part of FFC (Nayak 1999). The foster family may be changed if not satisfactory. However, frequent replacements should be avoided. The social worker also has to resolve if there are any conflicts between natural parents and foster parents with regard to the rearing of the child.

16.4.3.7 Psycho-educational Group Work

The social worker may conduct psycho-educational group sessions with groups of natural parents to develop their parenting skills and discuss their common problems. Similar group discussions may be undertaken for foster parents. Activities for foster children in groups may include, health check up, recreation, training in psychosocial skills and so on.

16.4.3.8 Child's Reunification with the Natural Family

Family reunification is defined by Pine et al. (1993, cited by Downs et al. 2009) as the "planned process of reconnecting children in out-of-home care with their families by means of a variety of services and supports to the children, their families and their foster parents or other service providers". For effective family reunification approach, the following are compiled by Downs et al. (2009) as useful:

- A wide variety of helping options
- A primary and continuing social work staff team
- Small caseloads
- Crisis intervention services round the clock
- Use of natural helping resources in the neighbourhood and the community
- Intensive counselling services
- Provision of transportation, health services, respite care and childcare
- Availability and use of substance abuse treatment

The help needed by the family may also include employment, health services, accommodation and so on. The social worker may provide information or may refer them to relevant agencies for getting the services. The social worker needs to judge the appropriate time when the natural family is ready to take the child back. Both the families and the child may then be assisted in the process of termination of placement and rehabilitation of the child in the natural family.

16.5 Child Adoption

16.5.1 Concepts of Child Adoption

As a child welfare service, adoption provides permanent substitute care for the child when his/her biological parents are unable or unwilling to take care of him or her, and have been legally freed of any ties to the child (Kadushin 1980). Adoption is thus a service for neglected children such as orphans, abandoned children or children whose parents are untraceable. Adoption involves becoming a parent through a legal and social process rather than through a biological process.

As adoption provides stability of intimate care, it is not appropriate in the following situations:

- When the child with close family ties has parents and/or relatives who might be helped to take care of the child adequately in his or her own family home.
- When an older child may face a problem of competing or conflicting loyalties and deprives the adoptive parents of the affectional contact with an infant and the satisfaction in shaping the child's life.
- When the child is so physically, mentally or emotionally handicapped that he or she cannot live in a normal family setting.

16.5.2 Child Rights in Adoption

Article 21 of the UNCRC states the following: State parties that recognise and/or permit the system of adoption shall ensure that the best interests of the child shall be the paramount consideration and they shall:

(a) Ensure that the adoption of a child is authorised only by competent authorities who determine, in accordance with applicable law and procedures and on the basis of all pertinent and reliable information, that the adoption is permissible in view of the child's status concerning parents, relatives and legal guardians and that, if required, the persons concerned have given their informed consent to the adoption on the basis of such counselling as may be necessary;
(b) Recognise that inter-country adoption may be considered as an alternative means of child's care, if the child cannot be placed in a foster or an adoptive family or cannot in any suitable manner be cared for in the child's country of origin;
(c) Ensure that the child concerned by inter-country adoption enjoys safeguards and standards equivalent to those existing in the case of national adoption;
(d) Take all appropriate measures to ensure that, in inter-country adoption, the placement does not result in improper financial gain for those involved in it;

(e) Promote, where appropriate, the objectives of the present article by concluding bilateral or multilateral arrangements or agreements, and endeavour, within this framework, to ensure that the placement of the child in another country is carried out by competent authorities or organs.

The UN Declaration on Social and Legal Principles relating to the Protection and Welfare of Children, with special reference to Foster Placement and Adoption Nationally and Internationally of 1986, states the following:

Article 13: The primary aim of adoption is to provide the child who cannot be cared for by his or her own parents with a permanent family.

Article 14: In considering possible adoption placements, persons responsible for them should select the most appropriate environment for the child.

Article 15: Sufficient time and adequate counselling should be given to the child's own parents, the prospective adoptive parents and, as appropriate, the child in order to reach a decision on the child's future as early as possible.

Article 16: The relationship between the child to be adopted and the prospective adoptive parents should be observed by child welfare agencies or services prior to the adoption. Legislation should ensure that the child is recognised in law as a member of the adoptive family and enjoys all the rights pertinent thereto.

Article 17: If a child cannot be placed in a foster or an adoptive family or cannot in any suitable manner be cared for in the country of origin, inter-country adoption may be considered as an alternative means of providing the child with a family.

Article 18: Governments should establish policy, legislation and effective supervision for the protection of children involved in inter-country adoption. Inter-country adoption should, wherever possible, only be undertaken when such measures have been established in the States concerned.

Article 19: Policies should be established and laws enacted, where necessary, for the prohibition of abduction and of any other act for illicit placement of children.

Article 20: In inter-country adoption, placements should, as a rule, be made through competent authorities or agencies with application of safeguards and standards equivalent to those existing in respect of national adoption. In no case should the placement result in improper financial gain for those involved in it.

Article 21: In inter-country adoption through persons acting as agents for prospective adoptive parents, special precautions should be taken in order to protect the child's legal and social interests.

Article 22: No inter-country adoption should be considered before it has been established that the child is legally free for adoption and that any pertinent documents necessary to complete the adoption, such as the consent of competent authorities, will become available. It must also be established that the child will be able to migrate and to join the prospective adoptive parents and may obtain their nationality.

Article 23: In inter-country adoption, as a rule, the legal validity of the adoption should be assured in each of the countries involved.

Article 24: Where the nationality of the child differs from that of the prospective adoptive parents, all due weight shall be given to both the law of the State of which the child is a national and the law of the State of which the prospective adoptive parents are nationals. In this connection due regard shall be given to the child's cultural and religious background and interests.

The Hague Convention on Protection of Children and Co-operation in Respect of Inter-country Adoption of 1995 contains provisions designed to ensure that consent for the adoption has not been obtained improperly, and requires that:

- Persons, institutions and authorities whose consent is necessary for adoption have been counselled as necessary and informed of the effects of their consent, in particular whether or not an adoption will result in the termination of the legal relationship between the child and his or her family of origin;
- Such persons, institutions and authorities have given their consent freely, in the required legal form, expressed or evidenced in writing;
- Consent has not been induced by payment or compensation of any kind and has not been withdrawn; and
- The consent of the mother, where required, has been given only after the birth of the child.

16.5.3 Intervention

The adoption worker has the following tasks:

- Counselling the natural parents
- Intake and assessment of the child and his/her natural family
- Study and selection of adoptive parents
- Placement of the child
- Counselling the adoptive parents
- Post-adoption services

16.5.3.1 Counselling the Natural Parents

Although the number of families seeking children to adopt is increasing, no adequate legal or social support system is available for the biological mothers to bring up their own children. Adoption should be used only after making adequate efforts to counsel and support parents to keep their babies rather than abandon them and explore the possibility to unite the abandoned children with their biological parents.

16.5.3.2 Study and Selection of Adoptive Parents

Child's welfare should be given priority to parents' welfare. Homes should, therefore, be selected for children, rather than children selected for homes. Adoptive parents should preferably be chosen from child's own racial, national, ethnic and religious community. Only if such families are not available, efforts should be extended outside the child's community. A thorough study should be made of the adoptive parents in terms of their financial stability, physical health, accommodation, neighbourhood and so on. Their emotional health, capacity for parenthood, marital relationship and motivation and attitude towards adoption should also be considered. The study may be carried out through home visits, individual and joint interviews and contacting references.

16.5.3.3 Counselling the Adoptive Parents

The social worker should provide counselling to the prospective adoptive parents in clarifying the implications of their decision, in considering anticipated problems, and in preparation for implementing the decision. Pertinent social history and background of the child may be shared with the adoptive parents. Adjustment of the child and the family should be supervised during a trial or probation period of 6 months–1 year before adoption is finalised.

16.5.3.4 Post-adoption Services

Lakin (1992, cited by Downs et al. 2009) identified the following issues that characterise the adoptive family experience: entitlement; unmatched expectations; separation, loss and grief; bonding and attachment; and identity formation. Entitlement is a sense of having a right to each other. Legal entitlement is granted with a court decree, but emotional entitlement is more complex and may take more time to appear. Both the parents and child may be confronted with a discrepancy between the expectations they had and the reality of the situation. The post-adoption services may address these issues and others through voluntary preventive as well as rehabilitative approaches, making use of support groups with and without professional input and offering specialised intensive services if the placement is at risk of disruption (Downs et al. 2009). The social worker may conduct psycho-educational group sessions with groups of adoptive parents to develop their parenting skills and discuss their common problems.

16.6 Institutional Childcare

16.6.1 Concepts of Institutional Childcare

16.6.1.1 History

Under the Elizabethan Poor Law, since the seventeenth century, the impotent poor, included children were placed in almshouses. In the nineteenth century, there was a movement to remove children from the almshouses and place them in orphanages, where it was believed they would receive more appropriate treatment to meet their needs (Jiminez 2010).

16.6.1.2 Definition

A children's institution is defined by Kadushin (1980) as a 24-hour residential group facility in which a group of unrelated children are living together in the care of a group of unrelated adults. It is the oldest and the main form of welfare service anywhere in the world.

16.6.1.3 Types

Kadushin and Martin (1988) list the following types of children's institutions as serving different children:

- Homes for dependent and neglected children (earlier known as orphanages)
- Institutions for the physically handicapped
- Institutions for the retarded children
- Institutions for the confinement and rehabilitation of 'juvenile delinquents'
- Institutions that provide treatment for emotionally disturbed children and their families, also known s residential treatment centres

16.6.1.4 Use

Because institutional living provides for a tight structure with rules and regulations, it can be useful for the following children:

- It can provide specialised care for children who have behavioural problems such that create conflict with law. The institution offers greater tolerance for behaviour that could not and would not be accepted in the community. It also offers such children the opportunity to work out their problems at their own tempo and spares them the pain of having to form substitute parental relationship for which they may have neither the desire nor the capacity (Banerjee 1962). On the other hand, group pressures may be applied in an institution to motivate the children to change their behaviour so as to be less deviant and more conforming.

- Institutional care permits planning and controlling child's daily living experience. As a result, it has the scope for providing a therapeutic environment to emotionally disturbed children.
- The institution can provide the supervision of specially trained personnel and special facilities necessary to meet the unusual needs of severely handicapped children.
- The institution offers opportunities for a diluted emotional relationship with parental figures and offers a greater variety and choice of parental figures. This situation makes it an appropriate placement for adolescents who are deprived of normal family life.
- It can also meet the need for temporary shelter before the child can return to his/her natural family or move to an adoptive family.

16.6.1.5 Disadvantages

Save the Children (No date) notes that the quality of life for children living in institutions in terms of their development and well-being may be adversely influenced by the following factors:

- Reduced potential to form secure, long-lasting attachments, and reduced access to individuals who take a real personal interest in the child's problems and achievements
- Overcrowding and lack of privacy
- Reduced or no possibility to maintain contact with family members and friends
- Stigmatisation in the local community
- A restricted choice of friends, especially from outside the institution
- The imposition of religious beliefs contrary to their family background
- A lack of preparation of future life when leaving the institution

Save the Children (No date) also observes that residential care is an expensive resource; its per capita cost can be 12 times the per capita cost of community-based care options.

A Joint Working Paper on Improving Protection for Children without Parental Care by International Social Service and UNICEF (2004) identified the following areas of concerns with reference to institutional care of children:

- *Conditions in residential care*: Many investigations undertaken worldwide have variously documented poor (sometimes inhuman) physical conditions, inadequate (sometimes life-threatening) nutrition, hygiene and health care, insufficient, unqualified and poorly remunerated staff, abuse and exploitation, harsh discipline, no review of the appropriateness of the placement, little or no contact with the family or others and no preparation for life outside.
- *Private residential facilities*: Residential care services of all kinds are increasingly being passed to the private sector. However, whether run by for-profit organisations or by voluntary associations, private residential facilities are frequently able to operate with little supervision by the authorities.

- *Preparing for deinstitutionalisation*: Deinstitutionalisation presupposes the creation or development of appropriate and operational alternatives. Far too many children are in residential care not because they need it but because suitable alternatives do not exist or are not promoted or exploited.

Save the Children (No date) notes that once the institutions are in place, backed by policy, laws and frameworks for the delivery of services, providing housing and employment, it is difficult to change them and to adapt to new functions in accordance with growing insight into what is best for children even with the argument of it being more expensive.

16.6.2 Intervention

16.6.2.1 Aims

With reference to child rights, there is a dire need to do the following:

- Prevent institutionalisation,
- Deinstitutionalise institutionalised children,
- Convert institutions into non-institutional centres for children, and
- Maintain minimum standards in the institutions.

Minimum standards in institutions need to be maintained in the following areas:

- Physical facilities
- Staff-training
- Intake and engagement
- Assessment of the child and his/her natural family
- Planning the child's placement in the institution
- Health and nutrition, education, and rest, recreation and cultural life of the child
- Psycho-educational group work for development of psychosocial skills
- Child's participation in the institution and the community life
- Child's safety and protection from neglect, abuse and commercial exploitation
- Child's contact and reunification with the natural family

16.6.2.2 Physical Facilities

All rooms shall be decorated in bright colours pleasing to children and provided with suitable and homelike decoration to make them comfortable. Security shall be provided by personnel, and bars and other prison-like forms of physical security shall not be permitted. Each child shall be provided with her/his own bed and secure, private storage space for clothing and other personal items. Children shall be allowed to personalise their personal living area with photographs, decorations, etc. within reason (Frederick 2005).

16.6.2.3 Staff-Training

Staff should be carefully selected and trained and adequately compensated.

16.6.2.4 Child's Participation in the Institution and the Community Life

Children and their families are asked their opinions and participate in decisions about the children's lives and their future. On intake, children receive orientation on the purpose and operation of the facility, the roles of the staff and the conditions of their residence. This is presented in child-friendly versions, in appropriate languages and explained to children who cannot read. The privacy and confidentiality of the child are ensured in all matters, and each facility has written policies on privacy and confidentiality (Frederick 2005).

Institutionalisation should not involve deprivation of liberty. Every effort should be made to avoid the isolation of children residing in institutions from the community (for example, by enrolment in community school and use of community recreation facilities), to maximise the chances of successful transition upon departure (UNICEF 2004).

Chart 16.2 Summary of Tertiary Prevention for Children

Goals of Tertiary Prevention

Goals of Tertiary Prevention of Abuse and Commercial Exploitation in Childhood

1. Prevention of
   - Further abuse and commercial exploitation of the same children,
   - Effects of abuse and commercial exploitation on mental and physical health of children,
   - Abused and commercially exploited children facing conflict with law and
   - The cycle of abuse by preventing the survivors of abuse and commercial exploitation growing up to be offenders of children as adults;
2. Promotion of their psychosocial skills;
3. Promotion of their age-appropriate developmental opportunities; and
4. Promotion of their rights to family care, development, participation and protection.

Goals of Tertiary Prevention of Conflict with Law in Childhood

1. Prevention of
   - First-time offence leading to more offences
   - Status offence leading to property crime, and
   - Property crimes leading to violent crimes;
2. Prevention of their vulnerability, neglect, abuse and commercial exploitation;
3. Promotion of their psychosocial skills;
4. Promotion of their age-appropriate developmental opportunities; and
5. Promotion of their rights to family care, development, participation and protection.

Chart 16.2 (continued)

Interventions for Tertiary Prevention

Child Advocacy Interventions for Restorative Justice	Supportive Interventions for Children	Integrated Substitute Childcare
• Facilitate child rights in the judicial proceedings. • Conduct victim–offender mediation. • Rehabilitate the child. • Treat and rehabilitate offenders of children.	• Case management: o Direct intervention for giving information and advice, teaching and training in psychosocial skills and counselling o Linking with natural support systems, self-help groups, flexitime supplementary childcare, integrated substitute childcare and other formal systems of state and voluntary organisations o Advocacy intervention for restorative justice through the juvenile justice system • Psycho-educational group work for enrichment of psychosocial skills of children and parents	• Foster Family Care • Child Adoption • Institutional Childcare

References

Banerjee, G. R. (1962). Requirements for development of foster home programmes in India. *The Indian Journal of Social Work*, 22(4), 403–408.

Bose, A. B. (1992). *The Disadvantaged Urban Child in India*. Innocenti Occasional Papers. Florence: UNICEF.

Burman, E. (2008). *Deconstructing Developmental Psychology* (2nd ed.). London: Routledge Taylor and Frances Group.

Child Welfare League of America, Inc. (1959). *Standards for Children's Organisations Providing Foster Family Care*. New York: CWLA.

Downs, S. W., Moore, E. and McFadden, E. J. (2009). *Child Welfare and Family Services: Policies and Practice* (8th ed.). Boston: Pearson A and B.

ECPAT International. (2008). *Questions and Answers About the Commercial Sexual Exploitation of Children*. http://www.ecpatusa.org/EcpatUSA_PDF/faq%20update%20from%20ecpat%20international.pdf. Accessed 4 July 2006.

Ferrara, F. F. (2002). *Childhood Sexual Abuse: Developmental Effects Across the Lifespan*. Pacific Grove, CA: Brooks/Cole.

Frederick, J. (2005). *Guidelines for the Operation of Care Facilities for Victims of Trafficking and Violence Against Women and Girls: Rationale, Basic Procedures and Requirements for Capacity Building. Kathmandu: Planète Enfants*. http://www.childtrafficking.com/Docs/planete_enfants_2005_guidelines_for_the_operation_of_care_facilities_20060223.pdf. Accessed 26 July 2009.

Goldson, B. (2002). Children, crime and the state. In B. Goldson, M. Lavalette and J. McKechnie (Eds.) *Children, Welfare and the State* (pp. 120–135). London: Sage.

Harding, L. F. (1991). *Perspectives in Childcare Policy*. London: Longman.

Hess, K. M. and Drowns, R. W. (2004). *Juvenile Justice*. Southbank, VIC: Thomson Wadsworth.

International Social Service and United Nations Children's Fund. (2004). *Joint Working Paper on Improving Protection for Children Without Parental Care: A Call for International Standards*. Geneva: International Social Service and United Nations Children's Fund.

Jiminez, J. (2010). *Social Policy and Social Change: Toward the Creation of Social and Economic Justice*. London: Sage.

Kadushin, A. (1980). *Child Welfare Services*. New York: Macmillan.

Kadushin, A. and Martin, J. A. (1988). *Child Welfare Services* (4th ed.). New York: Macmillan.

Maluccio, A. N., Fein, E. and Olmstead, K. A. (1986). *Permanency Planning for Children: Concepts and Methods*. New York: Tavistock Publications.

Mason, J. (1991). Foster care and permanency: An analysis of the context for practice. *Australian Journal of Social Issues*, 26(4), 242–256.

Nayak, N. P. (1999). India country paper, presented at the international conference on "Alternatives to Residential Care" held at Stockholm.

Save the Children. (No date). *A Last Resort: The Growing Concern About Children in Residential Care*. London. http://www.savethechildren.org.uk/en/54_5088.htm. Accessed 19 October 2008.

Save the Children. (2004). *Juvenile Justice: Modern Concepts of Working with Children in Conflict with the Law*. http://www.crin.org/docs/save_jj_modern_concepts.pdf. Accessed 27 July 2009.

SOS-Kinderdorf International. (2005). *Family-Based Childcare: The Experience, Learning and Vision of SOS Children's Villages: Position Paper*. Innsbruck: Schachinger, Claudia.

United Nations Children's Fund. (2004). *Child Protection: A Handbook for Parliamentarians*. Geneva: United Nations Children's Fund.

United Nations Children's Fund. (2005). *Combating Child Trafficking: Handbook for Parliamentarians*. Geneva and New York: United Nations Children's Fund.

United Nations Convention on the Rights of the Child. (1989). http://www.ohchr.org/english/law/pdf/crc.pdf. Accessed 3 March 2002.

Winton, M. A. and Mara, B. A. (2001). *Child Abuse and Neglect: Multidisciplinary Approaches*. Boston, MA: Pearson Allyn and Bacon.

Chapter 17
Abuse in Childhood and Tertiary Prevention

17.1 Concepts of Abuse in Childhood and Tertiary Prevention

17.1.1 Child Abuse

Child abuse is

- Any intentional non-accidental physical, emotional and psychological or sexual harm done to a child that endangers or impairs the child's physical, emotional and psychological or sexual health and development;
- By older children, parents, relatives, caretakers, neighbours, teachers, employers, police or strangers; in family, neighbourhood, street, school, institutions, site of occupation or police custody;
- Because of adult–child power imbalance due to adultism and patriarchy, psychosocial problems or socio-economic problems, and cycle of abuse.

The following factors differentiate family abuse from other types of abuse:

- It occurs within ongoing relationships that are expected to be protective, supportive and nurturing.
- The victim wants to escape the violence but also longs to belong to a family.
- Affection and attention may co-exist with violence and abuse.
- Ongoing family relationships create opportunities for repeat victimisation (American Psychological Association 1996, cited by Mignon, Larson and Holmes 2002).

The terms used to understand child abuse are defined by Doyle (1994) as follows:

Victim: Victim is the person who has been abused.
Co-victim: Co-victims are other siblings in the family or children in the vicinity who suffer because of the activities of the perpetrator.

M. Desai, *A Rights-Based Preventative Approach for Psychosocial Well-Being in Childhood*, Children's Well-Being: Indicators and Research 3,
DOI 10.1007/978-90-481-9066-9_17, © Springer Science+Business Media B.V. 2010

Survivor: Survivor is the term applied to adults who were victims of sexual abuse as children.

Abuser/Perpetrator/Offender: Abuser, perpetrator and offender are used interchangeably as the person who abuses.

17.1.2 Tertiary Prevention

17.1.2.1 Goals

Tertiary prevention of abuse of children may aim at the following goals:

1. Prevention of their abuse and commercial exploitation:
   - Further abuse and commercial exploitation of the same children,
   - Effects of abuse and commercial exploitation on mental and physical health of children,
   - Abused and commercially exploited children facing conflict with law, and
   - The cycle of abuse by preventing the survivors of abuse and commercial exploitation growing up to be offenders of children as adults;
2. Promotion of their psychosocial well-being;
3. Promotion of their age-appropriate developmental opportunities; and
4. Promotion of their child rights to family care, development, participation and protection.

17.1.2.2 Interventions

Tertiary prevention of abuse of children may be carried out through the following psychosocial interventions:

1. Child advocacy interventions for restorative justice:
   - Facilitate child rights in the judicial proceedings.
   - Conduct victim–offender mediation.
   - Rehabilitate the child.
   - Treat and rehabilitate offenders of children;
2. Case management for children and their families:
   - Direct intervention with children and abusers for giving information and advice, teaching and training in psychosocial skills and counselling
   - Linking children and their families with natural support systems, self-help groups, flexitime supplementary childcare, integrated substitute childcare, poverty alleviation programmes and other formal systems of state and voluntary organisations
3. Psycho-educational group work with children and abusers

17.2 Causes of Child Abuse

Causes of child abuse are explained by psychosocial and critical theories.

17.2.1 Psychosocial Theories of Child Abuse

17.2.1.1 Individual-Level Causes

Faller and Ziefert (1981, cited by Downs et al. 2009) have identified the following as the most common personality characteristics found in maltreating parents, most of which can be applied to other abusers also

- Low self-esteem
- Excessive dependency
- Poor impulse control
- Rigid superego structures
- Deficient superego development
- Social isolation
- Serious difficulty coping with the demands of parenting
- Lack of parenting skills and knowledge of child development

17.2.1.2 Family-Level Causes

Faller and Ziefert (1981, cited by Downs et al. 2009) have identified the following family dynamics in maltreating parents:

- Parental collusion: One or both parents may be the active abusers but in most instances there is a passive parent who gives covert permission for the other parent to abuse the child.
- Scapegoating: When there is a marital discord, the antagonism between husband and wife may be displaced on the child.
- Reorganised families: The resentment between members of the reconstituted households may result in the physical or sexual abuse of children.
- Single-parent status: Single-parenting in itself does not place children at risk of abuse or neglect, but poor single-parent families are overrepresented in child protection services.
- Adolescent parents
- Lack of extended family

Kendig and Lowry (1998) founded their model of child abuse treatment programme on the following beliefs:

- Parents do not want to hurt their children.
- Families have within them the answers to their problems.

- Abusive parents tend to be isolated from those around them. They need to be included in a community to reduce the risk of abuse.
- Child abuse is a community problem, requiring a coordinated community solution.

17.2.2 Critical Theories of Child Abuse

Critical theorists opine that people seem to be more comfortable thinking of abuse as individual or familial although it is systemic or structural (Burman 2008).

17.2.2.1 Poverty

Subsequent to psychosocial theories of abuse, attention was drawn to the link between the child abuser, on the one hand, and inequality and poverty, on the other. However, in doing so, the focus shifted from attending to the child victims to understanding the abuser as the victim. The Marxists emphasise that it is the powerless and deprived class who is most at risk of, both, engaging in crime and being victims of crime. Research shows a higher rate of abuse among the poor. However, abuse takes place across classes but the upper classes may be able to conceal it because of access to greater resources and less scrutiny by social services (Downs et al. 2009).

17.2.2.2 Patriarchy

The radical feminists criticise the class emphasis of the Marxists, as according to them, the oppression of women and children both are due to patriarchy. Women are more marginalised and poorer than men, yet women abuse less than men (Parton 1990). The feminist theorisation identifies male power, hegemony and socialisation as the key causal factors of child abuse, not only within the family but also outside of it, in a wide range of settings (Corby 2002).

17.2.2.3 Adultism

Adultism implies assumptions about the physical and mental incapability of children, which lead to role stereotypes of dependency, hierarchy, intolerance, discrimination and also justifies violence against them. Thus from an adultist perspective, child abuse is not an anomaly, it is built into the way in which we define childhood (Mason and Steadman 1996). When parents are given the authority to control their children for disciplining them, child abuse gets institutionalised in the family.

17.2.3 Cycle of Abuse

Children learn how to parent from their parents. Abused children develop low self-esteem, poor management of negative emotions and problem solving, and weak communication and social skills. Theses traits further make them abusers of children as adults, unless they can break the intergenerational transmission of abuse or the cycle of abuse.

17.3 Child Right to Protection from Abuse

According to Article 19 of the UNCRC,

1. State parties shall take all appropriate legislative, administrative, social and educational measures to protect the child from all forms of physical or mental violence, injury or abuse, neglect or negligent treatment, maltreatment or exploitation, including sexual abuse, while in the care of parent(s), legal guardian(s) or any other person who has the care of the child.
2. Such protective measures should, as appropriate, include effective procedures for the establishment of social programmes to provide necessary support for the child and for those who have the care of the child, as well as for other forms of prevention and for identification, reporting, referral, investigation, treatment and follow-up of instances of child maltreatment described heretofore, and, as appropriate, for judicial involvement.

According to Article 37 of the UNCRC state parties shall ensure that

(a) No child shall be subjected to torture or other cruel, inhuman or degrading treatment or punishment. Neither capital punishment nor life imprisonment without possibility of release shall be imposed for offences committed by persons below 18 years of age;
(b) No child shall be deprived of his or her liberty unlawfully or arbitrarily. The arrest, detention or imprisonment of a child shall be in conformity with the law and shall be used only as a measure of last resort and for the shortest appropriate period of time;
(c) Every child deprived of liberty shall be treated with humanity and respect for the inherent dignity of the human person, and in a manner which takes into account the needs of persons of his or her age. In particular, every child deprived of liberty shall be separated from adults unless it is considered in the child's best interest not to do so and shall have the right to maintain contact with his or her family through correspondence and visits, save in exceptional circumstances;
(d) Every child deprived of his or her liberty shall have the right to prompt access to legal and other appropriate assistance, as well as the right to challenge the legality of the deprivation of his or her liberty before a court or other competent, independent and impartial authority, and to a prompt decision on any such action.

According to Article 39 of the UNCRC: State parties shall take all appropriate measures to promote physical and psychological recovery and social reintegration of a child victim of any form of neglect, exploitation, or abuse; torture or any other form of cruel, inhuman or degrading treatment or punishment; or armed conflicts. Such recovery and reintegration shall take place in an environment, which fosters the health, self-respect and dignity of the child.

17.4 Assessment of Child Abuse

17.4.1 Types of Assessment

The abused child needs various types of assessment: medical, psychosocial/psychiatric, ecological and forensic that the social worker needs to coordinate as the trauma created by multiple interviews need to be minimised. Because of the child's fear of telling, and the lack of understanding or inability to expressively communicate abuse facts, the assessment often does not produce information found reliable for conviction of the offender (Winton and Mara 2001). The assessment of child abuse therefore needs to be carried out through the following multiple methods:

(1) Interview and observations of the child
(2) Interview and observations of the family members
(3) Interview of the abuser

Whoever is the informant, the following principles as given by Doyle (1994) are useful:

- Listen first, rather than firing direct questions, although occasional open questions may be useful in helping the person continue, to clarify or to demonstrate interest and understanding.
- Never stop a person who is freely recalling significant events, although a perpetrator may need to be reminded of the legal consequences of any admission.
- Make a note of the discussion, taking care to record the exact time, where it took place and who was present as well as what was said.
- Record carefully, and in detail, all subsequent events up to the time of any court proceedings or until the matter appears to be resolved.

17.4.2 Interview and Observation of the Child

The interview process with the abused child can be made less problematic in the following ways:

- According to Doyle (1994), ideally, the child victim should choose the sex of the interviewers, but as that is rarely feasible then in most cases at least one

investigator should be female. In seeking information the interview should be conducted in a way that is appropriate to the children's ages and abilities, as well as their culture. With young children, toys may be used to put them at their ease and to enable them to communicate.
- The number of interviews can be minimised, either by videotaping investigative interviews, having professionals who need to hear the child's account behind a one-way mirror, or having more than one professional in the room, usually with one asking the questions. Consent should be obtained from children before recording an interview. They should have an opportunity to see the camera. When a one-way mirror is used to enable others to view the proceedings, the children should again be consulted, as in most instances should parents. The tapes should be kept safely (Doyle 1994).
- Interviews should not be too long. It is tempting to keep a child in an interview until he or she discloses. This in itself is abusive; the child may not be ready to say anything or may have repressed and forgotten the abuse, or there may be nothing to disclose. It is sometimes better to have a few short interviews than one very long one, provided the child is protected in the interim (Doyle 1994).
- The use of a skilled and sensitive interviewer can minimise the negative effect of disclosure and even make it a cathartic or empowering experience. Allowing a support person to be with the child during part or the entire interview can diminish its traumatic impact. Conducting the interview in a facility that is private and designed to create comfort can be helpful (Faller 1993).

17.4.3 Interview and Observation of the Family Members

The investigative or assessment interview with the non-offending caretaker has several purposes:

- Gather additional information about the likelihood of the abuse;
- Determine whether the caretaker is protective and supportive of the victim;
- In some instances, to ascertain if the mother has had a role in prompting the child to make an allegation; and
- Understand the causes or dynamics leading to the abuse (Faller 1993).

Straus and Smith (1990, cited by Winton and Mara 2001) developed a Child Abuse Checklist that differentiates between abusive and non-abusive parents. Some of the variables listed in this List are

- Verbal aggression towards the child
- Verbal aggression between spouses
- Physical aggression between spouses

- High level of marital conflict
- Parent who was physically punished as a child/adolescent

Child abuse and violence against women generally occur together in the family. The major source of protection for the child is the mother so intervention with her is important for the child's rehabilitation into the family (Faller 1993).

17.4.4 Interview of the Abuser

The alleged perpetrators should be interviewed before they have time to destroy any evidence, intimidate witnesses or prepare a convincing story to contradict the victim (Doyle 1994).

17.5 Psychosocial Intervention in Child Abuse

As child abuse mainly takes place due to the adult–child power imbalance due to adultism and patriarchy, it has to be mainly dealt with by empowerment of children. As abuse mainly results in psychosocial impact on the child, psychosocial intervention with the child victims of abuse is extremely important to break the cycle of abuse.

17.5.1 Dealing with Guilt

Words of comfort to the child victim are important which include assurances that the child is not to blame for either the abuse itself or any of the consequences of disclosure. It can be acknowledged that by disclosing they may be helping others, but it is ultimately the task of adults to protect children. They cannot, however, be absolved from responsibility if they have in turn abused or bullied another child, unless they were forced to do so by the abuser (Doyle 1994).

17.5.2 Treating Fears and Anxiety

Experiences that evoke recollections of the abuse come to elicit anxiety and fear. In some children this anxiety and fear become pervasive and crippling because of the level of avoidance they engage in to reduce their stress. For treating the child's fears and anxiety, the social worker may use discussions, play therapy or interventions in the child's environment. For example, the victim may be encouraged to ventilate by talking about the abuse and accompanying feelings, thereby reducing the level of distress related to it (Faller 1993).

17.5.3 Treating Behavioural Problems

Some of the behavioural problems, for example, difficulties with sleep, eating, toileting and being alone, may be acute after disclosure but diminish over time and eventually disappear. Short-term intervention, labelling the behavioural problems as common reactions and helping the victim resolve the underlying emotional or cognitive issues is generally helpful. Treatment strategies for all behavioural problems include helping the victim understand the relationship between the behaviours and the abuse and emotional or cognitive reactions to it; helping the child develop insight into the self-destructive nature of some of these behaviours; assisting the victim in more appropriate expression of the emotions, for example, anger; and behavioural interventions to diminish and eliminate problematic behaviour (Faller 1993).

17.5.4 Rebuilding Trust

Being a victim of abuse can have a devastating effect on children's ability to trust other people. The social worker needs to create circumstances in which the child has positive experiences with trustworthy adults in order to ameliorate the damage to the child's ability to trust. This may involve rehabilitating the parents and/or creating opportunities for appropriate relationships with adults, for example, with foster parents, mentors or other relatives (Faller 1993).

17.6 Emotional and Psychological Abuse of Children

17.6.1 Concepts of Emotional and Psychological Abuse of Children

Emotional and psychological abuse of children is

- Any intentional non-accidental emotional and psychological harm done to a child, that endangers or impairs the child's emotional and psychological health and development;
- By older children, parents, relatives, caretakers, neighbours, teachers, employers, police or strangers; in family, neighbourhood, street, school, institutions, site of occupation or police custody;
- Because of adult–child power imbalance due to adultism and patriarchy or psychosocial problems, and cycle of abuse.

17.6.2 Types of Emotional and Psychological Abuse of Children

Following are the different types of emotional abuse identified by Hart, Brassard and Karlson (1996, cited by Downs et al. 2009, p. 213).

Spurning: Spurning includes belittling, degrading, shaming, ridiculing; singling out one child to do most of the household chores, or to criticise and punish, and public humiliation.

Terrorising: Terrorising includes threatening to hurt, kill or abandon a child; placing a child in recognisably dangerous situations; and threatening or perpetuating violence against a child's loved ones or objects.

Isolating: Isolating includes confining a child, or placing unreasonable limitations on the child's freedom of movement, or on social interactions, with peers and adults in the community.

Denying Emotional Responsiveness: Denying emotional responsiveness includes being detached and uninvolved, interacting only when absolutely necessary, and failing to express love and affection to the child.

17.6.3 Implications of Emotional and Psychological Abuse of Children

The psychosocial implications of emotional and psychological abuse include low self-esteem, negative view of the world, anxiety, destructive behaviours, depression, suicidal thoughts, impulsivity, feelings of inferiority, withdrawal, apathy and learning problems. The medical implications that follow the psychosocial impact of such abuse include developmental delays, speech delays, eating and sleep disorders, skin disorders, bed-wetting, suicidal gestures and so on (Winton and Mara 2001).

17.7 Physical Abuse of Children

17.7.1 Concepts of Physical Abuse of Children

Physical abuse of children is the most commonly known and widely prevalent form of child abuse which is

- Any intentional non-accidental physical harm done to a child, that endangers or impairs the child's physical, emotional and psychological health and development;
- By older children, parents, relatives, caretakers, neighbours, teachers, employers, police or strangers; in family, neighbourhood, street, school, institutions, site of occupation or police custody;

- Because of adult–child power imbalance due to adultism and patriarchy, psychosocial problems or socio-economic problems, and cycle of abuse.

Physical abuse is often used for disciplining the child and results in physical injuries as well as psychological damage (Winton and Mara 2001). Beating a child causes pain, injury, humiliation, anxiety, anger and vindictiveness that could have long-term psychological effects. It may reduce a child's sense of worth and increase vulnerability to depression. Even minor forms of violence can cause injuries, and in the worst case permanent disability and even death. Children subjected to repeated violence may exhibit dysfunctional behaviour such as poor communication and they may display aggressive behaviour towards themselves and others. Child abuse and physical punishment can produce feelings of guilt, violation, loss of control and lowered self-esteem. Sometimes the child may not clearly understand the reason for the punishment, or the punishment is inconsistently given, and in these cases, corporal punishment can lead to passivity or strong feelings of helplessness. While biological and various social factors interact in contributing to a child's development, studies show that child abuse and physical violence in the early years contribute significantly to a higher risk of children turning violent themselves (UNICEF 2001).

In schools, corporal punishment is often justified as a necessary mean to create classroom discipline. In fact, corporal punishment is the least effective method of discipline. Punishment reinforces uncertainty and an identity of failure. It reinforces rebellion, resistance, revenge and resentment. A common effect of corporal punishment is a growing fear of teachers among school children and therefore a dislike of school. Studies show that corporal punishment is a direct and significant reason for children dropping out of school. When driven by fear of punishment, children learn simply to please the teacher and not to acquire skills and knowledge for their own development. Physical punishment thus distorts a student's motivation and learning is influenced by fear. Children who are physically and emotionally abused develop anxiety that causes loss of concentration and poor learning. They tend to fear taking risks and being creative. It may not be only the children who are themselves subjected to physical punishment who are at risk of dropping out of school; children who are emotionally affected when others are beaten and humiliated in class may also refuse to return (UNICEF 2001).

17.7.2 Assessment of Physical Abuse of Children

Physical abuse requires medical assessment of physical injuries that are obvious or internal. There is a need to determine if the physical symptoms were caused intentionally and therefore abuse or non-intentional or accidental. Any injuries in different stages of healing, such as different colours of bruises, may be a sign of ongoing physical abuse. Physical abuse also requires psychosocial assessment that include inconsistent explanation of the injury, no explanation, unrealistic explanation of the child by the parent, delays in seeking medical attention, family isolation and so on (Winton and Mara 2001).

Straus and Smith (1990, cited by Winton and Mara 2001) developed a Child Abuse Checklist that differentiates between abusive and non-abusive parents. Some of the variables listed in this List are

- Verbal aggression towards the child
- Verbal aggression between spouses
- Physical aggression between spouses
- High level of marital conflict
- Parent who was physically punished as a child/adolescent

17.7.3 Intervention with Abusive Parents

According to Schellenbach (1998, cited by Thompson and Henderson 2007, p. 544), intervention with parents who physically abuse their children includes the following:

- Teach about normal child development to correct unrealistic expectations.
- Educate about appropriate discipline procedures and other child management practices.
- Help practice anger-control techniques and coping skills.
- Discuss stress management techniques.

17.8 Sexual Abuse of Children

17.8.1 Concept of Child Sexual Abuse

17.8.1.1 Definition

The UN has defined child sexual abuse (CSA) as contacts or interactions between a child and an older or more knowledgeable child or adult (a stranger, sibling or person in position of authority, such as a parent or a caretaker), when the child is being used as an object of gratification for the older child's or adult's sexual needs. These contacts or interactions are carried out against the child, using force, trickery, bribes, threats or pressure (UNICEF 2001).

Thus CSA is

- Any intentional non-accidental sexual harm done to a child, as an object of gratification, that endangers or impairs the child's physical, sexual, emotional and psychological health and development;
- By older children, parents, relatives, caretakers, neighbours, teachers, employers, police or strangers; in family, neighbourhood, street, school, institutions, site of occupation or police custody;
- Because of adult–child power imbalance due to adultism and male–female power imbalance due to patriarchy or psychosocial problems, and cycle of abuse.

It was a coalition of the women's movement and the child protection movement that established CSA as a social problem. The feminists believe that sexual abuse is essentially located within the patriarchal social structure and male socialisation (Parton 1990). Panchal and Sheikh (1997) observed that CSA is a social problem, not merely an individual crime. The cause of CSA cannot be located simply in psychopathology, but in social, economic, political and legal factors, mainly based in male–female and adult–child power imbalances. CSA is, therefore, carried out mainly against girls but against boys also, in early childhood, middle childhood as well as in adolescence.

Abuse does not exist where there is mutual consent and the activities are mutually satisfying. Children roughly of the same age, engaging in sexual games in which there is no coercion, shame or suffering, are not abusing one another. Sexual activities are abusive if one person with greater power, whether due to age, physique, or status, takes advantage of another person's vulnerability, fears, weaknesses, lack of understanding, helplessness or need. If the consent is not informed and not freely given, it is still abuse. Children cannot know the dangers and risks, whether emotional or physical, of engaging in sexual relationships where they are the vulnerable partner. In these circumstances, they cannot give informed consent (Doyle 1994). Sometimes the strong needs of the child for physical affection, attention and dependency lead to the child's apparent complicity and willingness to initiate and maintain abuse (Agarwal 2002). Thus there are three factors that are useful in clinically differentiating abusive from non-abusive sexual acts – power differential; knowledge differential and gratification differential (Faller 1993).

17.8.1.2 Types in the Order of Severity

Faller (1993) lists the types of CSA behaviour as follows, in the order of increasing severity:

- Non-Contact Acts: Sexual comments, exposing one's sex organs and persuading the child to do the same, voyeurism (peeping), showing pornographic material and masturbating self in the presence of the child.
- Sexual Contact: Touching the child's sex organs and inducing the child to do the same to one's own, and frottage or rubbing one's sex organs against the child's body or clothing.
- Digital or Object Penetration: Placing finger or an object in the child's vagina or anus and asking the child to do the same for self.
- Oral Sex: Tongue kissing, breast sucking, kissing, licking, biting, cunnilingus (licking, kissing, sucking, biting the vagina or placing the tongue in the vaginal opening), fellatio (licking, kissing, sucking, biting the penis) and anilingus (licking, kissing the anal opening).
- Penile Penetration: Vaginal and anal intercourse.

17.8.2 Child Sex Abusers

Child sex abusers may be grouped into preferential abusers or paedophiles, situational abusers and incestual abusers.

17.8.2.1 Paedophiles

The term paedophile refers to a sexual preference for pre-pubescent children (ECPAT International 2008). The *Diagnostic and Statistical Manual of Mental Disorders* describes paedophilia as "the act or fantasy of engaging in sexual activity with prepubertal children as a repeatedly preferred or exclusive method of achieving sexual excitement. . . Isolated sexual acts with children do not warrant the [clinical] diagnosis of paedophilia". The manual adds that a person who fits this diagnosis would have to be at least 16 years old and 5 years older than the child to whom their sexual fantasies are directed. Paedophiles may focus on either boys or girls, or have no gender preference. Not all paedophiles sexually abuse or harass children. Some may have fantasies about sex with children but they do not act them out with a child (although they may use child pornography). Others may abuse children in different ways, including non-physical sexual abuse and exploitation. Most clinically definable paedophiles are male; female paedophiles exist but are rare. Generally, paedophiles do not regard their sexual interaction with children as wrong (World Congress against... 1996).

N. Desai (2001) notes that organisations of paedophiles aggressively portray paedophilia as an issue of "sexual preference". According to these paedophile "theoreticians", children are ready to be initiated into sexual activity at the age of four "or even sooner". One of the slogans of the North American Men-Boy Love Association is " Sex Before Eight, Or Else It's Too Late". They claim that opponents of paedophilia not only violate the rights of children, but deprive children of their "sexual rights" – the opportunity of sexual expression and the right to sexual gratification. This, they say, can hamper a child's growth and development! Membership of paedophile networks presumably helps paedophiles to rationalise and normalise their understanding of their sexual preferences.

17.8.2.2 Incestual Sexual Abusers

Incestuous sexual abuse is abuse by close family members, which does not require force as it is facilitated by and couched within a trusted relationship between victim and perpetrator. Incestuous sexual abuse is not "sexual indiscretion" or "affection that went too far". It is often "planned, calculated and systematic". Those who commit this abuse frequently say that they did not intend to hurt the child. Whether or not this kind of abuse involves pain or injury, and whether or not the abuser intended to hurt the victim, it is a sexual violation (Poore 2002).

17.8.2.3 Situational Child Sex Abusers

Some men use children for sex not because they have a predisposition to do so but because they find themselves in a situation where it is possible to do so. Such abusers may be men with regular partners, living "normal" lives. For this reason, they are particularly difficult to identify and are often protected by those around them, who look upon their acts of sex with children as momentary lapses in an otherwise blame-free existence (ECPAT International 2001). These abusers also violate a relationship of trust with the child, taking advantage of their power and position (Sakshi 1999).

17.8.3 Vulnerability to and Pre-conditions of Child Sexual Abuse

Finkelhor (1993, cited by Winton and Mara 2001) identified the following risk factors for CSA to occur within the family:

- Age of victim (preadolescent)
- Gender of victim (female)
- Having a stepfather at home
- The absence of one or both natural parents in the home
- The absence of the mother due to disability, illness or employment
- Poor relationship between victim and parents
- The presence of parental conflict and violence

Finklehor (1984) proposed four pre-conditions that need to be met before CSA could occur, which are explained by Quinn (1992) as below:

1. *A potential offender needs to have some motivation to abuse a child sexually.* Factors influencing this may include such things as the belief that males must be sexually dominant, controlling and powerful in relationships while their partners must be passive, undemanding and weak.
2. *The potential offender has to overcome internal inhibitions against acting on that motivation.* This may be influenced by such factors as the individual's belief that children are seductive, the existence of child pornography and the sexualisaion of children in advertising and the belief in an exaggerated sense of entitlement of males in relation to women and children.
3. *The potential offender has to overcome external impediments to committing sexual abuse.* He has to create access and opportunity to sexually assault a child without getting caught, exposed or held accountable. This may be facilitated if the family is isolated from support networks and by belief in the privacy and sanctity of the family.
4. *The potential offender or some other factor has to undermine or overcome a child's possible resistance to the sexual abuse.* The offender must coerce, manipulate, threaten, bribe, force, frighten or trick the child into sexual activity and

into silence. This may be facilitated by such factors as the child's lack of sexual knowledge and the general powerlessness.

17.8.4 Impact of Child Sexual Abuse

The extent to which the experience of childhood sexual abuse impacts the child depends on the following factors as listed by Klausner and Hasselbring (1990):

Duration and Frequency of Abuse: The longer and more frequently the sexual abuse occurs, the more serious the later emotional and sexual consequences.

Type of Sexual Activity: Sexual abuse which involves penetration is the most damaging.

Use of Force and Aggression: The greater the use of physical force or violence, the greater the consequences.

Age at Onset: Some sexual abuse professionals believe the younger the child is when the sexual abuse occurs, the more damaging it is. Others believe that younger children are more emotionally insulated and that the most damage takes place in older abused children.

Age, Gender and Relationship to Abuser: The closer the relationship of the victim and the abuser and the greater the span of years that separates them, the more harm.

Passive Submission or Willing Participation of the Child: The child who willingly submits to the abuse and who actively participates in it suffers more negative effects.

Direct or Indirect Telling with No Support: When a child tells and is not helped, the consequences are more severe and long-lasting than when the child keeps the abuse a secret.

Parental Reaction: Children may suffer further trauma if parents react negatively to the truth by blaming the child or denying or minimising the abuse.

Institutional Response: Negative or ineffective responses by social service agencies to the child's sexual abuse serve to compound the negative effects of the abuse.

Children who have been sexually abused may or may not show physical symptoms. Finkelhor (cited by Faller 1993) divides the traumatogenic effects of CSA into four general categories, each having varied psychological and behavioural effects:

Traumatic Sexualisation: Included in the psychological outcomes of traumatic sexualisation are aversive feelings about sex, overvaluing sex and sexual identity problems. Behavioural manifestations of traumatic sexualisation constitute a range of hypersexual behaviours as well as avoidance of or negative sexual encounters.

Children who have been sexually abused may show a greater awareness of sexuality than would be expected of the child's developmental age. He/She may engage in excessive masturbation or inappropriate sex play with peers (Winton and Mara 2001).

Stigmatisation: Common psychological manifestations of stigmatisation are feelings of guilt and responsibility for the abuse or the consequences of disclosure. These feelings are likely to be reflected in self-destructive behaviours such as substance abuse, risk-taking acts, self-mutilation, suicidal gestures and acts, and provocative behaviour designed to elicit punishment.

Betrayal: Perhaps the most fundamental damage from sexual abuse is its undermining of trust in those people who are supposed to be protectors and nurturers. Other psychological impacts of betrayal include anger and borderline functioning. Behaviour that reflects this trauma includes avoidance of investment in others, manipulating others, re-enacting the trauma through subsequent involvement in exploitive and damaging relationships, and engaging in angry and acting-out behaviours.

Powerlessness: The psychological impact of the trauma of powerlessness includes both a perception of vulnerability and victimisation and a desire to control or prevail, often by identification with the aggressor. As with the trauma of betrayal, behavioural manifestations may involve aggression and exploitation of others. On the other hand, the vulnerability effect of powerlessness may be avoidant responses, such as dissociation and running away; behavioural manifestations of anxiety, including phobias, sleep problems, elimination problems and eating problems; and re-victimisation.

17.8.5 Child Right to Protection from Sexual Abuse

Article 34 of the UNCRC states that the state parties shall undertake to protect the child from all forms of sexual exploitation and sexual abuse. For these purposes, state parties shall in particular take all appropriate national, bilateral and multilateral measures to prevent the inducement or coercion of a child to engage in any unlawful sexual activity.

17.8.6 Medical Assessment of Child Sexual Abuse

The most obvious drawback of a medical examination for children who have undergone sexual abuse is that it can recreate the sense of being abused. The problem is exacerbated by the lack of women doctors, especially female police surgeons, although children may still be upset even when the doctor is of a preferred sex. The potentially traumatic effects of the medical examination can be decreased by obtaining the child's consent to the examination and by appointing a skilled and sensitive health professional. That person explains that the purpose of the examination is to ensure that the child is "okay"; usually does a complete physical, not just a genital examination, and both informs the child, at each step of the examination, what will happen next and allows the child some control over the process. If the child is resistant to the examination, even when properly undertaken, then serious consideration should be given to not doing it. Children have the right to refuse a medical examination. If it is deemed medically necessary, it might be rescheduled, when the child is less upset, or it might be done under anaesthesia (Faller 1993). Emergency powers may be granted through the courts if this is refused and the child is clearly at risk (Doyle 1994).

17.8.7 Intervention with Child Sexual Abuse

Sexually abused children require extra consideration, understanding and support from the counsellor. Empathetic listening, clarifications of words and non-verbal expressions are essential. They may need to be told that the adult's sexual or punishing behaviour was inappropriate (Thompson and Henderson 2007, pp. 546–547).

17.8.7.1 Facilitating Disclosure

Adults, who abuse children sexually, often warn the children to keep their secret. Sexually abused children are initially unable to discuss the problem with the counsellor also because of intense feelings of guilt, worthlessness and shame. They may further be affected by the questions and reactions that follow than by the act itself (Thompson and Henderson 2007). Robinson (2009) notes that many therapists believed that children usually pass through a sequence of stages while disclosing sexual abuse that they have experienced. Perhaps the most common model was that proposed by Rolland Summitt (1983, cited by Robinson 2009) and called the *Child Sexual Abuse Accommodation Syndrome*. The stages are secrecy, helplessness, entrapment, disclosure and retraction. Others use a different sequence: denial, reluctance, gradual disclosure, recantation and reaffirmation. This theory assumes that it is very difficult for children to discuss having been sexually abused. Special methods, like fantasy play, guided imagery, the use of anatomically direct dolls and other props, etc. help the child disclose. When children finally do reveal details of the abuse, they must be believed because children do not create false disclosures. Children who have not been abused lack the sexual experience to create such stories (Robinson 2009).

17.8.7.2 Treating Feelings of Guilt

An offender may make the victim feel responsible for the abuse, for the offender's well-being and/or for the consequences of disclosure. Victims of sexual abuse may also feel guilty for not having stopped the sexual abuse as well as for any positive aspects of the abuse, such as physical pleasure, the special attention given by the offender or an opportunity to have control over other family members because of "the secret". The role of the social worker is to help the child understand intellectually and accept emotionally that the child was not responsible. It was the adult's job – not the child's – to stop or prevent the abuse (Faller 1993).

17.8.7.3 Treating Altered Sense of Self and Self-Esteem

Guilt feelings as well as the invasive and intrusive nature of the sexual activity impact negatively on the child's sense of self and self-esteem. The effect is both physical, in that children have an altered sense of their bodies, and psychological, in that children may see themselves as markedly different from their peers. The task of the social worker is to make victims feel whole and good about themselves again. However, so are interventions that help children view themselves as more than merely victims of abuse. Normalising and ego-enhancing activities, such as doing well in school, participating in sports, getting involved in scouts or helping a younger victim, can be very important in victim recovery (Faller 1993).

17.8.7.4 Managing Traumatic Sexualisation

Children who have been sexually victimised may masturbate excessively and openly or sexually interact with other people. Sexual acting out may be controlled, for example, by teaching the child to masturbate privately. Behaviour management techniques, which can involve rewarding "sex-free" days and using "time-out" for sexual acting out, can be taught to the child's caretaker. In addition, the child's energies that might have gone into sexual behaviour can be channelled into more age-appropriate activities by having a caretaker monitor the child, interrupt any sexual acting out and provide opportunities for positive alternative behaviours. These interventions are conducted with the child's caretaker and/or in dyadic work with child and caretaker (Faller 1993).

17.8.7.5 Explanation of Child Sexual Abuse

An important part of the treatment of child victims of sexual abuse is to help them understand the meaning of CSA. This includes learning what is wrong about sexual activity between adults and children; why adults or a particular adult was sexual with them; and in some cases, why they were chosen as targets and what that means to them. How these issues are addressed will vary with the child's developmental stage. They may be more adequately dealt with in group treatment than individual therapy, and sometimes having the offender take full responsibility for the abuse in dyadic therapy with the victim is useful (Faller 1993).

17.8.7.6 Protection from Future Victimisation

Treatment of victimised children needs to include strategies for future protection. Teaching children to say "no" may be useful, especially if the material is presented in a group setting and there are opportunities to role-play resisting sexual advances. Specific protective strategies involving family members and helping professionals need to be developed in intra-familial sexual abuse situations. Additionally, the social worker must appreciate that placing even partial responsibility for self-protection on the victim is potentially an overwhelming burden (Faller 1993).

Children may need information about what is appropriate and inappropriate touching or treatment and to be assured that certain parts of their bodies are private. Children need help discerning when they should tell a secret and when information should be kept confidential, and also in deciding whom they should tell and what to do if the adult does not believe their story (Thompson and Henderson 2007).

17.8.7.7 Psycho-educational Group Work

Ferrara (2002) notes that PEG work helps the victims of child sexual abuse in the following ways:

- Emotional reactions that stem from the abuse are listened to, acknowledged and validated, leading to a greater sense of self-worth.
- Verbal feedback from group members can clarify distorted cognitions that may restrict healing or be a source of anxiety for the abused.
- The thought that they are the only ones this happened to gets disbanded.
- A shared experience fosters bonding between group members, based on trust, which in turn may serve as a bridge to expedite the healing process more efficiently than individual counselling.
- Role-playing helps to work through dysfunctional family issues.

17.8.7.8 Working with Men and Boys

Save the Children (2003) recommends working with men and boys to prevent CSA through the following ways:

- Calling on and organising boys and men in the society to protest against violence and CSA and to take initiatives for more equal gender roles and relationships.
- Promoting programmes for young men on parenting and stressing the benefits for all members in society of men playing a more active role in nurturing their children and abandoning the culture of violence and abuse as a proof of masculinity. Fathers should encourage both girls and boys to express and participate in decisions that affect them.
- Identifying boys and men who break with traditional stereotyped behaviour and internalise gender equality, and engaging them to support programmes that address violence and child abuse as good role models.

References

Agarwal, S. C. (2002). Computer ethics, child sexual abuse, pornography and the regulation of child pornography on the internet. *CBI Bulletin*, 11–17.

Burman, E. (2008). *Deconstructing Developmental Psychology* (2nd ed.). London: Routledge Taylor and Francis Group.

Corby, B. (2002). Child abuse and child protection. In B. Goldson, M. Lavalette and J. McKechnie (Eds.) *Children, Welfare and the State* (pp. 136–151). London: Sage.

Desai, N. (2001). *See the Evil: Tourism Related Paedophilia in Goa*. Mumbai: Vikas Adhyayan Kendra.

Downs, S. W., Moore, E. and McFadden, E. J. (2009). *Child Welfare and Family Services: Policies and Practice* (8th ed.). Boston, MA: Pearson Allyn and Bacon.

Doyle, C. (1994). *Child Sexual Abuse: A Guide for Health Professionals*. London: Chapman and Hall.

ECPAT International. (2001). *Documents for the Second World Congress Against the Commercial Sexual Exploitation of Children*. Yokohama: ECPAT International.

ECPAT International. (2008). *Questions and Answers About the Commercial Sexual Exploitation of Children*. http://www.ecpat.net/EI/Publications/About_CSEC/FAQ_ENG_2008.pdf. Accessed 20 July 2009.

Faller, K. C. (1993). *Child Sexual Abuse: Intervention and Treatment Issues*. Washington, DC: US Department of Health and Human Services.

Ferrara, F. F. (2002). *Childhood Sexual Abuse: Developmental Effects Across the Lifespan*. Southbank, VIC: Brooks/Cole.

Finklehor, D. (1984). *Child Sexual Abuse: New Theory and Research*. London: Collier Macmillan Publishers.

Kendig, B. and Lowry, C. (1998). *Cedar House: A Model Child Abuse Treatment Program*. New York: The Hayworth Maltreatment and Trauma Press.

Klausner, M. A. and Hasselbring, B. (1990). *Aching for Love: The Sexual Drama of the Adult Child: Healing Strategies for Women*. San Francisco, CA: Harpercollins.

Mason, J. and Steadman, B. (1996). *The Significance of the Conceptualisation of Childhood for Promoting Children's Contributions to Child Protection Policy*. Paper presented at the Fifth Australian Family Research Conference, organised by the Australian Institute of Family Studies, Brisbane.

Mignon, S. I., Larson, C. J. and Holmes, W. M. (2002). *Family Abuse: Consequences, Consequences, Theories, and Responses*. Boston, MA: Allyn and Bacon.

Panchal, T. and Shaikh, N. (1997). *Documentation of Police Cases of Sexually Abused Girls in Bombay City Between 1994–95*. Mumbai: The Special for Women and Children.

Parton, N. (1990). Taking child abuse seriously. In The Violence Against Children Study Group (Ed.) *Taking Child Abuse Seriously: Contemporary Issues in Child Protection Theory and Practice*. London: Unwin Hyman.

Poore, G. (2002). *What Is Incestual Sexual Abuse*? www.shaktiproductions.net/isa_whatis.html. Retrieved 15 June 2005.

Quinn, C. (1992). Protection and prevention: An integral approach to child sexual assault. In J. Breckenridge and M. Carmody (Eds.) *Crimes of Violence: Australian Responses to Child Sexual Assault*. Sydney: Allen and Unwin.

Robinson, B. A. (2009). *How Young Children Disclose Sexual Abuse*. http://www.religioustolerance.org/chil_int.htm. Accessed 22 July 2009.

Sakshi. (1999). *Child Sexual Abuse: Beyond Fear Secrecy and Shame*. New Delhi: Sakshi.

Save the Children. (2003). *Working with Boys and Men to End Gender Discrimination and Sexual Abuse of Girls and Boys*. Dhaka: Save the Children.

Thompson, C. L. and Henderson, D. A. (2007). *Counseling Children*. Southbank, VIC: Thomson/Brooks/Cole.

United Nations Children's Fund. (2001). *Summary Report on Commercial Sexual Exploitation of Children and Child Sexual Abuse in South Asia*. Kathmandu: United Nations Children's Fund.
United Nations Convention on the Rights of the Child. (1989). http://www.ohchr.org/english/law/pdf/crc.pdf. Retrieved 3 March 2002.
Winton, M. A. and Mara, B. A. (2001). *Child Abuse and Neglect: Multidisciplinary Approaches*. Boston, MA: Allyn and Bacon.
World Congress against Commercial Sexual Exploitation of Children. (1996). *15 Factsheets on Commercial Sexual Exploitation of Children*. Stockholm: World Congress against Commercial Sexual Exploitation of Children.

Chapter 18
Commercial Exploitation in Childhood and Tertiary Prevention

18.1 Concepts of Commercial Exploitation in Childhood and Tertiary Prevention

18.1.1 Commercial Exploitation in Childhood

In the context of increased consumerism among the rich and poverty among the poor, children from the poverty groups are commodified for begging, labour, sexual exploitation, adoption, marriage and entertainment to meet the needs of their poor parents and for consumption of the rich adults. Vitit Muntarbhorn, the Special Rapporteur on Sale of Children, Child Prostitution and Child Pornography, stated in his report (1994) that poverty alone does not lead to commercial exploitation of children. It relates to the supply side of the problem. The global demand is explained by customers and the criminal networks which benefit from it and by collusion and corruption in many national settings. Globalisation has also led to the expansion of the international organised crime, enlarging the scope for exploitation of children. Rehabilitation of the rescued children has become the most challenging issue for child protection due to the global nexus.

In commercial exploitation of children

- Child abuse is connected with cash or in-kind profit for the child and/or adult third person or persons;
- The child victims are generally neglected school dropouts from the poverty groups who are commodified mainly for labour or sexual consumption by the rich adults;
- The third person or persons who make profit out of this abuse, that is, the procurers or agents are part of the commercial and/or criminal nexus, comprised largely of men, but also women; and
- The result is not only impairment of the child's physical, emotional and psychological or sexual health and development, but also the child's right to health and nutrition, housing, education, rest and recreation, and participation (adapted from UNESCAP 1999, cited from UNICEF 2001).

M. Desai, *A Rights-Based Preventative Approach for Psychosocial Well-Being in Childhood*, Children's Well-Being: Indicators and Research 3,
DOI 10.1007/978-90-481-9066-9_18,

Commercial exploitation of children comprised of

1. *Exploitation of children for labour* takes place in organised hazardous industries and unorganised begging, domestic and hotel sectors; trafficked and bonded, unpaid or under-paid
2. *Commercial sexual exploitation of children* takes the forms of child prostitution, sex tourism and pornography
3. *Trafficking and sale of children* is gender- and age-specific, rural to urban, interstate and international, for begging, labour, prostitution, adoption, entertainment, sale of organs and marriage
4. *Substance abuse* among children

18.1.2 Tertiary Prevention

18.1.2.1 Goals

Tertiary prevention of commercial exploitation in childhood may aim at the following goals:

1. Prevention of children's abuse and commercial exploitation:
   - Further abuse and commercial exploitation of the same children,
   - Effects of abuse and commercial exploitation on mental and physical health of children,
   - Abused and commercially exploited children facing conflict with law and
   - The cycle of abuse by preventing the survivors of abuse and commercial exploitation growing up to be offenders of children as adults;
2. Promotion of their psychosocial well-being;
3. Promotion of their age-appropriate developmental opportunities; and
4. Promotion of their child rights to family care, development, participation and protection.

18.1.2.2 Intervention

Tertiary prevention of commercial exploitation in childhood may be carried out through the following psychosocial interventions:

1. Child advocacy interventions for restorative justice:
   - Facilitate child rights in the judicial proceedings.
   - Conduct victim–offender mediation.
   - Rehabilitate the child.
   - Treat and rehabilitate offenders of children;

2. Case management for children and their families:
   - Direct intervention with children for giving information and advice, teaching and training in psychosocial skills and counselling
   - Linking them with natural support systems, self-help groups, flexitime supplementary childcare, integrated substitute childcare, poverty alleviation programmes and other formal systems of state and voluntary organizations
3. Psycho-educational group work with children and offenders

18.2 Child Labour

18.2.1 Concepts of Child Labour

18.2.1.1 Child Work

In the pre-industrialised period, work was a natural part of life for children. Industrialisation was not responsible for children's entry into the workforce, but it extended children's employment opportunities out of domestic industries and in the factories, mills and mines. As home and work got separated, children were no longer employed by the parents but by strangers and in conditions that were not acceptable (Stack and McKechnie 2002).

Extension of childhood up to 18 years of age, sometimes isolates adolescents from productive activities that once conferred on them social standing and acceptance. Prolonged schooling does not assure employment that would have come more easily to them if they joined work early. In fact, prolonged schooling without vocational training may increase unemployment in young adults, who would then drift into idleness, substance use or crime. Work experience entails understanding how the adult labour market works, learning how to negotiate with adults other than parents, appreciating the value of money, developing a sense of responsibility and other good work habits. In situations where the quality of education is questionable, it is commonly thought preferable for children to leave school, so that they can focus their attention on work, which seems a more fruitful way of spending their time and brings immediate economic returns (Boyden and Levison 2000).

Thus, work is not necessarily bad for children. Children can help their parents in the home or in the family farm or business, as long as the work is not dangerous and does not interfere with school attendance and other normal childhood activities. This is often referred to as "light work".

18.2.1.2 Child Labour

The term "child labour" refers only to forms of employment or unpaid work that violate the rights of children, for example, under-age employment and hazardous employment (UNICEF 2004). According to the International Labour Organisation (2003), child labour includes children permanently leading adult lives, working long hours for low wages, under conditions damaging to their health and to their physical and mental development, sometimes separated from their families, and frequently deprived of meaningful educational and training opportunities that could open up for them a better future. Muntarbhorn (1994) noted that it is the exploitation of child labour rather than child labour per se that is objectionable.

18.2.1.3 Debt Bondage

Debt bondage is specifically defined as a practice similar to slavery. Debt bondage violates a range of basic human rights to which all persons are entitled, including the right to liberty and security of person; the right to free choice of employment; the right to equal pay for equal work; the right to an effective remedy by the competent national tribunal for acts violating their fundamental rights granted by law; and frequently, the right to health and the right to education (Anti-Slavery 2000).

18.2.2 Causes of Child Labour

Anti-Slavery (2007) identified the following causes of child labour:

- *Poverty*: Most children work because their families are poor and their labour is necessary for their survival. Being a result of poverty, child labour also perpetuates poverty. Many working children do not have the opportunity to go to school and often grow up to be unskilled adults trapped in poorly paid jobs, and in turn will look to their own children to supplement the family's income.
- *Discrimination*: Discrimination on grounds including gender, race or religion also plays its part in why some children work.
- *Profitability*: Children are often employed and exploited because, compared to adults, they are more vulnerable, cheaper to hire and are less likely to demand higher wages or better working conditions. Some employers falsely argue that children are particularly suited to certain types of work because of their small size and "nimble fingers".
- *Lack of Access to Education*: For many children, school is not an option. Education can be expensive and some parents feel that what their children will learn is irrelevant to the realities of their everyday lives and futures. In many cases, school is also physically inaccessible or lessons are not taught in the child's mother tongue, or both.

The international markets and consumer societies demand cheap products, compelling the developing world to employ child labour at a low cost to be able to compete in the global forum. Child labour allows goods to be sold at competitive prices, and emerging markets simply cannot employ adults for the same rates. Child labour thus increases with increased unemployment among adults, leading to further poverty in the families (Vikas Adhyayan Kendra 1998).

18.2.3 Child Right to Protection from Exploitation for Labour

Article 32 of the UNCRC states the following:

1. State parties recognise the right of the child to be protected from economic exploitation and from performing any work that is likely to be hazardous or to interfere with the child's education, or to be harmful to the child's health or physical, mental, spiritual, moral or social development.
2. State parties shall take legislative, administrative, social and educational measures to ensure the implementation of the present chapter. To this end, and having regard to the relevant provisions of other international instruments, State parties shall in particular

   (a) Provide for a minimum age or minimum ages for admission to employment;
   (b) Provide for appropriate regulation of the hours and conditions of employment;
   (c) Provide for appropriate penalties or other sanctions to ensure the effective enforcement of the present chapter.

The ILO Convention No. 138 establishes three age limits:

- 18 for hazardous work
- 15 for full-time employment in non-hazardous work
- 13 for "light" work that does not interfere with education

ILO Convention No. 182 lists the worst forms of child labour, namely, all forms of slavery or practices similar to slavery, such as the sale and trafficking of children, debt bondage and serfdom and forced or compulsory labour, including forced or compulsory recruitment of children for use in armed conflict; the use, procuring or offering of a child for prostitution, for the production of pornography or for pornographic performances; the use, procuring or offering of a child for illicit activities, in particular for the production and trafficking of drugs, which are to be eliminated as a priority.

18.2.4 Intervention

The strategies of the International Labour Organization (No date) are three-pronged:

1. Education in formal and non-formal settings is a crucial component of any effective effort to eliminate child labour. Non-formal or transitional education plays an instrumental role in the rehabilitation of former child labourers. Vocational education and training provide the skills needed for gainful employment, which in turn contributes to local and national development.

2. Child labour monitoring (CLM) is the active process that regularly checks the places where girls and boys may be working. Its overall objective is to ensure that children and young legally employed workers are safe from exploitation and hazards at work. The active scrutiny of child labour at the local level is supported by a referral system which establishes a link between appropriate services and ex-child labourers. In practice CLM involves the identification, referral, protection and prevention of child labourers through the development of a coordinated multi-sector monitoring and referral process that aims to cover all children living in a given geographical area. Its principal activities include regularly repeated direct observations to identify child labourers and to determine risks to which they are exposed, referral of these children to services, verification that they have been removed and tracking them afterwards to ensure that they have satisfactory alternatives.
3. ILO Convention No. 182 calls for the following time-bound measures to eliminate the worst forms of child labour:

    - Prevent the engagement of children in the worst forms of child labour;
    - Provide direct assistance for the removal of children from the worst forms of child labour and for their rehabilitation and social integration;
    - Ensure access to free basic education and appropriate vocational training for all children removed from the worst forms of child labour;
    - Identify and reach out to children at special risk; and
    - Take account of the special situation of girls.

18.3 Commercial Sexual Exploitation of Children

18.3.1 Concepts of Commercial Sexual Exploitation of Children

Commercial sexual exploitation of children (CSEC) commonly refers to using a child for sexual purposes in exchange for cash or in-kind favours between the client/customer and intermediary or agent who profits from such a trade. Those who profit include a wide range of persons, including parents, family members, and procurers/agents, community members, largely men, but also women (UNESCAP 1999, cited from UNICEF 2001). The Declaration and Agenda for Action against Commercial Sexual Exploitation of Children defines CSEC as a fundamental violation of children's rights that comprises sexual abuse by the adult and remuneration in cash or kind to the child or a third person or persons. The child is treated as a sexual object and as a commercial object. The commercial sexual exploitation of children constitutes a form of coercion and violence against children, and amounts to forced labour and a contemporary form of slavery (ECPAT International 2008).

Thus, in CSEC

- CSA is connected with cash or in-kind profit for the child and/or adult third person or persons;

- The third person or persons who make profit, that is, the procurers/agents are part of the commercial and/or criminal nexus comprising of largely men, but also women;
- The child victims are generally neglected school dropouts from the poverty groups who are commodified for sexual consumption of the rich adults;
- The result is not only impairment of the child's physical, emotional and psychological or sexual health and development, but also child right to health and nutrition, housing, education, rest and recreation, and participation (adapted from UNESCAP 1999, cited from UNICEF 2001).

The ECPAT International (2005, p. 21) differentiates CSEC from CSA as follows:

- In CSA, Child is inside the system – often still in school, whereas in CSEC the child is outside the system – not in school.
- In CSA, the wider community is sympathetic and supportive of the child victim, but in CSEC the wider community views such children's behaviour in a negative way.

The ECPAT International (2008) identifies the primary interrelated forms of CSEC as prostitution of children, child pornography and trafficking of children for sexual purposes. In other forms of CSEC they include child-sex tourism, and in some cases, child marriage. However, as the profit factor is an important characteristic of CSEC, child marriages do not fit into CSEC. As trafficking of children is carried out not only for commercial sex, it has been discussed in the next section. The forms of CSEC discussed in this Chapter are child prostitution, child pornography and child-sex tourism.

18.3.2 Causes of Commercial Sexual Exploitation of Children

Causes of commercial sexual exploitation of children can be seen as increase in the combination of the demand and the vulnerability of children. Hughes (2004) divides the demand for victims to be used for commercial sex acts into the following three components:

- The primary level of the demand is the men (and occasionally women) who seek out women, children and sometimes men for the purpose of purchasing sex acts. Men who solicit and buy sex acts are often called "customers", "clients", and "consumers", terms that normalise men's behaviour.
- The second level of demand is the profiteers in the sex industries. They include the traffickers, pimps, brothel owners and supporting corrupt officials who make money from sex trafficking and prostitution. They are criminals and often members of transnational organised crime networks.

- The third factor is the culture that indirectly creates a demand for victims by normalising prostitution. Media depictions of prostitution and other commercial sex acts suggest that prostitution is a victimless crime. In places where women and girls, or certain ethnicities or classes of women and girls are devalued, there is more acceptance of prostitution and the exploitation of a female relative in prostitution to financially support the family.

ECPAT International (2008) lists the following factors leading to vulnerability of children to CSEC:

- Societal acceptance/harmful traditions and customs
- Discrimination/ethnicity
- Irresponsible sexual behaviour and myths regarding benefits of having sex with virginity of young girls
- Poverty
- Family abuse and neglect of children
- Emergency situations such as disaster or conflict situations
- Living and working in the streets
- HIV/AIDS
- Consumerism in the middle class
- Guise of adoption
- Inadequate laws and corruption
- Information and communication technologies

18.3.3 Child Prostitution

18.3.3.1 Concept of Child Prostitution

The term "prostitution" is conventionally understood as an act of selling of sex, by a woman, against payment. According to Patkar and Patkar (No date), this term inaccurately conveys the woman as an independent actor acting on her own accord, for her own profits. They prefer the term "victims of commercial sexual exploitation", as it is sexual exploitation, carried out for the profit of the exploiter, by providing access to the victim's sexual faculties, to any customer who is ready to pay for it. According to Mehta (2002), adults in prostitution may be seen as victims or consenting parties, but there exists no two opinions that in child prostitution children are victims as they are powerless, innocent and dependent on adults for their well-being.

The Optional Protocol to the Convention on the Rights of the Child (CRC) on the Sale of Children, Child Prostitution and Child Pornography defines child prostitution as "the use of a child in sexual activities for remuneration or any other form of consideration". Most generally, it means that a party other than the child benefits from a commercial transaction in which the child is made available for sexual purposes – either an exploiter intermediary (pimp) who controls or oversees the child's activities for profit, or an abuser who negotiates an exchange directly with a child in order to receive sexual gratification.

18.3.3.2 Locations of Child Prostitution

Based on his work with child prostitutes in Goa, Pandey (2006) categorised the phenomenon of child prostitution into brothel-based, hotel and lodge-based, street-based and mobile nature:

Brothel-based Child Prostitution: In the brothel-based phenomenon the minor girls are housed in rooms and the perpetrators include brothel keepers and pimps who solicit the customers. They are mostly caged and do not have access to anyone other than the customers. The girls in this situation have to entertain all kind of customers brought by the traffickers. They do not have any choice as if they refuse they are physically abused. They are no different from bonded slaves.

Hotel and Lodge-based Child Prostitution: In the hotel and lodge-based phenomenon, minor girls are mostly locked in the rooms of a hotel/lodge and soliciting of the customers is done by the pimps, hotel staff, taxi drivers and traffickers. The girls are paraded before the customers for selection. Once the girl is selected by the customer she is sexually exploited by the customer in the same hotel. A large amount of earning from this kind of prostitution is taken by the hotel and lodge staff/owners.

Street-based Child Prostitution: In the street-based phenomenon, the traffickers/perpetrators force the minor girls to solicit customers on their own and then take the customers to a hotel/lodge with whom they already have an understanding. Sometimes they are even sexually exploited in isolated places such as jungles, vehicles and so on. A large amount of the earnings goes to the perpetrators and for renting rooms in hotels and lodges.

Mobile Child Prostitution: In the "mobile" phenomenon, victims are carried in vehicles by the traffickers and soliciting is done by the trafficker's agents. Most of the times, the victims are kept in the vehicle and the vehicle is parked in tourist areas. Once the traffickers' agents fix the deal with the customers they inform the traffickers sitting in the vehicle and the vehicle comes and drops the victim at the destination given by the agent. Once the job is over the vehicle comes back and collects the girl/s. It is found that this kind of exploitation is done in a very organised manner with the involvement of the traffickers who have control over the victims, taxi drivers and hotel and lodge staff. In this kind of phenomenon, the customers also directly contact the traffickers by mobile phones and girls are delivered at their desired location.

18.3.4 Child Pornography

According to the Optional Protocol to the Convention on the Rights of the Child on the Sale of Children, Child Prostitution and Child Pornography, child pornography is "any representation, by whatever means, of a child engaged in real or simulated explicit sexual activities or any representation of the sexual parts of a child for primarily sexual purposes".

Child pornography includes photographs, visual and audio representations and writing, and can be distributed through magazines, books, drawings, movies, videotapes, mobile phones and computer disks or files. Child pornography exploits children in many different ways:

1. Children may be tricked or coerced into engaging in sexual acts for the production of pornography or images may be made in the process of sexually exploiting a child without the child's knowledge. These images are then distributed, sold or traded.
2. Those who "consume" and/or possess pornographic depictions of children are also exploiting the children, especially as the demand for such materials maintains the incentive to their production and consequently to the sexual abuse of the child.
3. The makers of pornography commonly use their products to coerce, intimidate or blackmail the children used in the making of such material (ECPAT International 2008).

In certain parts of the world, there is a marked involvement of organised crime networks in the production and distribution of child pornography. The most obvious use of child pornography is sexual arousal and gratification. However, it is also used to validate certain beliefs and behaviour (for example, the notion that it is okay to have sex with children), establish trust among others interested in abusing children, gain entrance to private clubs and make a profit. At a societal level, child pornography, whether of real or simulated images of children, continues to cultivate a demand that involves sexual abuse and exploitation of children and is linked to prostitution of children, child-sex tourism and trafficking of children for sexual purposes (ECPAT International 2008).

The digital age has facilitated the production and dissemination of child pornography. Advances in computer technology have made the creation and distribution of child pornography easier, cheaper and more difficult to detect. It should be noted, however, that those who make and access child pornography are not only paedophiles or preferential abusers. It has developed into a multimillion-dollar industry that can be run from within the exploiter's home. It is virtually impossible to ensure the physical destruction of child pornography once it has been posted on the Internet. The International Conference on Combating Child Pornography on the Internet, held in Vienna in 1999, called for the worldwide criminalisation of the production, distribution, exportation, transmission, importation, intentional possession and advertising of child pornography, and stressing the importance of closer cooperation and partnership between governments and the Internet industry (UNICEF 2004).

18.3.5 Child-Sex Tourism

Child-sex tourism is the commercial sexual exploitation of children by people who travel from one location to another to engage in sexual acts with minors. Child-sex tourists often travel from a richer country to one that is less developed. However, child-sex tourists may also be travellers within their own countries or regions. Sex tourism preys on sexual and economic inequality, and fosters other forms of commercial sexual exploitation of children such as child trafficking for sexual exploitation. Child-sex tourists come from all walks of life: they may be married or single, male or female, wealthy tourists or budget travellers. Some child-sex tourists (preferential abusers and paedophiles) target children specifically; most, however, are situational abusers who do not usually have a sexual preference for children but take advantage of a situation in which a child is made available to them. Anonymity, availability of children and being away from the moral and social constraints that normally govern behaviour, facilitate abusive conduct in another country. Child-sex exploiters may try to rationalise their actions by claiming that sex with a child is culturally acceptable in the place they are visiting, or that the money or goods exchanged benefit the child and his or her community (ECPAT International 2008).

Sex tourism is an expression of massive and obscene economic inequalities between affluent and poor counties, as well as between affluent individuals in poor countries and the mass of poor people. Westerners' desire for sexual contact with local adults and children is often structured by their racist constructions of the exotic and erotic "primitive", while their racist assumptions about cultural difference are used to justify and defend their sexually exploitative acts (Davidson and Taylor 1996). Inadequate laws and inefficient judicial systems are among the main causes of child-sex tourism in developing countries, because they lead paedophiles to believe that they can go to these countries and abuse children without the risk of prosecution (UNICEF 2004).

18.3.6 Child Right to Protection from Commercial Sexual Exploitation

Article 34 of the UNCRC states that the state parties shall undertake to protect the child from all forms of sexual exploitation and sexual abuse. For these purposes, state parties shall in particular take all appropriate national, bilateral and multilateral measures to prevent

(a) The inducement or coercion of a child to engage in any unlawful sexual activity;
(b) The exploitative use of children in prostitution or other unlawful sexual practices;
(c) The exploitative use of children in pornographic performances and materials.

In 2000, an Optional Protocol to the CRC on the Sale of Children, Child Prostitution and Child Pornography was adopted and opened for signature, ratification and accession. The various rights guaranteed to children by this Protocol are the following: Right against exploitation and rights to information, be represented and heard, assistance, privacy and confidentiality, protection, speedy trial, rehabilitation and compensation.

The ILO C182, the Worst Forms of Child Labour Convention 1999, includes sale and trafficking of children; and the use, procuring or offering of a child for prostitution, for the production of pornography or for pornographic performances, in the term "worst forms of child labour", to be eliminated as a priority.

18.3.7 Intervention

To combat CSEC, ECPAT International (2008) calls for action to improve cooperation and coordination, provide health and educational programmes, strengthen law enforcement and legislation, adopt non-punitive rehabilitation measures and encourage child and youth participation. ECPAT International (2005) identifies the following three common settings for working with CSEC.

18.3.7.1 Street/Mobile Setting

The street or mobile approach works more towards encouraging less risky behaviour and contact with services, by making small changes to the environment (for example, providing condoms and needles) and offering health checks. This setting is sometimes criticised (by public, politicians and others) as sanctioning or encouraging the exploitative behaviour. However, it often acts as the "first step" to other, more comprehensive services.

18.3.7.2 Drop-in-Centre

A drop-in-centre provides support without placing too many demands and restrictions on young persons. It may be a bridge towards leaving the life of CSEC. The informal nature of the support offered at such centres, while being very useful to the child in terms of helping them make a break, can also lead to them not engaging with services, and just hop between providers (use of agreements and central registry might help reduce this).

18.3.7.3 Residential Care

Residential care provides place of safety, and regular ongoing support for children in a more structured and formal way. It may provide the bridge to reintegration of the children with their family (if appropriate). Children may initially find adjusting to life in care very difficult to cope with and as a result may present problems in behaviour (violence, anger and so on).

In 2004, ECPAT promoted launching of The Code of Conduct for the Protection of Children from Sexual Commercial Exploitation in Travel and Tourism. Suppliers of tourism services adopting the code commit themselves to implement the following six criteria:

1. Establish an ethical policy regarding commercial sexual exploitation of children.
2. Train the personnel in the country of origin and travel destinations.

3. Introduce a clause in contracts with suppliers, stating a common repudiation of commercial sexual exploitation of children.
4. Provide information to travellers by means of catalogues, brochures, in-flight films, ticket slips, home pages and so on.
5. Provide information to local key persons at the destinations.
6. Report annually.

18.4 Trafficking and Sale of Children

18.4.1 Child Trafficking

18.4.1.1 Concepts of Child Trafficking

According to the United Nations (UN) Protocol to Prevent, Suppress and Punish Trafficking in Persons, especially Women and Children (2000), and the United Nations Convention against Transnational Crime, 2000, trafficking in persons shall mean the recruitment, transportation, transfer, harbouring or receipt of persons; by means of threat or use of force or other forms of coercion, abduction, fraud, deception, abuse of power or a position of vulnerability or the giving or receiving of payments or benefits to achieve the consent of a person having control over another person; for the purpose of exploitation. However, the recruitment, transportation, transfer, harbouring or receipt of a child for the purpose of exploitation is considered trafficking, regardless of whether or not force, abduction, fraud and the other means mentioned above are employed. Exploitation includes, at a minimum, the exploitation of prostitution of others or other forms of sexual exploitation, forced labour or services, slavery or practices, similar to slavery, servitude or the removal of organs. Trafficking of human beings has been identified as a gross violation of human rights worldwide. The victims of trafficking are the most victimised, exploited, stigmatised and un-supported group.

Human trafficking has emerged as an issue of global concern in recent years. Facilitated by porous borders and advanced communication technologies, it has become increasingly transnational in scope and highly lucrative. People, particularly children, can be sold several times for various purposes – they are commodities in a business that generates billions of dollars and operates with impunity. Children are trafficked for sexual exploitation, labour, transplant of organs and illegal adoption. Regardless of the initial purpose, all child victims of trafficking are highly vulnerable to sexual abuse and exploitation because they are removed from support structures such as their families and communities (ECPAT International 2008).

The Optional Protocol to the Convention on the Rights of the Child on the Sale of Children, Child Prostitution and Child Pornography of 2000 notes the significant increase in international traffic in children for the purpose of sale of children, child prostitution and child pornography, and the widespread and continuing practice of sex tourism, to which children are especially vulnerable, as it directly promotes the sale of children, child prostitution and child pornography.

Population Council (2002) clarifies the distinction between trafficking and migration and smuggling, all of which refer to movements within or across border. Migration is free, with consent, for the purpose of improvement of livelihood, and legal. Smuggling is also with consent and for the purpose of improvement of livelihood, but illegal, with a brokerage fee. On the other hand, trafficking is slavery because traffickers use violence, threats and other forms of coercion to force their victims to work against their will. This includes controlling their freedom of movement, where and when they will work and what pay, if any, they will receive (Anti-Slavery No date).

18.4.1.2 Factors Leading to Trafficking

According to a United Nations Development Programme Report (1999), factors contributing to the increase in trafficking of women include globalisation and economic liberalisation, increased demand and supply of trafficked persons, professionalisation of the traffickers and syndicates, modern transport, technology and the Internet, growth of sex tourism, feminisation of poverty, trading in human organs, changing nature of prostitution and erosion of social capital. UNICEF (2005) notes the following factors that make children vulnerable to trafficking:

Poverty: Victims of trafficking often come from poor families and lack economic opportunities. Children who have minimal education, lack vocational skills or have few prospects for job opportunities are most at risk. With promises of employment opportunities abroad, families in extreme poverty may send their children away to work.

Gender Inequality: Where women and girls are objectified and seen as commodities, a climate is created in which girls can be bought and sold. Girls are frequently abused within their families, making the lure of traffickers seem like an escape from domestic exploitation and violence.

Low School Enrolment: Children who are not in school can easily fall prey to traffickers. Uneducated children have few opportunities for their future, and are therefore more vulnerable to traffickers' promises of money and a "better life".

Children without Care-givers: Children without parental protection, or those placed in institutions, are targets for traffickers. Without guidance, a sense of belonging or opportunities, they may be at an increased risk of trafficking.

Lack of Birth Registration: Children who are not registered are more susceptible to trafficking. When children are without a legal identity it is easier for traffickers to "hide" them.

Humanitarian Disasters and Armed Conflict: During conflicts, children may be abducted by armed groups and forced to participate in hostilities. Cataclysmic events that disrupt livelihoods or result in the death of one or both parents make children vulnerable to trafficking.

Demand for Exploitative Sex and Cheap Labour: Trafficking and the skyrocketing demand for exploitative labour and sexual services are inexorably linked. The drive for rising profits too often trumps ethics, resulting in children being exploited in factories and sweatshops.

18.4.1.3 Modus Operandi of Trafficking

There are three phases in the trafficking process; the recruitment phase, the transit phase and the destination phase, but these phases can overlap. Some victims are trafficked over and over again. As with adult victims, traffickers get hold of children and young people in many different ways. It is a complex crime, and not always easy to recognise as such. The traffickers themselves might be part of a well-organised criminal network, or they might be individuals taking part in only one or more of the various stages of the operation, such as the provision of false documentation, transport or a "safe house". These criminals are frequently highly dangerous and willing to commit serious crimes of violence to avoid detection and protect their financial interests (ECPAT International 2006).

At the time of recruitment, the family members are instrumental or at least aware of the trafficking. Earlier forcible and coercive methods were used and now, increasingly, deception and false promises are used to lure children and their families for trafficking (Communication material of Joint Women's Programme). They are, therefore, active participants in their own trafficking, as far as recruitment and transportation are concerned. This dimension adds to the difficulty of developing methodologies to ascertain the actual number of trafficked persons and creating effective protections against the phenomenon (UNICEF 2001).

ECPAT International (2006) notes the following common ways in which traffickers keep young people submissive:

- Confiscation of their identity documents
- Threats of reporting them to the authorities
- Violence or threats of violence
- Threats of violence towards members of the young person's family
- Social isolation
- Keeping the young person locked up or limiting their freedom in another way
- Claiming that the young person owes a debt of money
- Depriving the young person of money

18.4.1.4 Impact of Trafficking

UNICEF (2005) notes that child trafficking victims are subjugated and physically abused by the perpetrators: traffickers, employers, pimps, madams and "customers". The report describes the following physical, emotional and social impact of trafficking on children.

Sexually Transmitted Infections: Children trafficked into the sex industry are susceptible to contracting sexually transmitted infections, including HIV/AIDS. Many women and girls report that "customers" pay more for sex without a condom, and they – especially girls – are rarely in a position to insist upon condom use. Domestic workers, street children, child labourers and children in detention are vulnerable to rape and sexual exploitation and are at high risk of contracting HIV/AIDS.

Emotional Impact: Children who have been trafficked have reported feelings of shame, guilt and low self-esteem and are frequently stigmatised. They often feel betrayed, especially if the perpetrator was someone they had trusted. These factors as well as the experience itself can cause nightmares, sleeplessness, feelings of hopelessness and depression. Some children who have been trafficked turn to substance abuse to numb their psychic pain, and others attempt suicide.

Social Impact: Children who are trafficked typically suffer adverse effects to their social and educational development. Many have no family life and are forced to work at young ages. Without access to school or family support, and cut off from normal social activities, they fail to develop their potential. Also, under constant surveillance and restriction, they have little contact with the outside world and often do not have the possibility to seek help.

Re-victimisation: For children who have been trafficked and "rescued", the repatriation process can be traumatic. Children are often treated as criminals and even sometimes imprisoned, either in the country to which they have been trafficked or subsequently in their home country on return. They may also be vulnerable to re-victimisation or re-trafficking if appropriate care and protection is not available (ECPAT International 2001).

Anti-Slavery International (2002) looked at measures to protect trafficked people in 10 countries. It reported that increasingly governments have responded to trafficking through restrictive immigration policies. These not only render migrants more vulnerable to traffickers, but often lead to trafficked persons being swiftly returned to their home countries as undocumented migrants. They return to the very same conditions from which they left, rather than being identified as victims of crime. This fails to give trafficked persons opportunities for recovery and redress, and further deprives them of access to justice, through the possibility of criminal or civil action against traffickers.

Population Council (2002) notes that children are more expensive and difficult to care for once they are rescued and more problematic to reintegrate or repatriate. States experience many difficulties in assuming responsibility for non-citizen minors and are therefore often reluctant to assume any responsibility for their protection and care.

18.4.2 Sale of Children

According to the Optional Protocol to the Convention on the Rights of the Child on the Sale of Children, Child Prostitution and Child Pornography of 2000, sale of children means "any act or transaction whereby a child is transferred by any person or group of persons to another for remuneration or any other consideration". The Protocol states that the purpose of sale of children ranges from sexual exploitation of the child, transfer of organs of the child for profit, engagement of the child in forced labour or for the adoption of a child. The concept of sale overlaps with that of trafficking, except that trafficking implies a practice whereby a child is moved (UNICEF 2004).

Based on her work in Goa, Almeida (No date) recommends that sale of children cannot simply be defined in terms of money obtained. According to her, sale of children should be construed as having taken place in the following situations:

1. There is sale or purchase of a child;
2. A child travels alone to a foreign country without valid reason or written permission or justification from the child's parents or legal guardians;
3. A pregnant woman is made to execute an affidavit of consent for adoption for a consideration;
4. A person, agency, establishment or child-caring institution recruits women or couples to bear children for the purposes of child trafficking;
5. A doctor, hospital or clinic official or employee, nurse, midwife, local civil registrar or any other person simulates birth records for the purpose of child trafficking; or
6. A person engages in the act of finding children of women who are vulnerable or from among low-income families, hospitals, clinics, nurseries, day-care centres or other child-caring institutions who can be offered for the purposes of child trafficking or who can be raised for the purpose of offering them for the sale of their body parts or blood.

18.4.3 Child Right to Protection from Trafficking and Sale

The 2000 Protocol to Prevent, Suppress and Punish Trafficking in Persons, especially Women and Children, supplements the United Nations Convention against Transnational Organized Crime. It aims at preventing and combating trafficking in persons, paying particular attention to women and children; protecting and assisting the victims of such trafficking, with full respect for their human rights; and promoting cooperation among state parties in order to meet those objectives. It protects and promotes the following rights to the trafficked persons: Right against exploitation, rights to non-discrimination, privacy and confidentiality, information, be represented and heard, assistance, safety, compensation and voluntary repatriation and right against forceful deportation.

The ILO C182, the Worst Forms of Child Labour Convention 1999, includes sale and trafficking of children; and the use, procuring or offering of a child for prostitution, for the production of pornography or for pornographic performances, in the term "worst forms of child labour" to be eliminated as a priority.

The Optional Protocol to the Convention on the Rights of the Child on the Sale of Children, Child Prostitution and Child Pornography of 2000 prohibits the sale of children, child prostitution and child pornography.

18.4.4 Intervention

18.4.4.1 Identification and Rescue

Population Council (2002) noted that suspected trafficking cases are quite difficult to identify at border crossings particularly if the trafficked person is not yet aware of the deception or fraud. The application of a definition of trafficking requires specific parameters for identifying victims that can be linked with appropriate operational responses by border agents. Only highly contextualised, individualised responses to the needs of trafficking victims succeed. The limited ability of children to provide consent for themselves coupled with agreed upon international guidelines governing child labour make it easier to identify situations where children (as opposed to adults) are living and working in servile status.

UNICEF (2005) recommends the following tasks at the time of identification and rescue of trafficked children:

Proactive and Preemptive Identification: Proper procedures for rapidly identifying trafficked children need to be established. This requires coordination among law enforcement, border and immigration authorities, health, education and social welfare agencies, and non-governmental organisations, all of which should be on the lookout for trafficked children. There is a need to establish procedures for a rapid referral and coordination mechanism so children expeditiously receive the care they need. Help lines for children to call if they become victims of abuse or exploitation are effective tools. Such phone numbers should be given to all children arriving in a destination country under a special visa.

Rescue: From time to time, "rescue operations" are needed to remove children from places where they are being exploited, particularly in brothels. Depending on the circumstances that brought them there, rescued children often return to the sex industry because they see no alternative. For some children, considerable time and support are needed to adapt to life outside the brothel. Attempts to rescue such children should be part of a holistic approach that also ensures safe reintegration into a family and community. Additionally, rescue operations need to be sensitive to children's needs. For instance, it is extremely problematic to use an all-male police operation to aid a girl or to interview a child in front of a madam or pimp.

Appointment of a Guardian: As soon as a child victim is identified, a legal guardian should be appointed to accompany the child throughout the process. The guardian should oversee the child's welfare (housing, health care, education and psychosocial and language support) and cooperate with service providers on behalf of the child. The legal guardian needs to have a good understanding of child rights, the specific needs of child victims and the legal issues surrounding child trafficking.

Interim Care and Protection: Trafficked children need interim care and protection that include separate, safe housing, medical care, education, psychosocial rehabilitation, and reintegration and repatriation assistance. In identifying appropriate services, attention to a child's cultural identity/origin, gender, age and such specific needs as disabilities, psychosocial distress, illness or pregnancy is essential. Special assistance is necessary for children who have been sexually exploited.

18.4.4.2 Standards for the Treatment of Trafficked Persons

The Human Rights Standards for the Treatment of Trafficked Persons (Global Alliance Against Trafficking in Women 1999) mandate the following State obligations towards trafficked persons:

Principle of Non-Discrimination: States shall not discriminate against trafficked persons in substantive or procedural law, policy or practice.

Safety and Fair Treatment: States shall recognise that trafficked persons are victims of serious human rights abuses, protect their rights notwithstanding any irregular immigration status and protect them from reprisal and harm.

Access to Justice: The police, prosecutors and court shall ensure that their efforts to punish traffickers are implemented within a system that respects and safeguards the rights of the victims to privacy, dignity and safety.

Access to Private Actions and Reparations: States must ensure that trafficked persons have a legal right to seek reparations from traffickers as well as assistance in bringing such actions, if necessary.

Residential Status: States shall provide trafficked persons with temporary residence visas (including the right to work) during the pendency of any criminal, civil or other legal actions and shall provide trafficked persons with the right to seek asylum and have the risk of retaliation considered in any deportation proceedings.

Health and Other Services: States shall provide trafficked persons with adequate health and other social services during the period of temporary residence.

Repatriation and Reintegration: States shall ensure that trafficked persons are able to return home safely, if they so wish, and when they are able to do so.

Recovery: Recovery includes medical and psychological care as well as legal and social services to ensure the well-being of trafficked persons.

State Cooperation: States must work cooperatively in order to ensure full implementation of these standards.

Legislation is also needed that would allow the State to confiscate or garnish all proceeds derived from the crime of trafficking. Confiscated proceeds can be applied towards satisfying any civil remedies sought and be used to pay for social services for trafficking victims. In the case of proceeds derived from child trafficking, the State should create a mechanism to hold the proceeds in trust for the trafficked child (UNICEF 2005).

18.4.4.3 Rehabilitation

According to the Global Alliance Against Trafficking in Women (2000), the social workers could carry out the following tasks towards support and rehabilitation of child victims of international trafficking:

- Provide a general orientation of the society (legal system, cultural practices, travel information, political system, language and so on) in which the trafficked person is a stranger.
- Facilitate contacts, when desired, with community groups or voluntary organisations, for example, women's organisations, civic organisations and so on, or own community groups in the host country.
- Undertake proper preparation for an eventual return to their own country, in accordance with the wishes of the person concerned, especially regarding communications with agencies and other persons, including family members, in the country of origin.
- Facilitate voluntary, humane and safe repatriation of migrants.
- Facilitate the application of longer term stay visa, if the trafficked person cannot return to his/her own country or prefers to stay on in the host country.
- Facilitate the application for a stay visa and obtaining the right of citizenship for children born in the host country.

References

Almeida, A. (No date). *Trafficking for Sale of Children*. Bailancho Saad: A Women's Collective. Goa.

Anti-Slavery. (No date). *Human Trafficking Q and A*. www.antislavery.org/homepage/antislavery/trafficking.htm#qanda. Accessed 5 August 2005.

Anti-Slavery. (2000). *Debt Bondage in India, Nepal and Pakistan*. Geneva: Anti-Slavery. www.antislavery.org/archive/submission/submission2000-BondLabour.htm. Accessed 5 August 2005.

Anti-Slavery. (2007). *Child Labour*. http://www.antislavery.org/homepage/antislavery/child labour.htm#what. Accessed 30 June 2008.

Anti-Slavery International. (2002). *Human Traffic, Human Rights: Redefining Victim Protection*. London: Anti-Slavery International.

Boyden, J. and Levison, D. (2000). *Children as Economic and Social Actors in the Development Process*. Stockholm: Ministry of Foreign Affairs.

Davidson, J. O. and Taylor, J. S. (1996). *Child Prostitution and Sex Tourism in Goa*. Bangkok: ECPAT International.

ECPAT International. (2005). *The Psychosocial Rehabilitation of Children Who Have Been Commercially Sexually Exploited: A Training Guide*. Bangkok: ECPAT International.

ECPAT International. (2006). *Combating the Trafficking in Children for Sexual Purposes: Questions and Answers*. http://www.ecpat.net/EI/Publications/Trafficking/Trafficking_FAQ_ENG.pdf. Accessed Retrieved 20 July 2009.

ECPAT International. (2008). *Questions and Answers About the Commercial Sexual Exploitation of Children*. http://www.ecpatusa.org/EcpatUSA_PDF/faq%20update%20from%20ecpat%20international.pdf. Accessed 4 July 2006.

Global Alliance Against Trafficking in Women. (1999). *Human Rights Standards for the Treatment of Trafficked Persons*. Bangkok: Global Alliance Against Trafficking in Women.

Global Alliance Against Trafficking in Women. (2000). *Human Rights and Trafficking in Persons: A Handbook*. Bangkok: Global Alliance Against Trafficking in Women.

Hughes, D. M. (2004). *Best Practices to Address the Demand Side of Sex Trafficking*. http://www.uri.edu/artsci/wms/hughes/demand_sex_trafficking.pdf. Accessed 7 May 2008.

International Labour Organisation. (2003). *Investing in Every Child, An Economic Study of the Costs and Benefits of Eliminating Child Labour*. Geneva: International Labour Organisation.

International Labour Organization. (No date). *International Programme on the Elimination of Child Labour*. http://www.ilo.org/ipec/Action/lang–en/index.htm. Accessed 21 July 2009.

International Programme on the Elimination of Child Labour. (No date). http://www.ilo.org/ipec/Action/lang–en/index.htm. Accessed 21 July 2009.

Mehta, L. (2002). Social profile of child sex workers. *Social Welfare*, 49(8), 3–7.

Muntarbhorn, V. (1994). *Report of the Special Rapporteur on Sale of Children, Child Prostitution and Child Pornography*. Geneva: Office of the United Nations High Commissioner for Human Rights.

Pandey, A. (2006). *Trafficking and Sale of Children and Child Prostitution*. Paper submitted for the Assessment and Recommendations for Mainstreaming Child Rights in Goa, by the Goa Initiative for Mainstreaming Child Rights, Panjim.

Patkar, P. and Patkar, P. (No date). *Frequently Asked Questions on Commercial Sexual Exploitation and Trafficking*. Mumbai: Prerana.

Population Council. (2002). *Anti-trafficking Programs in South Asia: Appropriate Activities, Indicators and Evaluation Methodologies*. New Delhi: Population Council.

Stack, N. and McKechnie, J. (2002). Working children. In B. Goldson, M. Lavalette and J. McKechnie (Eds.) *Children, Welfare and the State* (pp. 87–101). London: Sage.

United Nations. (2000). *Protocol to Prevent, Suppress and Punish Trafficking in Persons, especially Women and Children, Supplementing the United Nations Convention Against Transnational Organized Crime*. http://www.uncjin.org/Documents/Conventions/dcatoc/final_documents_2/convention_%20traff_eng.pdf Accessed 14 June 2008.

United Nations Children's Fund. (2001). *Summary Report on Commercial Sexual Exploitation of Children and Child Sexual Abuse in South Asia*. Kathmandu: UNICEF.

United Nations Children's Fund. (2004). *Child Protection: A Handbook for Parliamentarians*. Geneva and New York: IPU and UNICEF.

United Nations Children's Fund. (2005). *Combating Child Trafficking: Handbook for Parliamentarians*. Geneva and New York: IPU and UNICEF.

United Nations Development Programme. (1999). *AIDS in Southwest Asia: A Development Challenge*. New Delhi: United Nations Development Programme.

Vikas Adhyayan Kendra. (1998). Labouring under delusion the myths on child labour. *Facts Against Myths*, 3(8/96).

Chapter 19
Conflict with Law in Childhood and Tertiary Prevention

19.1 Concepts of Conflict with Law in Childhood and Tertiary Prevention

19.1.1 Conflict with Law in Childhood

19.1.1.1 Status Offenders

Status offenders who are children who commit an act that violates a law or ordinance designed to regulate his or her behaviour because of his or her age or status. Status offences are solely based on the offender's age and are unique to juveniles. Anyone above the legal age who engages in the same behaviours would not be committing an offence. Examples of a status offence are truancy and early substance abuse (Hess and Drowns 2004).

19.1.1.2 Juvenile Delinquents

The term "juvenile" refers to any person under the legal age of majority. In general, "juvenile delinquency" is legally defined as any act which, if committed by adults, would be a crime. However, generally children under the age of 7 are exempted from legal responsibility for any deviant behaviour. In relation to "delinquency", therefore, the terms "juvenile" and adolescent are virtually interchangeable (Bynum and Thompson 1996). Among "juvenile delinquents", there are two sub-groups: those who commit property crimes and those who commit violent crimes such as murder and rape (Hess and Drowns 2004). Save the Children (2005) states that the overwhelming majority of children in conflict with the law (over 90 per cent) are petty offenders, who mainly commit offences against property and four out of five children who commit an offence only commit one in their lifetime. School bullying and juvenile gangs are manifestations of violent crimes.

19.1.1.3 Bullying

Sampson (2002, cited by Hess and Drowns 2004, p. 184), "Bullying has two key components: repeated harmful acts and an imbalance of power. It involves repeated

M. Desai, *A Rights-Based Preventative Approach for Psychosocial Well-Being in Childhood*, Children's Well-Being: Indicators and Research 3,
DOI 10.1007/978-90-481-9066-9_19,

physical, verbal, or psychological attacks or intimidation directed against a victim who cannot properly defend him or herself because of size or strength, or because the victim is outnumbered or less psychologically resilient." According to Ericson (2001, cited by Hess and Drowns 2004, p. 184), "Bullying can affect the social environment of a school, creating a climate of fear among students, inhibiting their ability to learn, and leading to other antisocial behaviour..."

19.1.1.4 Gangs

A gang is an ongoing group of people that have a common name or common identifying sign or symbol, form an allegiance for a common purpose and engage in unlawful or criminal activity. A street gang is a group of individuals who meet over time, have identifiable leadership, claim control over a specific territory in the community and engage in criminal behaviour. The youth gang is a sub-set of the street gang (Hess and Drowns 2004). Children normally seek gang involvement for the following reasons: structure, nurturing, a sense of belonging, economic opportunity and excitement (Allender 2001, cited by Hess and Drowns 2004).

19.1.1.5 Children in Conflict with Law

"Juvenile delinquent" is a term that labels a child. In labelling theory, it is important to differentiate between primary deviance and secondary deviance. Primary deviance is the initial criminal act and secondary deviance is accepting the criminal label and consequently committing other crimes like a self-fulfilling prophecy (Hess and Drowns 2004).

According to Goldson (2002), research and practice showed that most juvenile offending was petty, opportunistic and transitory and that the majority of children grow out of it. However, he observed that entry of these children into the juvenile justice system results in application of criminal labels that stigmatise them, trigger negative social reaction to them and compound the likelihood of further delinquency. The UNCRC does not use the term "juvenile delinquency", however, it does not mention avoidance of labelling language. According to the United Nations Guidelines for the Prevention of Juvenile Delinquency (The Riyadh Guidelines) adopted and proclaimed by General Assembly in 1990, "...in the predominant opinion of experts, labelling a young person as "deviant", "delinquent" or "pre-delinquent" often contributes to the development of a consistent pattern of undesirable behaviour by young persons. It is important to restrict the labelling to specific behaviours rather than the person (Hess and Drowns 2004).

"Child in conflict with law" is a broad term that describes the situation in which the child is rather than describing the child himself/herself. Conflict with law in childhood thus includes the following:

- Status offences
- Property offences
- Violent offences

19.1.2 Tertiary Prevention

19.1.2.1 Goals

Tertiary prevention of conflict with the law in childhood may aim at the following goals:

1. Prevention of
   - First-time offence leading to more offences
   - Status offence leading to property crime, and
   - Property crimes leading to violent crimes;
2. Prevention of their vulnerability, neglect, abuse and commercial exploitation;
3. Promotion of their psychosocial well-being;
4. Promotion of their age-appropriate developmental opportunities; and
5. Promotion of their child rights to family care, development, participation and protection.

19.1.2.2 Interventions

Tertiary prevention of conflict with law in childhood may be carried out through the following psychosocial interventions:

1. Child advocacy interventions for restorative justice:
   - Facilitate child rights in the judicial proceedings.
   - Conduct victim–offender mediation.
   - Rehabilitate the child.
   - Treat and rehabilitate offenders of children; and
2. Case management:
   - Advocacy intervention for restorative justice through the juvenile justice system
   - Linking with natural support systems, self-help groups, integrated supplementary and substitute childcare and other formal systems of state and voluntary organisations
   - Direct intervention for giving information and advice, teaching and training in psychosocial skills and counselling
3. Psycho-educational group work

19.2 Causes of Conflict with Law in Childhood

Besides labelling children as "juvenile delinquents", the causes of conflict with law in childhood is comprised of the following:

- Scientific Construction of "Normal" Childhood
- Social Construction of Adolescence and Testing of Boundaries
- Neglect and Abuse
- Poverty and Class Conflict
- Neuro-Behavioural Disorders

19.2.1 Scientific Construction of "Normal" Childhood

The sciences of developmental psychology, child/human development and social work have developed norms of "normal" childhood development, based on the Western, white, middle class, male constructs of normality. These are based on adultist notions of childhood as a basically biologically driven "natural" phenomenon in which children are distinguished from adults by specific physical and mental (as opposed to social) characteristics. Children are seen as separated from the world of work and devoting their time to learning and play and thus are economically worthless, apolitical and asexual. Another feature of this model is the emphasis on the child as an individual (rather than a member of a social group), and on parents and nuclear family as the "natural" immediate vehicles of protection, socialisation and control (White 2003).

Since childhood is constructed as a time of innocence, of purity and lack of responsibility, when children do not live up to these expectations, our societies respond with particular vindictiveness, as if in shock that the image we created, the childhood we want to believe in does not exist (Save the Children 2005). These mythical norms of childhood are being transferred to the world's children, a majority of whom are growing up in poverty groups of the developing nations. The transfer of these "normal" norms to them makes their life seem deviant, inferior or pathological (White 2003). The world's children are then vulnerable to services that control and work on them to attain measures that bring them inside the bands of "normal" (EU Canada Project 2003).

19.2.2 Social Construction of Adolescence and Testing of Boundaries

Baethge (1989, cited by Saraswathi 1999) noted that adolescence emerged as a life stage in the twentieth century, under the following conditions: learning process that is divorced from practice, delayed experience of one's own social usefulness, later choice of job or career, prolonged economic dependence on parents, more leisure time that can be spent with the same age group members and longer time spent in individual development rather than in a collective code of performance. The prolonged emotional, psychological and economic dependency led to a century-long enduring mythology of adolescence, depicted as a period of storm and stress subject to hormonally induced mood swings. Those, who did not meet these norms of dependency in this stage, got to be termed "juvenile delinquents" (Ruddick 2003).

Growing up is a period when children are learning to test boundaries and develop their own sense of right and wrong. Adolescents adopt "risky behaviour" and they do so at a time when their lives and behaviour are particularly regulated by their families, schools and society (Save the Children 2005).

19.2.3 Neglect and Abuse

Save the Children (2005) notes that most of the children who come into conflict with the law are children who are facing challenges in their care and protection and in their relationships with their families, communities and society. Their lives, choices and opportunities are affected to a great extent by the social, economic and political realities in which they live. These include communities increasingly fragmented through urbanisation, chronic poverty, social and interpersonal violence, and increased pressure from commercialisation and materialism. Yet, somehow we expect children to remain outside of all this and be better (Downs et al. 2009).

Children who originally come to the attention of the child welfare system because of neglect or abuse later appear in system for committing offences. This reappearance suggests that the earlier interventions of the child welfare system were not successful (Downs et al. 2009).

19.2.4 Poverty and Class Conflict

Large numbers of children in conflict with the law are socio-economic victims, denied their rights to education, health, shelter, care and protection. Many of them have had little or no access to education; many are working children. Some children have left their homes and taken to the streets to escape from violence and abuse at the hands of their families. Some are forced to make a living on the streets in order to survive. Others have been abandoned by their families and left to fend for themselves and sometimes for younger siblings. These children, who are abandoned and destitute, are at high risk of sexual exploitation, trafficking and becoming involved in substance abuse and the drug trade through peer influence or the influence of adult criminals (Save the Children 2004). These children coming into conflict with the law are children who are criminalised for simply trying to survive (Downs et al. 2009).

The conflict theories that originated with the writings of Karl Marx, suggest that laws are established to keep the dominant class in power. This theory explains the over-representation of racial and ethnic minorities in arrest, prosecution, imprisonment and capital punishment (Hess and Drowns 2004). According to the conflict theory, the criminal justice system and criminal law are thought to be operating on behalf of the rich and powerful social elites, with resulting policies aimed at controlling the poor. The criminal justice establishment aims at imposing standards of morality and good behaviour created by the powerful on the whole of society. Their focus is on separating the haves from the have-nots who would steal from others and protecting themselves from physical attacks. In the process the legal rights of poor folks might be ignored. The middle class are also co-opted; they side with the elites rather the poor, thinking they might themselves rise to the top by supporting the status quo (Criminological Theory 2005).

19.2.5 Neuro-behavioural Disorders

Educational disability does not cause delinquency, but learning and behavioural disorders place youth at greater risk of involvement with the juvenile courts and for incarceration. School failure, poorly developed social skills, and inadequate school and community supports are associated with the over-representation of youth with disabilities at all stages of the juvenile justice system (The National Center on Education, Disability and Juvenile Justice No date).

According to the National Mental Health Association (2004), youth who are involved in the juvenile justice system have substantially higher rates of mental health disorders (60 per cent) than children in the general population (22 per cent), and they may have rates of disorder comparable to those among youth being treated in the mental health system.

19.3 Review of the Retributive Justice for Children

The classical world view holds that humans have free will and are responsible for their own actions. Proponents of this view advocate that punishment, deterrence and incapacitation are the ways to deal with delinquency (Hess and Drowns 2004). Save the Children (2005) states that the overwhelming majority of children in conflict with the law who are petty offenders are considered "juvenile delinquents" and arrested and detained by police, tried by magistrates and sent to institutions, including prisons, under systems of justice which in many cases are set up for adults. The processes of arrest, trial and custody destroy their childhood as a result of being denied their right to, for example, family life, education, care, protection and play. Many of them have little chance of rehabilitation and reintegration into society: discrimination against children who have been in conflict with the law, together with deprivation and poverty, limit their opportunities for developing into active and contributing adult citizens (Save the Children 2004).

19.3.1 Police Violence

Save the Children (2005) notes that children's experiences of coming into conflict with the law tend to begin with their first encounters with police or local security officers, and these are often brutal. From immediate violence upon arrest, attempted extortion in exchange for promises of release, torture to extract a confession, regular beatings and further violence, including sexual abuse, when in police custody, the continuum of violence that many children experience at the hands of law enforcement agencies means that the agencies are "all powerful" as far as these children are concerned. Usually isolated from the protection of families, who in some cases even view the use of violence by the police as part of "teaching a lesson" to the child, often with no other adults to intervene on their behalf, these children are particularly vulnerable to violent and corrupt police officers. In addition to violence, rampant corruption within some police forces, often compounded by low levels of salaries, leave children at the mercy of unscrupulous officers who use the round-ups, curfews and other restrictions on children's use of public spaces as an easy means of supplementing their meagre incomes.

19.3.2 Detention

In the juvenile justice system, children in conflict with law are incarcerated and their opportunity to learn to be respectful and respected members of societies and communities is removed. They are expected to learn responsibility by being exposed to the totally artificial environment of detention, where choices are made for them, imposed rules define their everyday living and decide their every move, and where all the challenges they faced in the real world are temporarily removed but not dealt with. And then, when the sentence is over, they are plunged back into the same context and environment that led to their offending in the first place, hoping that they have learnt their "lessons" (Save the Children 2005).

While the period of arrest and interrogation is often one of the most dangerous for children, detention brings its own set of added dangers. Conditions in detention are usually overcrowded, often inhumane and always traumatising. Violations of international standards in relation to the detention of children are rife, with fundamental principles such as the total separation of minors from adults continuing to be violated in a majority of countries, despite overwhelming evidence that this invariably exposes children to violence, including sexual abuse by adults. Even where the conditions of incarceration are in accordance with international law, and children are segregated from adults and provided with educational and recreational facilities, detention as a last resort and for the shortest appropriate time is rarely practised anywhere in the world. That such a high percentage of children in detention are awaiting trial and that the overwhelming majority of children in jail are accused of non-serious and non-violent offences point to a fundamental flaw in the way juvenile justice is administered. The screening process and the required determination that a particular child is a genuine risk to the security of others or seriously at risk of flight while awaiting trial are usually totally non-existent or flawed, resulting in detention on remand being the rule rather than the exception (Save the Children 2005).

19.4 Child Rights in the Juvenile Justice System

19.4.1 United Nations Convention on the Rights of the Child

Article 37 of the UNCRC states that the state parties shall ensure the following:

(a) No child shall be subjected to torture or other cruel, inhuman or degrading treatment or punishment. Neither capital punishment nor life imprisonment without possibility of release shall be imposed for offences committed by persons below 18 years of age;
(b) No child shall be deprived of his or her liberty unlawfully or arbitrarily. The arrest, detention or imprisonment of a child shall be in conformity with the law and shall be used only as a measure of last resort and for the shortest appropriate period of time;
(c) Every child deprived of liberty shall be treated with humanity and respect for the inherent dignity of the human person, and in a manner which takes into account the needs of persons of his or her age. In particular, every child deprived of liberty shall be separated from adults unless it is considered in the child's best interest not to do so and shall have the right to maintain contact with his or her family through correspondence and visits, save in exceptional circumstances;
(d) Every child deprived of his or her liberty shall have the right to prompt access to legal and other appropriate assistance, as well as the right to challenge the legality of the deprivation of his or her liberty before a court or other competent, independent and impartial authority, and to prompt decision on any such action.

Article 40 states the following:

1. State parties recognise the right of every child alleged as, accused of, or recognised as having infringed the penal law to be treated in a manner consistent with the promotion of the child's sense of dignity and worth, which reinforces the child's respect for the human rights and fundamental freedoms of others and which takes into account the child's age and the desirability of promoting the child's reintegration and the child's assuming a constructive role in society.
2. To this end, and having regard to the relevant provisions of international instruments, state parties shall, in particular, ensure that

   (a) No child shall be alleged as, be accused of, or recognised as having infringed the penal law by reason of acts or omissions that were not prohibited by national or international law at the time they were committed;
   (b) Every child alleged as or accused of having infringed the penal law has at least the following guarantees;

      (i) To be presumed innocent until proven guilty according to law;
      (ii) To be informed promptly and directly of the charges against him or her, and, if appropriate, through his or her parents or legal guardians, and to have legal or other appropriate assistance in the preparation and presentation of his or her defence;

(iii) To have the matter determined without delay by a competent, independent and impartial authority or judicial body in a fair hearing according to law, in the presence of legal or other appropriate assistance and, unless it considered not to be in the best interest of the child, in particular, taking into account his or her age or situation, his or her parents or legal guardians;
(iv) Not to be compelled to give testimony or to confess guilt; to examine or have examined adverse witnesses and to obtain the participation and examination of witnesses on his or her behalf under conditions of equality;
(v) If considered to have infringed the penal law, to have this decision and any measures imposed in consequence thereof reviewed by a higher competent, independent and impartial authority or judicial body according to law;
(vi) To have the free assistance of an interpreter if the child cannot understand or speak the language used;
(vii) To have his or her privacy fully respected at all stages of the proceedings.

3. State parties shall seek to promote the establishment of laws, procedures, authorities and institutions specifically applicable to children alleged as, accused of, or recognised as having infringed the penal law, and, in particular

   (a) The establishment of a minimum age below which children shall be presumed not to have the capacity to infringe the penal law;
   (b) Whenever appropriate and desirable, measures for dealing with such children without resorting to judicial proceeding, providing that human rights and legal safeguards are fully respected.

4. A variety of dispositions, such as care, guidance and supervision orders; counselling; probation, foster care; education and vocational training programmes and other alternatives to institutional care shall be available to ensure that children are dealt with in a manner appropriate to their well-being and proportionate both to their circumstances and the offence.

19.4.2 United Nations Standard Minimum Rules for the Administration of Juvenile Justice

Following are some excerpts from the Standard Minimum Rules for the Administration of Juvenile Justice, adopted by the UN in 1985:

- Basic procedural safeguards such as the presumption of innocence, the right to be notified of charges, the right to remain silent, the right to counsel, the right to the presence of a parent or guardian, the right to confront and cross-examine witnesses and the right to appeal, shall be guaranteed to children in conflict with the law, at all stages of proceedings.

- Detention pending trial shall be used only as a last resort and for the shortest possible period of time. When possible, detention pending trial shall be replaced by alternative measures, such as close supervision or placement with a family. Juveniles under detention pending trial shall be kept separate from adults.
- Efforts shall be made to provide semi-institutional arrangements, such as halfway houses, educational homes and daytime training centres, to assist juveniles in their reintegration into society.

19.4.3 United Nations Rules for the Protection of Juveniles Deprived of Their Liberty

Some of the main principles of the UN Rules for the Protection of Juveniles Deprived of their Liberty, which set forth a comprehensive approach to the rehabilitation of juvenile offenders, inspired by the UNCRC, are listed below (cited from UNICEF 2004):

- Facilities should be decentralised, to prevent juveniles from being detained far from their families and communities, and small enough to allow for individualised attention.
- The system should include open or semi-open facilities, to meet the needs of children who require a residential setting but do not pose a serious danger to the community.
- Treatment should begin with an evaluation of the needs of the individual, and should include appropriate forms of education, work, spiritual and psychosocial counselling, recreation and care of medical problems, including drug or alcohol dependency.
- Respect for the rights of the child is essential to rehabilitation, because it encourages respect for the rights of others.

19.5 Child Advocacy Intervention for Restorative Justice

19.5.1 Child Advocacy Interventions for Restorative Justice

Advocacy interventions with children in conflict with law for restorative justice include the following:

- Prevention of Conflict with Law
- Decriminalisation of Status Offences
- Community-based Diversion for Petty Offences
- Regulating Detention for Violent Offences
- Reintegration and Rehabilitation of Children in Conflict with Law.

19.5.2 Prevention of Conflict with Law

The section on causes for children in conflict with law shows that conflict with law has its roots in labelling, scientific construction of "normal" childhood, social construction of adolescence and tendency to test boundaries in this stage, neglect and abuse, poverty and class conflict, and learning disabilities and other mental health problems. If so, the prevention of conflict with law in childhood should comprise of the following:

- Prevention of the labelling language of "juvenile delinquency"
- Deconstruction and contextualisation of "normal" childhood
- Deconstruction of adolescence and psycho-educational group work in this stage
- Prevention of neglect and abuse
- Alleviation of poverty and class conflict
- Use of alternative educational strategies for the learning disabled
- Psycho-educational group work to prevent mental health problems.

Save the Children (2005) emphasises that children should be prevented from coming into conflict with the law in the first place by properly addressing the care and protection challenges they face. Prevention strategies supporting children within their families, communities and societies should be prioritised and developed, with the participation of children themselves. Early intervention with a holistic, multi-sectoral and community-based approach, involving at the very minimum the education, health and protection sectors, must be undertaken to prevent children coming into conflict with the law.

According to UNICEF (2004), there is a need for effective programmes that help adolescents involved in crime overcome their problems, to the extent possible, and assist them in preparing for life as law-abiding members of society. Exposing them to further violations of their rights when they come into conflict with the law is always both wrong and counter-productive. Rose and Fatout (2003) note that social programmes designed to keep children from turning to crime include positive after-school, weekend and holiday activities; positive role models and mentors; school-based community services and so on. The expression of aggression can be constructively utilised within athletic and other physical activities.

19.5.3 Decriminalisation of Status Offences

Save the Children (2005) believes that the following children should be decriminalised or that the criminal system should never be used to deal with them and, instead, supportive services should be provided to them

- Children who have care issues or are deprived of good parental care for whatever reason.

- Children who are victims of violence, including children who are trafficked, children in commercial sexual exploitation, children who have been sexually abused, children fleeing forced marriages or who have married without the consent of their parents and eloped.
- Children who have not committed a criminal offence but whose behaviour is deemed socially unacceptable should never be dealt with through the justice system.
- Status offenders and survival behaviours such as truancy, running away from home, begging, loitering, vagrancy.

19.5.4 Community-Based Diversion for Petty Offences

According to Save the Children (2005), children who have committed petty offences, usually first offences and whose behaviour has been criminalised – who represent the overwhelming majority of children in conflict with the law – should be diverted away from the criminal justice system through community-based alternative diversion mechanisms. The formal criminal justice system should only deal with the small minority of children who have committed very serious crimes, usually involving violence, and who represent a threat to themselves and/or their society. Diversion must take place at every given opportunity, including informal diversion mechanisms at the community level and in the justice system. Resources and priorities must be refocused away from an expensive, ineffective and often dangerous criminal justice system to developing a range of sustainable and localised community-based options focused on reintegration, guidance and support. A focus on community-based diversion and alternatives to detention can free the system and its resources from a backlog of petty offending by children that is only made worse by the use of incarceration, as this is shown to usually lead to more serious offending by young people.

19.5.5 Regulating Detention for Violent Offences

Save the Children (2005) recommends alternatives to detention with an overarching aim of social reintegration. Detention should *always* be a measure of last resort and should be for the shortest appropriate period of time. Specific measures, including proper screening mechanisms, should be in place to ensure that. Detention represents the most dangerous and isolating period for a child coming into conflict with the law and it is often the place where he or she is exposed to the highest risk of violence. Regulating conditions of detention is a fundamental requirement for preventing violence, including ensuring the segregation of children away from adults, the separation of boys from girls and the convicted from those awaiting trial. The investigation and prosecution of perpetrators of violence and those who abuse the system, including officials responsible for condoning arbitrary and unlawful detention, should be a priority for governments.

The juvenile justice system is not well equipped to screen, assess or treat a young person who has special mental, emotional or behavioural needs. Incarceration presents potential risks for these children, including victimisation, self-injury and suicide. For these reasons, children should be diverted from incarceration whenever possible with community-based alternatives. Because some children with emotional disorders commit serious and violent offences, it is not always possible to divert them from incarceration. Nevertheless, these children need treatment for their disorders, and juvenile facilities and programmes should have adequate policies and procedures for identifying and treating these youth. Children who need help must be identified before their behaviours escalate and/or create problems for juvenile authorities (National Mental Health Association 2004).

19.5.6 Reintegration and Rehabilitation

According to Save the Children (2005), it is vital that reintegration and rehabilitation in the community and society should be clearly stated as the overall aim of all interventions with children in conflict with the law. The most marginalised children should be supported and encouraged to be part of, and play a positive and constructive role in, the society and community that will ensure that these children have a stake in abiding by the social rules. Children are the key in finding effective solutions to the problems and challenges they face. Children, including those who have already come into conflict with the law, must be involved in developing preventative strategies to minimise them coming into conflict with the law in the first place, as

Chart 19.1 Summary of Conflict with Law in Childhood and Tertiary Prevention

Causes of Conflict with Law in Childhood	**Prevention of Conflict with Law**
• Labelling children as "juvenile delinquents"	• Prevention of the labelling language of "juvenile delinquency"
• Scientific construction of "normal" childhood	• Deconstruction and contextualisation of "normal" childhood
• Social construction of adolescence and testing of boundaries	• Deconstruction of adolescence and psycho-educational group work in this stage
• Neglect and abuse	• Prevention of neglect and abuse
• Poverty and class conflict	• Alleviation of poverty and class conflict
• Neuro-behavioural disorders and other mental health problems	• Use of alternative educational strategies for the learning disabled • Psycho-educational group work to prevent mental health problems
Types of Conflict with Law in Childhood	**Child Advocacy Interventions for Restorative Justice**
• Status Offences	Decriminalisation of Status Offences
• Property Offences	• Community-based Diversion for Property Offences
• Violent Offences	• Regulating Detention for Violent Offences

well as in the reform of the justice system and the development of community-based alternatives. Children need the opportunity to be recognised not just as victims or as perpetrators, but as social actors and members of families, communities and societies. The aim and focus of interventions with these children should be to empower and support them to respond to these challenges and to make better choices for themselves and their communities.

References

Bynum, J. E. and Thompson, W. E. (1996). *Juvenile Delinquency: A Sociological Approach*. Boston, MA: Allyn and Bacon.

Criminological Theory. (2005). *Conflict*. http://www.criminology.fsu.edu/crimtheory/conflict.htm. Accessed 27 November 2007.

Downs, S. W., Moore, E. and McFadden, E. J. (2009). *Child Welfare and Family Services: Policies and Practice* (8th ed.). Boston, MA: Pearson Allyn and Bacon.

EU Canada Project. (2003). *Child Welfare Across Borders*. www.sws.soton.ac.uk/cwab/index.htm. Accessed 19 July 2006.

Goldson, B. (2002). Children, crime and the state. In B. Goldson, M. Lavalette and J. McKechnie (Eds.) *Children, Welfare and the State* (pp. 120–135). London: Sage.

Hess, K. M. and Drowns, R. W. (2004). *Juvenile Justice*. Southbank, VIC: Thomson Wadsworth.

The National Center on Education, Disability and Juvenile Justice. (No date). *Resources on Prevention of Delinquency*. http://www.edjj.org/focus/prevention/. Accessed 27 November 2007.

National Mental Health Association. (2004). *Mental Health Treatment for Youth in the Juvenile Justice System: A Compendium of Promising Practices*. www.nmha.org/children/JJCompendiumofBestPractices.pdf. Accessed 7 October 2005.

Rose, S. R. and Fatout, M. F. (2003). *Social Work Practice with Children and Adolescents*. Boston, MA: Allyn and Bacon.

Ruddick, S. (2003). The politics of aging: Globalization and the restructuring of youth and childhood. *Antipode: A Radical Journal of Geography*, 35(2), 334–362.

Saraswathi, T. S. (1999). Adult–child continuity in India: Is adolescence a myth or an emerging reality? In T. S. Saraswathi (Ed.) *Culture, Socialization and Human Development* (pp. 213–232). New Delhi: Sage.

Save the Children. (2004). *Juvenile Justice: Modern Concepts of Working with Children in Conflict with the Law*. http://www.crin.org/docs/save_jj_modern_concepts.pdf. Accessed 27 July 2009.

Save the Children. (2005). *The Right Not to Lose Hope: Children in Conflict with the Law*. London: Save the Children.

United Nations Children's Fund. (2004). *Child Protection: A Handbook for Parliamentarians*. Geneva and New York: IPU and UNICEF.

United Nations Convention on the Rights of the Child. (1989). http://www.ohchr.org/english/law/pdf/crc.pdf. Accessed 3 March 2002.

Wellford, C. F. and Triplett, R. A. (No date). *The Future of Labeling Theory: Foundations and Promises*. http://www.criminology.fsu.edu/crimtheory/blomberg/thefuture.html. Accessed 27 November 2007.

White, B. (2003). *A World Fit for Children?* Dies Natalis address delivered on the occasion of the 51st anniversary of the Institute of Social Studies, The Hague, The Netherlands.

Index

M. Desai, *A Rights-Based Preventative Approach for Psychosocial Well-Being in Childhood*, Children's Well-Being: Indicators and Research 3, DOI 10.1007/978-90-481-9066-9, © Springer Science+Business Media B.V. 2010

Lightning Source UK Ltd.
Milton Keynes UK
15 February 2011

167590UK00005B/27/P

9 789048 190652